Challenging Concepts in Cardiovascular Medicine:
A Case-Based Approach with Expert Commentary

Forthcoming titles in the Challenging Concepts in series

Anaesthesia (Edited by Dr Phoebe Syme, Dr Robert Jackson, and Dr Timothy Cook)

Emergency Medicine (Edited by Dr Sam Thenabadu, Dr Fleur Cantle, and Dr Chris Lacy)

Neurosurgery (Edited by Mr Robin Bhatia and Mr Ian Sabin)

Obstetrics and Gynaecology (Edited by Dr Natasha Hezelgrave, Dr Danielle Abbott, and Professor Andrew Shennan)

Oral and Maxillofacial Surgery (Edited by Mr Matthew Idle and Group Captain Andrew Monaghan)

Respiratory Medicine (Edited by Dr Lucy Schomberg and Dr Elizabeth Sage)

Challenging Concepts in Cardiovascular Medicine:
A Case-Based Approach with Expert Commentary

Edited by

Aung Myat

SpR Cardiology and NIHR Clinical Research Fellow
West Midlands Deanery and The Rayne Institute, St Thomas' Hospital,
King's College London, UK

Shouvik Haldar

SpR Cardiology and Electrophysiology Research Fellow
London Deanery and The National Heart & Lung Institute, Royal Brompton Hospital,
Imperial College London, UK

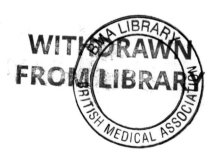

Simon Redwood

Professor of Interventional Cardiology and Honorary Consultant Cardiologist
King's College London and Guy's and St Thomas'
NHS Foundation Trust London, UK

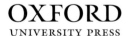

OXFORD
UNIVERSITY PRESS

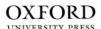

OXFORD
UNIVERSITY PRESS

Great Clarendon Street, Oxford OX2 6DP

Oxford University Press is a department of the University of Oxford.
It furthers the University's objective of excellence in research, scholarship,
and education by publishing worldwide in

Oxford New York

Auckland Cape Town Dar es Salaam Hong Kong Karachi Kuala Lumpur
Madrid Melbourne Mexico City Nairobi New Delhi Shanghai Taipei Toronto

With offices in

Argentina Austria Brazil Chile Czech Republic France Greece Guatemala
Hungary Italy Japan Poland Portugal Singapore South Korea Switzerland
Thailand Turkey Ukraine Vietnam

Oxford is a registered trade mark of Oxford University Press
in the UK and in certain other countries

Published in the United States
by Oxford University Press Inc., New York

British Library Cataloguing in Publication Data

Data available

Library of Congress Cataloguing in Publication Data

Data available

Typeset in Slimbach by Cenveo, Bangalore, India
Printed in Italy on acid-free paper
by L.E.G.O. S.p.A.—Lavis TN

ISBN 978-0-19-969554-6

10 9 8 7 6 5 4 3 2 1

FOREWORD

The authors are to be congratulated on producing an innovative and informative text on the management of common cardiovascular conditions. By presenting facts through the vehicle of a series of case presentations the text comes alive and has relevance and immediacy for anyone having to deal with patients with heart disease. Rather than cite references to publications in the conventional way, the authors provide up to date commentaries on the published evidence with additional, personalized opinions from an impressive array of distinguished specialists from around the UK with each case representing a virtual 'grand round' on a particular topic.

Although not exhaustive, the book covers most of the clinical presentations that are likely to be encountered by a trainee in their day-to-day practice, whether in the A & E department, on the wards or in the catheterization laboratory. Not only does it provide invaluable reading for the relatively inexperienced cardiologist, it also serves as a highly palatable update for those of us who have been around somewhat longer.

In a modern clinical practice setting dominated by guidelines, protocols and directives it is refreshing to encounter a text that brings all aspects of case management together in such an informative and entertaining way.

I can thoroughly recommend it to all cardiologists, whether established or in training, as well as any healthcare professional wishing to keep abreast of modern, evidence-based management of heart disease.

Professor Peter Weissberg
Medical Director, British Heart Foundation

A REVIEW FROM THE BRITISH CARDIOVASCULAR SOCIETY

There are many books published in cardiovascular medicine but few that offer a practical patient based approach. The authors should be congratulated for producing a highly readable, unique, and memorable educational experience suitable for a wide audience: medical students, trainees, trained cardiologists, allied professionals, and GPs.

This book presents 25 'real world' cases of the common, and some not so common, cardiac diagnoses. Each scenario, written by a Specialist Registrar, follows the patient pathway through their presenting complaint, history, examination findings, investigation and treatment options. Along the way, there are highlighted sections of 'clinical tips' to aid the diagnosis and 'learning points'. These 'learning points' range from basic facts to the ever important evidence base and this is where this book excels. With the growing evidence base from clinical trials, with all their acronyms to remember, and increasing number of clinical guidelines, the authors pick out, and summarise, those relevant to the case in hand. This information becomes far easier to remember simply by association with the case. In addition a distinguished expert in the relevant field adds an 'expert commentary' and a 'final word' after the case discussion to complete the tutorial. I am sure the information held in each of these case scenarios will be recalled frequently in clinical practice and beyond.

The British Cardiovascular Society, through its education strategy, supports the delivery of high quality education and this book, through its knowledge based learning, certainly provides that. It comes highly recommended by the Society.

Dr Sarah Clarke
Vice President Education and Research
British Cardiovascular Society

PREFACE

Cardiovascular medicine in the 21st Century continues to be a dynamic and continually evolving landscape with high impact journals rapaciously churning out trial after landmark trial, alongside the emergence of novel translational techniques and discoveries at the cellular level. We as healthcare professionals must critically appraise and selectively plunder this evidence base and apply it to everyday clinical practice so that we can give our patients the very best possible care biomedical science will allow. Local, national and international guidelines help, as do the expert consensus of opinion leaders and the advice of our colleagues and peers on the ground. We have tried to encapsulate this contemporary scheme of patient-focussed care, with its foundation supported by guidelines and an evidence base, in this publication.

We present 25 real-world clinical scenarios, each aiming to provide the reader with an holistic approach to dealing with a variety of challenging concepts in cardiovascular medicine. It has been our deliberate intention to include detailed reviews centred around individual cases which we may all encounter either in the emergency department, outpatient clinic, catheterisation laboratory or on the coronary care unit. Indeed we have tried to avoid presenting a compendium of the rare, weird or wonderful. Each case has been written by a UK Specialty Trainee(s) and is punctuated by "Learning Points", "Clinical Tips," and "Landmark Trial Summaries". These highlighted boxes are embedded in the main body of the case text and should help to aid memory and provoke thought. We have then sought the peer review of an internationally-renowned Expert for each of the clinical scenarios and have asked them to provide a narrative as the case proceeds in the form of "Expert Comments" boxes. These should provide the reader with a unique insight into how today's opinion leaders deal with the very same clinical scenarios we all manage day in and day out.

We very much hope this text will appeal, first and foremost, to all specialty trainees in cardiology and to some degree those in acute and general internal medicine. Allied to this our aim has been to make this book stimulating, transferable, and accessible to all those with an interest in cardiovascular medicine so in that respect general practitioners (particularly those with a specialist interest in cardiology), clinical electrophysiologists, specialist cardiac nurses and physicians' assistants may all find the content applicable to their everyday practice. It is now standard practice to explore the management of clinical scenarios both in specialist training post interviews and fellowship exams. We would therefore expect our junior colleagues preparing to navigate these career milestones to find this text particularly relevant too.

We, the Editors, very much hope you enjoy the read.

Aung Myat
Shouvik Haldar
Simon Redwood

ACKNOWLEDGEMENTS

We would like to thank our faculty of Experts for their fantastic contribution, indeed without which this book would not have been possible. This text has also witnessed a collaboration of UK Specialty Trainees and the knowledge and innovation they have had to offer. We are extremely grateful to them for their time and dedication. And last, but certainly not least, we express our sincere gratitude to the publishing team at Oxford University Press, namely: Susan Crowhurst, Charles Haynes, and Helen Liepman for their trust, guidance, and supervision.

Aung Myat
Shouvik Haldar
Simon Redwood

In addition, I would like to thank Dr David Gareth Jones, whose expert opinion was hugely appreciated. I would like to thank my parents, Ganes and Manju, and my two sisters, Sananda and Shreya, for all their support during the writing of this book. Finally, I am truly indebted to Dr Elizabeth Caswell, for her invaluable encouragement and advice throughout this whole process.

Shouvik Haldar

CONTENTS

EXPERT FACULTY PROFILES

Case 1 Coronary artery bypass graft surgery vs percutaneous coronary intervention Professor Simon Redwood

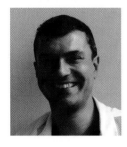

Professor Simon Redwood is Professor of Interventional Cardiology, King's College London and Honorary Consultant Cardiologist at Guy's and St Thomas' NHS Foundation Trust in London. He attained Fellowship of the American College of Cardiology (ACC) in 2001 and became a Fellow of the Royal College of Physicians (RCP) in 2003. He was previously Honorary Treasurer to the British Cardiovascular Intervention Society (BCIS) and is an International Editorial Board Member for the journal *Heart*. Professor Redwood has published widely in several top line cardiovascular journals on subjects ranging from post-infarction left ventricular remodelling; warm-up angina and ischaemic preconditioning to coronary collateral flow, left ventricular support during high-risk PCI and use of the pressure wire in practice.

Case 2 Can a rash cause stent thrombosis? Professor Tony Gershlick

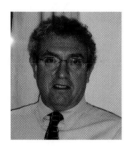

Professor Tony Gershlick is Professor of Interventional Cardiology at the University Hospitals of Leicester NHS Trust. He currently sits on the International Editorial Board of the *European Heart Journal* and leads the Research and Development arm of BCIS as a Council Member. He is a world-renowned expert on chronic total occlusion angioplasty and has been Principal Investigator for a number of landmark clinical trials including CLASSICS and REACT; the former demonstrating the superior tolerability of clopidogrel over ticlopidine after coronary stenting and the latter representing the seminal study proving the benefit of coronary angioplasty after failed thrombolysis for acute ST-elevation myocardial infarction.

Case 3 Triple antithrombotic therapy after coronary stenting for chronically anticoagulated patients: too much of a good thing? Professor Gregory Lip

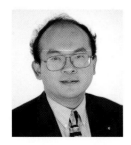

Professor Gregory Lip is Professor of Cardiovascular Medicine at the University of Birmingham, and Visiting Professor of Haemostasis, Thrombosis and Vascular Sciences at the University of Aston in Birmingham. He is based at the Centre for Cardiovascular Sciences, City Hospital in Birmingham. Professor Lip has a major interest in the epidemiology of atrial fibrillation, as well as the pathophysiology of thromboembolism in this arrhythmia. Furthermore, he has been researching stroke and bleeding, risk factors, and improvements in clinical risk stratification. The CHA_2DS_2 – VAS_c and HAS-BLED scores – for assessing stroke and bleeding risk, respectively – were first proposed and independently validated following his research, and are now incorporated into international guidelines.

Case 4 A closer look at lipid management following an acute coronary syndrome **Dr Anthony Wierzbicki**

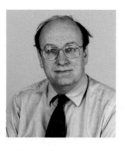

Dr Anthony Wierzbicki is a Consultant in Metabolic Medicine and Chemical Pathology and Director of the Lipid and Cardiovascular Prevention Unit at Guy's and St Thomas' NHS Foundation Trust and Honorary Reader (Assistant Professor) of Lipids and Cardiometabolic Disease at King's College London. His pre-clinical training was completed at Cambridge University. He then moved to Oxford University to finish clinical training having graduated in 1986 and later completing a Medical Research Council (MRC) Fellowship there. He is a Fellow of the National Association of Clinical Biochemistry in the United States and a Fellow of the American Heart Association. He is credited with over 250 publications in the field of atherosclerosis and lipid biology. He has sat on the panels of many national and international societies of cardiovascular disease and is a member of the technology appraisal panels of the National Institute of Health and Clinical Excellence.

Case 5 Management of prosthetic heart valves in pregnancy **Dr Fiona Walker**

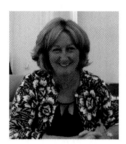

Dr Fiona Walker is the lead for the Adult Congenital Heart Disease service and maternal cardiology service at University College London Hospital. This unit provides all aspects of care for over 6000 patients and has given specialist antenatal care to 600 + women with all forms of heart disease with excellent outcome. Specific research areas include the impact in patients with single ventricle physiology. She is also interested in education and training and represents Grown Up Congenital Heart Disease on the ESC working group nucleus so contributes to training and guidelines Europe-wide.

Case 6 Symptomatic aortic stenosis: new horizons in management **Dr Martyn Thomas**

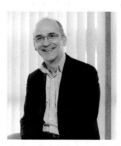

Dr Martyn Thomas is Consultant Interventional Cardiologist and Director of Cardiothoracic Services at Guy's and St Thomas' NHS Foundation Trust in London. Dr Thomas was President of BCIS from 2004 to 2008 and performed the first case of intra-coronary radiation (brachytherapy) to treat in-stent restenosis in the UK in 1998. More recently he has become one of the leading exponents of trans-catheter aortic valve implantation (TAVI) in the UK and speaks on this new interventional technology across the world.

Case 7 Assessment and management of mitral regurgitation
Professor Petros Nihoyannopoulos

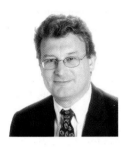

Professor Petros Nihoyannopoulos is Professor of Cardiology at the National Heart and Lung Institute in London. He is a fellow of the ACC, AHA, RCP and the European Society of Cardiology (ESC). He served as President of the British Society of Echocardiography (BSE) between 2001 and 2003 and is a past President of the European Association of Echocardiography of the ESC (2006–2008). His particular area of research is in the study of ventricular function; a field in which he pioneered the use of stress echocardiography in the UK in the early 80s, as well as leading the development of contrast microbubbles in clinical practice. He has published over 200 full papers in peer-review journals along with 350 abstracts, and written 2 books (*Echocardiography*, and *Non-invasive imaging of myocardial ischaemia*) and contributed to more than 20 book chapters.

Case 8 *Streptococcus mutans* endocarditis: a cautionary tale
Dr Bernard Prendergast

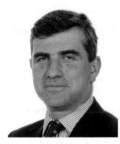

Dr Bernard Prendergast is the Clinical Director of Cardiology at the John Radcliffe Hospital in Oxford where he is also the clinical lead for the TAVI programme and director of the OxVALVE research programme. He is Honorary Secretary of the British Cardiovascular Society (BCS) and a leading authority on the management of and prophylaxis against infective endocarditis having recently published articles in both *The Lancet* and *Heart*. He is also the Chairman Elect of the ESC Valvular Heart Disease Working Group.

Case 9 A word to the wise: not all chest pain is ischaemic   Dr Iqbal Malik

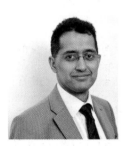

Dr Iqbal Malik is a Consultant Cardiologist and Honorary Senior Lecturer at St Mary's and Hammersmith Hospital, Imperial College Healthcare NHS Trust. He is a specialist in complex coronary angioplasty and since 2003, has lead the primary percutaneous coronary intervention team setting up a Heart Attack Treatment centre at Imperial College Healthcare NHS Trust. He has also recently become the National Clinical Lead in Web-based transfer systems. His research is focused on interventional cardiology: the role of patent foramen ovale closure in stroke, comparison of carotid artery stenting and surgery to prevent stroke and treatment of coronary heart disease with interventional techniques. He is also the Commissioning Editor for the journal *Heart*.

Case 10 Assessment and management of the breathless patient
Professor Theresa McDonagh

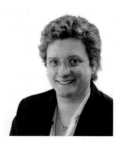

Professor Theresa McDonagh is Professor of Heart Failure and Consultant Cardiologist at King's College Hospital, London. She is a world-renowned expert on all aspects of heart failure including its epidemiology, the role of novel biomarkers and left ventricular dysfunction. She is a past Chair of the British Society for Heart Failure; a member of the Specialist Advisory Committee for Cardiology; and sits on the ESC Heart Failure Association committee for patient care. Professor McDonagh has published extensively on heart failure in several leading peer-reviewed journals and is on the editorial board for the journal *Heart*. She has also co-authored the *Oxford Specialist Handbook of Heart Failure*, and the *Oxford Textbook of Heart Failure*, and contributed numerous chapters to many other textbooks.

Case 11 Cardiac transplantation ### Dr Jayan Parameshwar

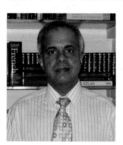

Dr Jayan Parameshwar is a Consultant Transplant Cardiologist at Papworth Hospital in Cambridge. He has research interests in all aspects of this field. He has published extensively with over 40 peer-reviewed articles to his credit and is currently on the board of directors of the International Society for Heart and Lung Transplantation.

Case 12 Young patients with hypertrophic cardiomyopathy: how to decide on implantable defibrillators ### Professor Michael Frenneaux

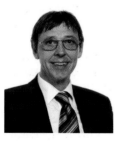

Professor Michael Frenneaux was appointed the Regius Professor of Medicine at the University of Aberdeen in 2009 having moved from his post as British Heart Foundation Chair in Cardiovascular Medicine at the University of Birmingham. He qualified from London and has previously held Chairs in Brisbane and Cardiff. His research is wide-ranging but is best described as integrated physiology with particular emphasis on investigating pathophysiological mechanisms in heart failure and in heart muscle diseases. He also has an interest in the physiological and potential therapeutic rates of nitrite.

Case 13 Myocarditis: an inflammatory cardiomyopathy
Dr Rakesh Sharma

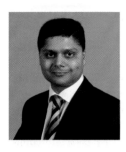

Dr Rakesh Sharma is Consultant Cardiologist at the Royal Brompton and Harefield NHS Foundation Trust. His specialist interests include heart failure and cardiac imaging. He is an expert in advanced pacing including biventricular pacemakers and implanted defibrillators. Dr Sharma is a regular speaker at national and international conferences including those of the BCS, ESC, and AHA. He is the author of more than 50 peer-reviewed articles, numerous editorials, abstracts and has written five book chapters.

Case 14 Arrhythmogenic right ventricular cardiomyopathy
Dr Elijah Behr

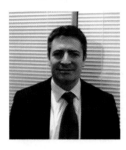

Dr Elijah Behr is a Senior Lecturer and Honorary Consultant Cardiologist specialising in Electrophysiology at St George's Hospital, London. He is a leading expert in sudden cardiac death in the young; drug-induced arrhythmia; families with a history of Sudden Arrhythmic Death Syndrome (SADS); ion channel diseases including the long QT and Brugada syndromes and cardiomyopathies including arrhythmogenic right ventricular cardiomyopathy (ARVC). He has published papers in several leading journals including *The Lancet*, *Heart* and *Heart Rhythm* and has presented at many national and international meetings. He has also worked with charities, particularly Cardiac Risk in the Young (CRY) and the BHF.

Case 15 The sparkly heart Dr Simon Dubrey

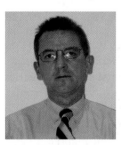

Dr Simon Dubrey is a Consultant Cardiologist at the Hillingdon and Mount Vernon Hospitals. He is also Honorary Senior Lecturer at the Imperial College School of Medicine and has an Honorary Consultant Cardiologist contract at the Royal Brompton & Harefield NHS Foundation Trust. He worked for 2 years in the American healthcare system. His clinical interests include atrial fibrillation and heart failure. He is an international expert on amyloid heart disease and has a particular interest in sarcoid and other 'infiltrative' cardiomyopathies. He has published in several leading cardiovascular journals on diabetic and amyloid heart disease.

Case 16 Paroxysmal atrial fibrillation **Professor John Camm**

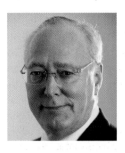

Professor John Camm is Professor of Clinical Cardiology at St George's University of London and Chairman of the Division of Cardiac and Vascular Sciences. His specialist interests include clinical cardiac electrophysiology, pacing, risk stratification post myocardial infarction and the inherited aspects of cardiac arrhythmias. He is a Fellow of the RCP, AHA, ACC and the ESC. At present he is also the President of the Arrhythmia Alliance. Professor Camm has written extensively and has over 1000 peer-reviewed papers, 250 book chapters and 22 books (as editor/author or both) to his credit. He has served as associate editor, guest editor or reviewer for many prestigious cardiovascular journals and is currently Editor-in-Chief of Europace.

Case 17 Ventricular tachycardia in a 'normal' heart **Dr Anthony Chow**

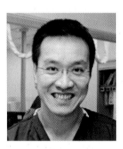

Dr Anthony Chow is Consultant Cardiac Electrophysiologist at University College Hospital in London having graduated from the Royal Free Hospital School of Medicine and later completing his specialist training at St. Mary's Hospital in London. His specialist interests include cardiac electrophysiology as well as heart failure and complex cardiac device therapy. He is engaged in active research programmes in arrhythmia and device treatment and has published a number of peer-reviewed articles as well as books on these subjects. He holds a number of BHF and substantial industry-funded research grants. He is a fellow of the RCP and is the joint clinical lead for the Arrhythmia and Sudden Cardiac Death Subgroup in The Thames Valley, London.

Case 18 Dual-chamber vs single-chamber pacing: the debate continues **Dr Vias Markides**

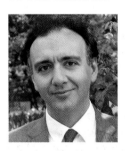

Dr Vias Markides was awarded the University of London Gold Medal in 1992, having received Honours in Medicine, Surgery, Clinical Pharmacology and Therapeutics, Obstetrics and Gynaecology, and Pathology. He is Consultant Cardiac Electrophysiologist at the Royal Brompton and Harefield NHS Foundation Trust and specialises in radiofrequency ablation of simple and complex rhythm problems, implantation of pacemakers, defibrillators, and devices for heart failure. His main research interest focuses around atrial fibrillation and other complex arrhythmias on which he has published numerous peer-reviewed articles. Dr Markides was also a member of the writing group for the National Service Framework (NSF) on arrhythmias and sudden cardiac death in the UK. He has also written or contributed to numerous book chapters.

Case 19 Reflex syncope: to pace or not to pace? **Professor Richard Sutton**

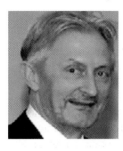

In the 1970s Professor Richard Sutton pioneered dual chamber pacing and in the 1980s introduced tilt testing for the diagnosis of vasovagal or neurally-mediated syncope. This work became the subject of an ACC Consensus document in 1996 and an ESC Task Force report in 2001 and later in 2004. Professor Sutton continues to research in the field of vasovagal syncope as well as cardiac resynchronization therapy for the treatment of advanced heart failure. During 1976–1993 he was a Consultant Cardiologist at Westminster Hospital (London) and from 1993 to 2007 at the Royal Brompton Hospital. His current appointment is at St Mary's Hospital (London). He is a past President of the British Pacing and Electrophysiology Group and Chairman of the ESC Working Group on Cardiac Pacing.

Case 20 Cryptogenic stroke **Dr Michael Mullen**

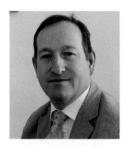

Dr Michael Mullen is a Consultant Cardiologist at University College Hospital in London. His main interests centre on the interventional treatment of structural and adult congenital heart disease. He specialises in both patent foramen ovale (PFO) and atrial septal defect closure and percutaneous aortic and pulmonary valve replacement. He was a leading contributor to the Migraine Intervention with STARFlex Technology (MIST) study that examined the role of PFO closure on the management of migraine and has now moved on to be the principal investigator of the BioStar evaluation study. He is also on the International Editorial Board of the journal *Heart* and has written several chapters for a variety of medical textbooks.

Case 21 Surgically-corrected tetralogy of Fallot and associated arrhythmias **Professor Michael Gatzoulis**

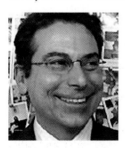

Professor Michael Gatzoulis is the academic head of the ACHD Centre and the Centre for Pulmonary Hypertension at the Royal Brompton Hospital and Professor of Cardiology and ACHD at the National Heart & Lung Institute, Imperial College, London. He is the past president of the International Society for Adult Congenital Cardiac Disease (ISACCD), and also holds executive or advisory board positions in other professional bodies, including the International Committee of the ACC. He is also the author of over 150 peer-reviewed publications including papers in *Nature*, the *New England Journal of Medicine*, *The Lancet* and *Circulation*. Professor Gatzoulis has also written the thorax section of the 40th edition of Gray's Anatomy: The Anatomical Basis of Clinical Practice, published in 2008.

Case 22 A case of refractory systemic hypertension
Professor Gareth Beevers

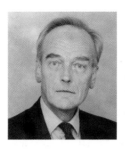

Professor Gareth Beevers qualified from The London Hospital in 1965. After working in district hospitals, in 1972 he moved to the MRC Blood Pressure Unit at the Western Infirmary Glasgow to research into the epidemiology of hypertension and the renin-angiotensin-aldosterone system. In 1977 he moved to a senior lectureship at the University of Birmingham, based at what is now the City Hospital. In Birmingham research was conducted on the role of salt, alcohol, and nutrition in hypertension. Subsidiary interests include ethnic differences in cardiovascular disease and hypertension in pregnancy. He was appointed professor of medicine in 1994 and emeritus professor in 2010. He finally retired from NHS clinical practice in 2011. Professor Beevers was the founder and Editor-in-Chief of the Journal of Human Hypertension and a past president of the British Hypertension Society.

Case 23 Syncope secondary to pulmonary arterial hypertension an ominous sign? **Dr Gerry Coghlan**

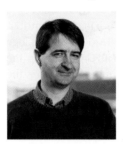

Dr Gerry Coghlan is a Consultant Cardiologist at the Royal Free Hospital in London and a Director of the National Pulmonary Hypertension Unit at the same institution where he has become an international authority on this particular disease process. He specialises in the management of connective tissue disorders associated with pulmonary arterial hypertension and has published extensively in this field.

Case 24 Cardiovascular preoperative risk assessment: a calculated gamble? **Dr Derek Chin**

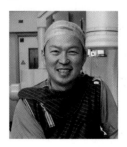

Dr Derek Chin is a graduate of the Royal Free Hospital School of Medicine, University of London. He specialised in Cardiovascular and General Internal Medicine at King's College Hospital, London and the Royal Sussex County Hospital, Brighton. He is now Consultant Cardiologist and Honorary Senior Lecturer at the University Hospitals of Leicester NHS Trust, providing one of the highest volume stress and intra-operative echocardiography services in the UK. He is a member of the Accreditation Committee of the BSE and was chief examiner of the inaugural UK Transoesophageal Echocardiography examination in 2003. His interests centre on resynchronising heart failure, revascularising hibernating myocardium, remodelling/regenerating cardiomyopathy and repairing/replacing diseased valves. He is part of the team that introduced TAVI to the UK and is currently developing other percutaneous catheterization laboratory therapies.

Case 25 The role of cardiac rehabilitation following cardiac surgery
Dr Jane Flint

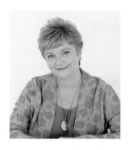

Dr Jane Flint is Consultant Cardiologist and Medical Service Head in the Dudley Group of Hospitals, and since 1988 Medical Director of the Beacon Award winning Action Heart Rehabilitation and Prevention programme since 1988. She has championed Nuclear Cardiology since her MD, District Cardiology services (RCP then BCS Council 2000-2004), Women in Cardiology (BCS Report and first BCS Council Representative 2005-2009), and chairs the BCS Joint Working group for Women's Heart Health since 2006. She also co-founded and is Clinical Lead for the BCS Patient Voice, Heart Care Partnership UK. As President of the British Association of Cardiac Rehabilitation 1997-1999 she was on the External Reference Group for the NSF for Coronary Heart Disease, was Clinical Director of The Black Country Cardiovascular Network 2003-2008, and is now National Clinical Advisor for Cardiac Rehabilitation to the NHS Improvement Heart Team. She is also a professional Trustee of the BHF.

Speciality Trainee Contributors

Dr Sarah Bowater, SpR in Cardiology, West Midlands Deanery

Dr Badrinathan Chandrasekaran, SpR in Cardiology, Wessex Deanery

Dr Imogen Clarke, SpR in Acute Medicine, West Midlands Deanery

Dr Owais Dar, SpR in Cardiology, East Midlands South Deanery

Dr Shouvik Haldar, SpR in Cardiology, London Deanery

Dr Ali Hamaad, SpR in Cardiology, West Midlands Deanery

Dr Arif Khan, SpR in Cardiology, London Deanery

Dr Jamal Khan, SpR in Cardiology, West Midlands Deanery

Dr Kate von Klemperer, SpR in Cardiology, London Deanery

Dr Pipin Kojodjojo, SpR in Cardiology, London Deanery

Dr William Moody, SpR in Cardiology, West Midlands Deanery

Dr Martina Muggenthaler, SpR in Cardiology, London Deanery

Dr Amal Muthumala , SpR in Cardiology, Oxford Deanery

Dr Aung Myat, SpR in Cardiology, West Midlands Deanery

Dr Bejal Pandhya, SpR in Cardiology, London Deanery

Special Trainee Contributors

Dr Ricardo Petraco, SpR in Cardiology, West Midlands Deanery

Dr Chris Steadman, SpR in Cardiology, West Midlands Deanery

Dr Joseph Tomson, SpR in Cardiology, West Midlands Deanery

Dr Ali Vazir, SpR in Cardiology, London Deanery

Dr Lynne Williams, SpR in Cardiology, West Midlands Deanery

ABBREVIATIONS

°C	degree Celsius
≥	equal to or greater than
≤	equal to or less than
=	equal to
κ	kappa
λ	lambda
<	less than
6MWT	6-minute walk test
>	more than
Ω	Ohm
%	per cent
π	pi
2D	two-dimensional
3D	three-dimensional
AA	arachidonic acid
AAD	anti-arrhythmic drug
AAS	acute aortic syndromes
ACC	American College of Cardiology
ACCP	American College of Chest Physicians
ACE	angiotensin-converting enzyme
ACEi	angiotensin-converting enzyme inhibitor
ACHD	adult congenital heart disease
ACS	acute coronary syndrome
ACT	activated clotting time
ADP	adenosine diphosphate
A&E	Accident and Emergency
AF	atrial fibrillation
AHA	American Heart Association
ALP	alkaline phosphatase
ALT	alanine aminotransferase
AMI	acute myocardial infarction
APA	aldosterone-producing adenoma
APCR	activated protein C resistance
APET	aortic pre-ejection time
APTT	activated partial thromboplastin time
AR	aortic regurgitation
ARB	angiotensin receptor blocker
ARC	Academic Research Consortium
ARVC	arrhythmogenic right ventricular cardiomyopathy
AS	aortic stenosis
ASA	atrial septal aneurysm

ASCS	agitated saline contrast study
ASD	atrial septal defect
ASH	asymmetric septal hypertrophy
AST	aspartate aminotransferase
ATP	Acute Treatment Panel
AV	aortic valve
AVNRT	atrioventricular nodal re-entrant tachycardia
AVR	aortic valve replacement
BACR	British Association for Cardiac Rehabilitation
BARI	Bypass Angioplasty Revascularization Investigation
BAV	balloon aortic valvuloplasty
BCSH	British Committee for Standards in Haematology
BCT	broad complex tachycardia
bd	*bis die* (twice daily)
BHS	British Hypertension Society
BMI	body mass index
BMS	bare-metal stent
BNP	B-type/brain natriuretic peptide
BP	blood pressure
bpm	beats per minute
BSA	body surface area
CABG	coronary artery bypass grafting
CAD	coronary artery disease
cAMP	cyclic adenosine monophosphate
CCB	calcium channel blocker
CCS	Canadian Cardiovascular Society
CCU	Coronary Care Unit
CDU	Clinical Decisions Unit
CHB	complete heart block
CHD	coronary heart disease
CI	confidence interval
CK	creatine kinase
cm	centimetre
CMR	cardiac magnetic resonance
CMV	cytomegalovirus
COX	cyclooxygenase
CPAP	continuous positive airway pressure

CPET	cardiopulmonary exercise test		FFP	fresh frozen plasma
CR	cardiac rehabilitation		FH	familial hypercholesterolaemia
CRP	C reactive protein		fL	femtolitre
CRT	cardiac resynchronization therapy		FVC	forced vital capacity
CRT-D	cardiac resynchronization therapy with a defibrillator		g	gram
CRT-P	cardiac resynchronization therapy-pacemaker		GFR	glomerular filtration rate
			GI	gastrointestinal
CRY	Cardiac Risk in the Young		GP	general practitioner
CSA	cross-sectional area		GRACE	Global Registry of Acute Coronary Events
CSH	carotid sinus hypersensitivity		GTN	glyceryl trinitrate
CSM	carotid sinus massage		GTP	guanosine triphosphate
CSS	carotid sinus syncope/syndrome		GUCH	grown-up congenital heart
CT	computed tomography			
CTPA	computed tomography pulmonary angiogram		h	hour
			HAD	Hospital Anxiety and Depression
CTT	Cholesterol Treatment Trialists		Hb	haemoglobin
CV	cardiovascular		HCM	hypertrophic cardiomyopathy
CVA	cerebrovascular accident		HCO_3^-	bicarbonate
CXR	chest X-ray		HDL-C	high-density lipoprotein cholesterol
			HF	heart failure
d	day		HFNEF	heart failure with normal ejection fraction
DAPT	dual antiplatelet therapy		HIT	heparin-induced thrombocytopenia
DCCV	direct current cardioversion		HIV	human immunodeficiency virus
DES	drug-eluting stent		HLA	human leucocyte antigen
dL	decilitre		HPR	high on-treatment platelet reactivity
DVLA	Driving and Vehicles Licensing Authority		HPS	Heart Protection Study
			HR	heart rate
EAPCI	European Association of Percutaneous Coronary Interventions		HRS	Heart Rhythm Society
			HRUK	Heart Rhythm UK
EBV	Epstein Barr virus		hsCRP	high sensitivity C reactive protein
ECG	electrocardiogram			
ED	Emergency Department		IABP	intra-aortic balloon pump
EDV	end-diastolic volume		ICD	implantable cardioverter-defibrillator
EEG	electroencephalogram		ICMA	mycotic aneurysm in intracranial arteries
EF	ejection fraction		i.e.	*id est* (that is)
e.g	*exempli gratia* (for example)		IE	infective endocarditis
eGFR	estimated glomerular filtration rate		IgG	immunoglobulin G
EHRA	European Heart Rhythm Association		IHA	idiopathic hyperaldosteronism
EMB	endomyocardial biopsy		IHD	ischaemic heart disease
ERO	effective regurgitant orifice		ILR	implantable loop recorder
ESC	European Society of Cardiology		INR	international normalized ratio
ESV	end-systolic volume		IPA	inhibition of platelet aggregation
ETT	exercise tolerance test		iPAH	idiopathic pulmonary arterial hypertension
			IQ	intelligence quotient
FBC	full blood count		IRAD	International Registry for acute Aortic Dissections
FCH	familial combined hyperlipidaemia			
FDA	Food and Drug Administration		ISR	in-stent restenosis
FEV1	forced expiratory volume in first second		IU	international unit

IUGR	intrauterine growth retardation
IV	intravenous
IVD	interventricular delay
IVUS	intravascular ultrasound
J	Joule
JVP	jugular venous pressure
K	potassium
kg	kilogram
kPa	kilopascal
L	litre
LA	left atrial
LAA	left atrial appendage
LAD	left anterior descending
LBBB	left bundle branch block
LCx	left circumflex
LD	loading dose
LDH	lactate dehydrogenase
LDL-C	low-density lipoprotein cholesterol
LDLR	low-density lipoprotein receptor
LIMA	left internal mammary artery
LMCA	left main coronary artery
LMS	left main stem
LMWH	low molecular weight heparin
LSVC	left superior vena cava
LTA	light transmittance aggregometry
LV	left ventricular
LVAD	left ventricular assist device
LVEF	left ventricular ejection fraction
LVH	left ventricular hypertrophy
LVOT	left ventricular outflow tract
LVSD	left ventricular systolic dysfunction
m	metre
MA	mycotic aneurysm
MACE	major adverse cardiac events
MACCE	major adverse cardiovascular and cerebrovascular events
MADIT-CRT	Multicentre Automated Defibrillator Implantation Trial with Cardiac Resynchronization Therapy
MAU	Medical Admissions Unit
mcg	microgram
MCV	mean corpuscular volume
MD	maintenance dose
MDRD	Modification of Diet in Renal Disease
MDT	multidisciplinary team

MET	metabolic equivalent
mg	milligram
MI	myocardial infarction
MIBG	meta-iodobenzylguanidine
min	minute
mm	millimetre
MMF	mycophenolate mofetil
mmHg	millimetre mercury
mmol	millimole
micromol	micromole
mo	month
mPAP	mean pulmonary arterial pressure
MR	mitral regurgitation
MRA	magnetic resonance angiography
MRI	magnetic resonance imaging
ms	millisecond
MS	mitral stenosis
mV	millivolt
MV	mitral valve
MVD	multivessel disease
MVR	mitral valve replacement
Na	sodium
NAC	National Amyloid Centre
NACR	National Audit for Cardiac Rehabilitation
NCEP	National Cholesterol Education Programme
NCT	narrow complex tachycardia
ng	nanogram
NICE	National Institute for Health and Clinical Excellence
NSAID	non-steroidal anti-inflammatory drug
NSF	National Service Framework
NSTEMI	non-ST-elevation myocardial infarction
NSVT	non-sustained ventricular tachycardia
NT	N-terminal
NYHA	New York Heart Association
OAC	oral anticoagulation
OCT	orthotopic cardiac transplantation
od	*omni die* (once daily)
OGD	oesophagogastroduodenoscopy
OM	obtuse marginal
OM1	first obtuse marginal
p	probability
PA	pulmonary arteries
PAD	peripheral arterial disease
PAF	paroxysmal atrial fibrillation
PAH	pulmonary arterial hypertension

PAP	pulmonary arterial pressure	SIGN	Scottish Intercollegiate Guidelines Network
PCC	prothrombin complex concentrate	SND	sinus node dysfunction
PCI	percutaneous coronary intervention	SNP	sodium nitroprusside
PCM	physical countermeasure	SNS	sympathetic nervous system
PCO_2	partial pressure of carbon dioxide	STEMI	ST-elevation myocardial infarction
PCWP	pulmonary capillary wedge pressure	STS	Society of Thoracic Surgeons
PDA	posterior descending artery	SV	stroke volume
PFO	patent foramen ovale	SVG	saphenous vein graft
PGE_1	prostaglandin E_1	SYNTAX	Synergy between Percutaneous Coronary Intervention with Taxus and Cardiac Surgery
PISA	proximal isovelocity surface area		
PLAX	parasternal long axis		
pmol	picomole		
PMVL	posterior mitral valve leaflet	TAPSE	tricuspid annular plane systolic excursion
PO_2	partial pressure of oxygen		
POBA	plain old balloon angioplasty	TAVI	trans-catheter aortic valve implantation
PPCI	primary percutaneous coronary intervention	TC	total cholesterol
		TCD	transcranial Doppler
PPM	permanent pacemaker	TDI	tissue Doppler imaging
PR	pulmonary regurgitation	tds	*ter die sumendus* (three times daily)
PV	pulmonary vein	TG	triglycerides
PVC	premature ventricular complexes	TIA	transient ischaemic attack
PVI	pulmonary vein isolation	TIMI	Thrombolysis In Myocardial Infarction
PVR	pulmonary vascular resistance	TLR	target lesion revascularization
		TOE	transoesophageal echocardiography
QRSd	QRS duration	ToF	tetralogy of Fallot
QT_c	QT corrected	TR	tricuspid regurgitation
		TSH	thyroid stimulating hormone
RACPC	Rapid Access Chest Pain Clinic	TT	triple therapy
RAAS	renin-angiotensin-aldosterone system	TTE	transthoracic echocardiogram
RATG	rabbit anti-thymocyte globulin	TTP	thrombotic thrombocytopaenic purpura
RAVI	right atrial volume index	TTR	transthyretin
RBBB	right bundle branch block	TXA_2	thromboxane-A_2
RBC	red blood cells		
RCA	right coronary artery	U	unit
RCT	randomized controlled trial	UA	unstable angina
RITA	Randomized Intervention Treatment of Angina	U&E	urea and electrolytes
		UFH	unfractionated heparin
RV	right ventricular	UK	United Kingdom
RVFRS	right ventricular failure risk score	ULN	upper limit of normal
RVOT	right ventricular outflow tract	US	United States
RWMA	regional wall motion abnormalities	TVR	target vessel revascularization
s	seconds	V	volt
SA	sinoatrial	VA	ventriculo-atrial
SAECG	signal-averaged electrocardiogram	VASP-P	vasodilator-stimulated phosphoprotein phosphorylation
SAM	systolic anterior motion		
SAP	serum amyloid protein	VF	ventricular fibrillation
SC	subcutaneous	VIP	vasoactive intestinal peptide
SCD	sudden cardiac death	VKA	vitamin K antagonist

VLDL-C	very low density lipoprotein cholesterol		WCC	white cell count
VO$_2$	volume of oxygen		WHO	World Health Organization
VPB	ventricular premature beat		WPW	Wolff–Parkinson–White
vs	versus		WT	wild type
VSD	ventricular septal defect			
VT	ventricular tachycardia		y	year
VTE	venous thromboembolism			
VTI	velocity time integral			

Coronary artery bypass graft surgery vs percutaneous coronary intervention

Aung Myat

ⓘ **Expert commentary** Professor Simon Redwood

Case history

A 65-year-old gentleman presented to his general practitioner (GP) with a 2-month history of exertional central chest discomfort. He described it as a squeezing, vice-like sensation. As time had passed, the effort required to precipitate this pain had gradually reduced to the point where simply walking a few yards in a stiff breeze would precipitate an episode. Apart from feeling clammy, there were no other associated symptoms. Resting would relieve the discomfort which was then often followed by a 'second wind' that would allow him to finish whatever task he was performing. He had previously had unlimited effort tolerance and would normally complete a round of golf without any problems. There was no history of pain at rest.

There was a history of treated hypertension and hypercholesterolaemia. He was taking ramipril (5 mg once daily) and simvastatin (40 mg nocte). There was a family history of coronary heart disease (CHD) in a first-degree relative. He had smoked socially for a few years in his early twenties. He drank alcohol within recommended limits and perhaps drank three caffeine-containing drinks per day.

At the GP surgery, the patient was pain-free and haemodynamically stable. There was nil of note on examination and an electrocardiogram (ECG) revealed no evidence of acute ischaemia. The last episode of pain was reported to have occurred 24 hours prior to the consultation. The GP recommended the patient make his way to the local Emergency Department (ED) to be formally assessed.

On arrival, the patient was seen by an ED doctor who took a thorough history and examination, ordered a chest X-ray (CXR), and took routine bloods, including a troponin T. The patient was again pain-free and an admission ECG demonstrated no acute ischaemia. The patient was referred to the medical team on-call and transferred to the Clinical Decisions Unit (CDU) to rule out an acute coronary syndrome (ACS). Antithrombotic therapy, however, was not commenced.

On the CDU, observations remained essentially unchanged and routine blood tests, including troponin T, were all reported as normal (Table 1.1). A postero-anterior CXR demonstrated clear lung fields with no evidence of focal consolidation or pneumothorax and a normal cardiothoracic ratio.

The patient was assessed by the general medical registrar who deemed the patient at low risk of further adverse cardiovascular events. A repeat ECG with the patient free of pain again confirmed normal sinus rhythm. The doctor reassured the patient that he had not had a heart attack in light of the negative troponin and a normal resting ECG and a plan was made to discharge the patient back to the care of the GP with a view to a direct referral to cardiology if symptoms were to recur. No new medication was initiated.

Table 1.1 Routine blood test results and observations on the Clinical Decisions Unit

Haematology		Biochemistry		Observations	
Hb	14.4 g/dL	Na	138 mmol/L	BP	135/88 mmHg
WCC	7.85 × 10⁹/L	K	4.2 mmol/L	O₂ saturations	98% on air
Platelets	300 × 10⁹/L	Urea	7.2 mmol/L	Temperature	36.5°C
		Creatinine	138 micromol/L		
INR	1.1	Random glucose	6.4 mmol/L	Total cholesterol	3.2 mmol/L
		TSH	2.3 mIU/L	LDL-C	2.1 mmol/L
		CRP	<3 mg/L	HDL-C	1.2 mmol/L
		Troponin T	<0.01 ng/mL	Triglycerides	1.0 mmol/L

⊕ **Learning point** The Thrombolysis In Myocardial Infarction (TIMI) risk score for UA/non-ST-elevation myocardial infarction (NSTEMI) [1]

Patients admitted with cardiac-sounding chest pain present with a spectrum of risk of death and subsequent ischaemic cardiac events. Previous attempts to establish a gradient of risk amongst this cohort of patients tended to focus primarily on one or two variables such as elevated serum cardiac markers or the presence or absence of ECG changes. The TIMI risk score, however, utilizes seven independent variables which, if present, serve to indicate the severity of risk and, therefore, the degree of urgency with which intervention should be instigated. The test cohort for development of this risk assessment tool came from the 1,957 patients assigned to receive unfractionated heparin (UFH) in the TIMI 11B trial [2]. The risk score was then validated using the enoxaparin arm of TIMI 11B (n = 1,953) and both the UFH and enoxaparin arms of the ESSENCE trial (n = 3,171) [3].

The seven variables are as follows and each is assigned a single point:

- Age ≥65 years;
- ≥3 risk factors for coronary artery disease (CAD) (i.e. diabetes mellitus, hypertension, hyperlipidaemia, current smoker, and family history of CAD);
- Known CAD (significant coronary stenosis >50% on previous angiography);
- Aspirin use within the last seven days;
- Severe anginal symptoms (e.g. ≥2 anginal events in the last 24 hours);
- ST deviation ≥0.5 mm on ECG;
- Elevated serum cardiac markers.

The percentage risk of the primary endpoint (all-cause mortality, myocardial infarction (MI), or urgent revascularization) occurring by 14 days in the UFH test cohort of the TIMI 11B trial according to the accumulated TIMI risk score was as follows:

Risk score	Death or MI (%)	Death, MI, or urgent revascularization (%)
0/1 points	3	5
2 points	3	8
3 points	5	13
4 points	7	20
5 points	12	26
6/7 points	19	41

The patient in this case scored two points at initial presentation and, therefore, was certainly at an increased risk of deleterious cardiac events if no therapeutic intervention was instigated. Of note, a meta-analysis of the TIMI 11B and ESSENCE trials demonstrated the superior efficacy of enoxaparin over UFH in UA/NSTEMI, giving rise to a 20% lower risk of death and major adverse cardiovascular and cerebrovascular events (MACCE) with similar rates of bleeding between the two strategies [4].

> **☼ Learning point** The Global Registry of Acute Coronary Events (GRACE) risk score for ACS [5]
>
> Unlike the 7-point TIMI risk score, the GRACE model covers the entire spectrum of ACS, from UA through to ST-elevation myocardial infarction (STEMI), and can be used to predict both in-hospital and 6-month mortality. It also takes into account patients with comorbidities such as renal dysfunction and heart failure at acute presentation. It has been derived from a multinational registry of ACS patients from 94 hospitals in 14 different countries that enrolled a total of 13,708 patients in a 2-year period between 1 April 1999 and 31 March 2001.
>
> The authors identified eight parameters that could be used to predict clinical outcome and, therefore, aid the therapeutic decision-making process:
>
> - Age;
> - Heart rate;
> - Systolic blood pressure (BP);
> - Creatinine level;
> - Congestive heart failure at presentation (Killip class):
>   - Killip class I: no heart failure;
>   - Killip class II: presence of rales and/or jugular venous distension;
>   - Killip class III: pulmonary oedema;
>   - Killip class IV: cardiogenic shock;
> - Cardiac arrest at admission;
> - ST-segment deviation (i.e. elevation or depression in the anterior, inferior, or lateral lead groups of at least 1 mm);
> - Elevated cardiac enzymes/markers.
>
> Each parameter is scored and the cumulative risk corresponds to an estimated probability of all-cause mortality from hospital discharge through to six months. The GRACE risk score calculator is available online (available from: www.outcomes-umassmed.org/grace/) and is a readily accessible and easy-to-use tool that will calculate the risk of an individual patient for you.

Following discharge, the patient suffered further chest pain on walking to his local supermarket 200 yards away from his home. He became sweaty and, more worryingly to him, quite breathless for the first time. He rested and the symptoms spontaneously resolved. He called his GP for advice who subsequently contacted the medical registrar on-call to request direct admission to the CDU for further assessment that day.

On arrival, the patient was pain-free with a BP of 148/79 mmHg and a heart rate (HR) of 88 beats per minute (bpm). An ECG was again normal, but given the history, previous admission the day before with similar symptoms, and multiple risk factors for CHD, the patient was immediately commenced on an ACS therapeutic protocol consisting of loading doses of aspirin and clopidogrel (300 mg of each stat) (see CURE trial) and a weight-adjusted treatment dose of enoxaparin (1 mg/kg twice daily) (see TIMI 11B and ESSENCE Trials) alongside his regular ramipril and simvastatin. The patient was referred for a specialist cardiology opinion and a plan was made to check a 12-hour troponin T which was subsequently found to be negative. The cardiologist agreed with the diagnosis of troponin-negative UA and arranged for a doctor-led exercise stress test that day. This was subsequently found to be abnormal (Figure 1.1).

In light of the positive stress test, the decision was made to proceed to coronary angiography with a view to performing percutaneous coronary intervention (PCI), if indicated, the next day. Bisoprolol (2.5 mg od) was commenced at this point.

A coronary angiogram was conducted via the right femoral artery. It revealed severe 3-vessel CAD. The left main coronary artery (LMCA) was normal. The left anterior

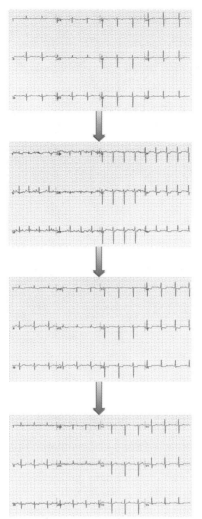

Resting ECG confirms normal sinus rhythm with no acute ischaemic changes.

In stage 2 of the Bruce protocol, the patient complains of central chest discomfort and dyspnoea. There is corresponding ST-segment depression in the anterolateral leads (i.e. V3–V6, I. and aVL). At 5.30 minutes, the decision is made to abort the test. The patient has displayed appropriate increases in both BP and heart rate.

In the first recovery stage, the patient reports improvement in his symptoms. There are still persistent ischaemic changes anterolaterally.

In the final recovery stage, both heart rate and BP are back to baseline levels. The patient is symptom-free and the anterolateral changes have almost resolved. There is, however, a hint of ischaemia developing in the inferior leads (i.e. II, III, and aVL).

Figure 1.1 Exercise stress test ECGs demonstrating significant anterolateral and inferior ST depression following stage 2 of the Bruce protocol.

⊘ Landmark trial TIMI 11B trial [2]

- Enoxaparin (n = 1,953) vs UFH (n = 1,957) in 3,910 UA/NSTEMI patients;
- Randomized, double-blind, double-dummy (in-hospital), placebo-controlled (out-of-hospital), parallel group design;
- In hospital: enoxaparin 30 mg intravenous (IV) bolus, then 1 mg/kg bd subcutaneously (SC) for eight days or until hospital discharge; UFH 70 U/kg IV bolus, then 15 U/kg/h IV for three days according to activated partial thromboplastin time;
- Out of hospital: enoxaparin 4–60 mg SC bd (previous enoxaparin patients) or placebo SC bd (previous UFH patients);
- Death, MI, or urgent revascularization at 8 days: enoxaparin 12.4% vs UFH 14.5% (p = 0.048); at 43 days: enoxaparin 17.3% vs UFH 19.7% (p = 0.048);
- No significant difference in the incidence of major haemorrhage at 72 hours and at hospital discharge.

> **⊘ Landmark trial** ESSENCE trial [3]
>
> - Enoxaparin (n = 1,607) vs UFH (n = 1,564) in 3,171 UA/NSTEMI patients;
> - Randomized, double-blind, double-dummy, parallel group design;
> - Enoxaparin 1 mg/kg bd plus UFH placebo or UFH 5,000 U IV bolus, then continuous infusion plus enoxaparin placebo for ≥48 hours and ≤8 days;
> - Risk of death, MI, or recurrent angina significantly lower in enoxaparin arm at 14 and 30 days;
> - Need for revascularization also significantly lower in enoxaparin arm at 30 days;
> - Findings in favour of enoxaparin extended to one year.

> **⊘ Landmark trial** CURE trial [6]
>
> - Clopidogrel plus aspirin vs aspirin alone in 12,562 patients presenting within 24 hours of ACS without ST elevation;
> - Randomized, double-blind, placebo-controlled;
> - Clopidogrel: 300 mg loading dose, then 75 mg/day; all patients received 75–325 mg/day aspirin;
> - 20% risk reduction in cardiovascular (CV) death, MI, or stroke with clopidogrel;
> - 14% risk reduction in CV death, MI, stroke, or refractory ischaemia with clopidogrel;
> - Significant increase in major bleeding episodes with clopidogrel although post hoc analysis of the results would show this was actually related to increasing doses of aspirin [7];
> - No significant difference in life-threatening bleeds.

> **✪ Learning point** What to look for when assessing exercise stress tests along with parameters associated with an adverse prognosis and multivessel CAD
>
> *(adapted from Braunwald's Heart Disease: A Textbook of Cardiovascular Medicine, Elsevier Saunders, 2005)*
>
> - ST-segment changes
>   - Exercise-induced ST elevation; or
>   - Downsloping or planar depression ≥2 mm, starting at <5 metabolic equivalents (METs), involving ≥5 leads
>   - Persisting ≥5 min into recovery;
> - Blood pressure
>   - Failure to increase systolic BP ≥120 mmHg;
>   - Sustained reduction ≥10 mmHg, repeatable within 15 seconds; or
>   - Sudden reduction below standing rest levels when the BP has otherwise been appropriately rising;
> - Maximal work capacity
>   - Amount of work performed is measured in METs (not the duration of exercise in minutes)
>   - Symptom-limiting exercise of <5 METs achieved is associated with an adverse prognosis
> - Heart rate response
>   - Aim to increase HR above 75% of age-predicted maximum and ideally >85–90% to ensure a valid diagnostic test result;
>   - **Chronotropic incompetence** refers to an inability to increase HR to 85% of age-predicted maximum;
>   - **Chronotropic index** refers to an increase in HR per stage of exercise below that of normal;
>   - Chronotropic index of ≤80% is associated with an increased CV mortality and may indicate autonomic dysfunction, sinus node disease, myocardial ischaemia, or simply HR-limiting drug therapy;
>   - Abnormal HR rate recovery, i.e. an attenuated deceleration of HR in recovery may suggest decreased vagal tone and is also associated with adverse outcomes;
> - Arrhythmias
>   - Reproducible, sustained (>30 s), or symptomatic ventricular tachycardia can indicate multivessel CAD;
> - Chest pain
>   - Typical angina at low exercise workloads is an ominous sign.

descending (LAD) artery had a 95% proximal stenosis involving the ostium of the first diagonal artery which itself had an 80% proximal lesion. The left circumflex (LCx) artery was a large, dominant vessel with a 90% proximal stenosis and a proximally occluded first obtuse marginal (OM1) branch which appeared to be serving a wide myocardial territory. The right coronary artery (RCA) was small, recessive, and subtotally occluded in its proximal segment. Subsequent left ventriculogram confirmed good systolic function with no evidence of mitral incompetence (Figure 1.2).

There were lesions amenable to PCI: the proximal LAD stenosis, for instance, and an attempt could be made at opening the proximally occluded OM1 vessel. The RCA would be too narrow to attempt stent insertion. The patient, however, was relatively young, had little in the way of limiting comorbidity, had preserved left ventricular systolic function, and normal renal function on a background of severe 3-vessel CAD. Hence, the opinion of a cardiac surgeon was sought.

The cardiac surgeon on-call accepted that the patient was a valid candidate for coronary artery bypass grafting (CABG), but also suggested that PCI would be a reasonable alternative. Quoting the medical literature, he stated there was little difference in overall mortality between CABG and PCI in patients of this age with preserved left

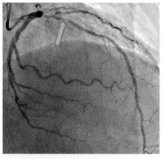

Right anterior oblique (RAO) cranial view revealing a tight proximal LAD stenosis (blue arrow).

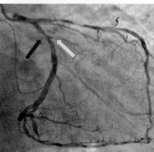

RAO caudal view demonstrating a significant proximal LCx lesion (red arrow) at the bifurcation with a proximally occluded first obtuse marginal branch artery (yellow arrow).

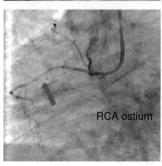

RCA ostium

Left anterior oblique (LAO) caudal view revealing a small, recessive RCA subtotally occluded in its mid-segment (green arrow).

Figure 1.2 Coronary angiogram images confirming multivessel coronary artery disease.

ventricular function and no history of diabetes. He also felt that the patient's preferred revascularization strategy should be taken into consideration. Since the patient was still on the table and had a femoral sheath *in situ*, it was deemed inappropriate to make any definitive decisions there and then. The situation was explained to the patient and the femoral sheath removed with haemostasis achieved through manual pressure. A vascular closure device was not instituted since recannulation of the right femoral artery may have been required if PCI was the chosen strategy.

The patient was discharged to the ward armed with British Heart Foundation brochures detailing the pros and cons of both PCI and CABG. The weekly multidisciplinary meeting was later convened and the case discussed amongst cardiac surgeons, interventional, and non-interventional cardiologists. A consensus decision for CABG surgery as the best revascularization strategy for the patient was made. The patient was also in agreement with this decision, having had the time and information provided by cardiothoracic and cardiac specialist nursing staff to discuss the matter fully with his family.

Maintenance dose clopidogrel was stopped and the patient proceeded to semi-urgent inpatient CABG surgery a week later. He received saphenous vein grafts to his distal RCA and OM1 and a left internal mammary artery graft to his LAD. He made an uneventful recovery and was home within six days post-operatively.

Discussion

This case highlights an all too familiar treatment dilemma posed to both clinician and patient when faced with symptomatic CAD amenable to both PCI and CABG surgery. Each has been shown to be an effective and a safe revascularization strategy for multivessel disease (MVD). In recent times, however, there has been a dramatic upsurge in the volume and scope of PCI procedures and alongside this, a concurrent plateau in CABG numbers which have remained relatively constant since 1997 in the United Kingdom (UK); indeed in 2008, over 80,000 PCI were undertaken in comparison to approximately 25,000 isolated CABG procedures [8]. This disparity must take into account those patients with 1- or 2-vessel CAD, predominantly discrete *de novo* lesions not involving the LMCA, for which PCI is often the preferred method of revascularization. There is less clinical risk with PCI, a comparatively shorter hospital stay, and good evidence that it reduces angina burden and myocardial ischaemia in this patient cohort [9]. In contrast, patients with significantly impaired left ventricular function found to have either LMCA or triple-vessel disease tend to do better with CABG when compared with medical therapy [10,11]. It is over those patients that sit between these two extremes and for whom either revascularization option is technically feasible that the debate continues as to which strategy is 'better'.

There have been numerous randomized controlled trials (RCT) specifically designed to answer this question. They have tended to enrol, however, a highly selective MVD patient cohort which may not be representative of the general CAD population. For instance, of the 8,826 patients screened in 15 RCT of PCI (balloon angioplasty and/or bare-metal coronary stenting) vs CABG for MVD (ERACI, EAST, GABI, CABRI, MASS, BARI, SIMA, LAUSANNE, RITA, TOULOUSE, AWESOME, ERACI II, ARTS, SOS, and MASS II), only 5% went on to be randomized to either revascularization strategy [12]. All had ejection fractions greater than 50% and only 35% had documented triple-vessel disease, thus nullifying the perceived benefit of CABG in higher-risk groups (i.e. diabetics, significantly impaired left ventricular (LV) function, and triple-vessel CAD).

Clinical tip Essential preoperative tick boxes prior to CABG surgery

- Ensure irreversible P2Y$_{12}$ antagonists (i.e. clopidogrel, ticlopidine or, more latterly, prasugrel) are stopped at least five days prior to CABG surgery;
- Look for abnormal dentition and refer appropriately;
- Organize ultrasound carotid Dopplers to ensure no evidence of significant stenoses;
- Arrange full lung spirometry; and
- Ensure up-to-date blood tests are performed, including a full blood count, urea and electrolytes, and a full clotting screen.

Expert comment

I would also stop the angiotensin-converting enzyme (ACE) inhibitor; cardiac surgeons like to have all vasoactive medications stopped prior to surgery.

Some may argue this screening process is a true reflection of the gradation in the extent of CAD and LV function in the CHD population at large and that only with RCTs do you negate selection bias and potential confounders through the workings of independent core laboratories, clinical events committees, and data safety monitoring boards. On the other hand, it is essential that we do not and, therefore, cannot apply these results to those who may have less or more extensive CAD.

The early RCTs of CABG vs PCI were conducted in the pre-stent era when plain old balloon angioplasty (POBA) was the single percutaneous mode of coronary revascularization available (see RITA 1 and BARI trials). A meta-analysis of 13 RCTs of CABG vs PCI by Hoffman et al. [17], including the RITA 1 and BARI trials, demonstrated a small 1.9% absolute survival advantage favouring CABG for all trials at five years ($p < 0.02$), but not at one, three, or eight years. Four of the trials (SIMA, ERACI II, ARTS, and SOS) used stents as their initial mode of PCI. The trend favouring CABG for survival at three years in the POBA trials was no longer evident in the stent era. The positive impact of coronary stenting was also revealed in the need for subsequent revascularizations which had halved from a 34% risk difference for POBA against CABG to 15% in trials using stents at 3-year follow-up. Furthermore, stents gave rise to a significant decrease in non-fatal MI compared to CABG at three years. CABG was shown to significantly reduce the incidence of angina at 1- and 3-year intervals, but this difference had converged by five years and was no longer statistically significant. Again approximately two thirds of all patients enrolled in these RCT had double-vessel disease and all had ejection fractions within the normal range. Those high-risk individuals (i.e. triple-vessel disease with LV systolic dysfunction and diabetics) were excluded from these trials, thus perhaps creating an environment in which PCI could achieve relative parity with CABG in terms of survival.

Landmark trial The Randomized Intervention Treatment of Angina (RITA) 1 trial [13,14]

- Seminal UK RCT comparing balloon angioplasty in the pre-coronary stent era against CABG surgery in patients with 1-, 2- or 3-vessel CAD;
- 1,011 patients with CHD randomized to PTCA (n = 510) or CABG (n = 501);
- Included patients with impaired LV function or recent MI;
- No significant difference in the combined primary endpoint of death or non-fatal MI at 2 years;
- Significantly more PTCA patients required a second revascularization procedure (PTCA 38% vs CABG 11%, p < 0.001);
- No treatment difference in terms of primary endpoint or in deaths alone at 5 years;
- Most reinterventions occurred within a year of randomization; from 3 years onwards, the rate of repeat revascularizations averaged 4% for PTCA and 2% for CABG;
- PTCA patients consistently suffered more angina with an absolute average excess of 10% over CABG (P < 0.001);
- No significant difference in total health service costs between the two strategies.

Landmark trial The Bypass Angioplasty Revascularization Investigation (BARI) trial [15,16]

- North American multicentre RCT;
- 1,829 patients with MVD and clinically severe angina or objective evidence of reversible ischaemia randomized to PTCA or CABG over a 3-year period;
- Initial revascularization procedure conducted within two weeks of randomization;
- Coronary stents were available, but not used for the index procedure;
- No significant difference in primary endpoint of all-cause mortality or Q-wave MI at five years;
- PTCA group required significantly greater subsequent revascularization procedures (PTCA 54% vs CABG 8%);

continued

- Ad hoc subgroup analysis demonstrated improved 5-year survival amongst diabetics randomized to CABG arm (PTCA 80.6% vs CABG 65.6%, p = 0.003);
- At ten years, overall survival rates remained similar; additional revascularization procedures much greater for PTCA patients (PTCA 76.8% vs CABG 20.3%, p < 0.001) and survival advantage had persisted for diabetics randomized to CABG (PTCA 45.5% vs 57.8%, p = 0.025).

A more recent meta-analysis of 23 RCTs by Bravata et al. published in 2007 looked at 5,019 patients randomly assigned to PCI and 4,944 to CABG. Trials included both POBA and coronary stenting vs standard and/or minimally invasive forms of CABG [18]. It should be remembered that as PCI has improved, CABG techniques and outcomes have also evolved over time. Contemporary CABG can be performed off-pump and via minimally invasive keyhole techniques which obviate the need for median sternotomy. Enhanced myocardial preservation, increasing use of arterial conduits, and improvements in post-operative care have all helped to reduce morbidity, mortality, and incidence of graft occlusion. There was no significant difference in survival between the two revascularization modalities at 10-year follow-up. As demonstrated previously, the rate of subsequent revascularizations was significantly greater with PCI, although this did improve in the stent trials. CABG also conferred an improved angina burden. Interestingly, and not eluded to by the meta-analysis from Hoffman et al., procedure-related strokes were significantly more common after CABG. Furthermore, in the six trials (AWESOME, BARI, EAST, ERACI II, MASS II, and RITA) that reported outcome data on a diabetic subgroup, CABG did not confer an *overall* survival advantage over PCI. This is in contrast to the individual BARI trial findings [15,16], which have been the cause of much debate and have ultimately led to the initiation of ongoing RCTs comparing CABG to PCI in diabetics.

Diabetic patients tend to be associated with smaller vessel calibre, greater plaque burden, longer lesion lengths, and possibly a different restenotic cascade when compared to non-diabetic patients. This makes them more prone to atherothrombosis and a greater need for repeat revascularization.

The CARDia trial was the first randomized trial of coronary revascularization in 510 diabetic patients with either MVD or complex single-vessel disease. Individuals received either PCI (29% bare-metal stents (BMS) and 71% drug-eluting stents (DES)) or on- or off-pump CABG [19]. The purpose of the study was to demonstrate that PCI was non-inferior to CABG in this patient subset. The trial was stopped early due to slow enrolment and as such, the event rates used for sample size calculations could not be achieved. Nevertheless, the incidence of the primary endpoint of death, non-fatal MI, and non-fatal stroke at one year was similar for both strategies although non-inferiority could not be proven. There was again a significant reduction in the incidence of repeat revascularization for those having had CABG. As intimated by the Bravata meta-analysis, however, there was a trend towards a greater stroke incidence with CABG. Longer-term follow-up to assess the durability of these data is eagerly anticipated as are data from the much larger FREEDOM RCT which is again looking at coronary revascularization in diabetics.

Similar long-term survival rates following PCI and CABG demonstrated by the RCTs analyzed by Bravata et al. are in contrast to the data collected from many large-scale clinical registries. Registry data are observational, non-randomized, and prone to significant selection bias and as such, cannot be as reliable as RCT data. Some may argue, however, that an observational approach reflects a more 'real-world' viewpoint of clinical practice and should be considered a supportive adjunct to RCT data.

For instance, Hannan et al. looked at 37,212 individuals with MVD undergoing CABG against 22,102 MVD patients receiving PCI (with stenting) during a 3-year period between 1 January 1997 and 31 December 2000 in New York State [20]. The authors reported a significantly improved 'risk-adjusted' survival rate for those having had CABG in all of the anatomical subgroups studied along with, as expected, a much higher repeated revascularization rate for patients having had PCI as their index procedure. These results, however, should be taken with a note of caution. Risk adjustment had to be performed since the patient cohorts contained a number of differences that would have made subsequent comparisons non-robust and highly questionable. Indeed the unadjusted hazard ratios showed no difference in outcome, irrespective of the number of diseased vessels treated or involvement of the LAD artery, the revascularization modalities only diverging once hazard ratios were 'adjusted' to attempt to equalize differences between the groups [21]. Furthermore, closer inspection of such registries only confirm what we already know: most patients with single-vessel disease on the whole receive PCI and most patients with triple-vessel disease receive CABG [18]. It is the patients with coronary disease intermediate to these extremes that have been enrolled by the RCTs and interestingly enough, the clinical registries analyzed by Bravata et al. have also shown similar outcomes between CABG and PCI in this patient subset.

The introduction of DES has led to a significant reduction in the need for repeat revascularizations after PCI. Coronary stenting causes significant local trauma to the vessel wall and exposure of the sub-endothelium, thereby increasing the risk of thrombotic and occlusive complications. Exposure of the stent struts can stimulate further platelet activation, aggregation, and adherence to a non-endothelialized vessel wall. PCI can also potentiate the release of vasoactive agents from the platelet-rich thrombus, thus adding to the pro-thrombotic milieu already present. The two potential clinical sequelae that reduce best outcomes after stenting are in-stent restenosis (ISR) secondary to intimal hyperplasia and stent thrombosis due to the processes described above. Much of the literature suggests that an intact and functionally viable endothelium is not only non-thrombogenic, but also prevents the smooth muscle cell proliferation that leads to the late luminal loss and addtional deleterious effects caused by intimal hyperplasia, hence the trial-driven clinical success of DES which reduces restenosis by inhibiting smooth muscle proliferation. Although these refinements in PCI technique have reduced the need for repeat revascularization, they have not, nor do they claim to, reduce the rate of mortality or MI.

The ERACI III registry was a multicentre, prospective, non-randomized, open-labelled study designed to evaluate outcomes in patients with MVD who received DES [22]. The aim was to compare outcomes with the BMS and CABG arms of the ERACI II trial which had previously demonstrated no survival benefits from either strategy, although patients initially treated by CABG had greater freedom from repeat revascularization and major adverse cardiovascular and cerebrovascular events (MACCE) at 5-year follow-up [23]. At one year ERACI III-DES patients were shown to have greater freedom from MACCE compared to ERACI II-CABG and ERACI II-BMS patients as a consequence of a reduced incidence of death and anterior MI and a lower rate of target vessel revascularization (TVR), respectively. By three years, however, MACCE rates had converged between the DES and CABG arms, signifying a trend towards increased late death and non-fatal MI in addition to a greater late requirement for TVR in DES patients. The incidence of MACCE at three years remained lower in the DES cohort compared with ERACI II-BMS individuals, primarily as a result of a sustained avoidance of the need for repeat TVR. Pertinently, MACCE rates in diabetic ERACI III-DES patients were significantly lower compared to BMS patients and similar to those of CABG patients, the rate of TVR being the predominant differentiator.

The ARTS II trial utilized a similar format to that of ERACI III by comparing 607 patients who underwent multivessel PCI using sirolimus-eluting stents with the BMS and CABG arms of the ARTS I trial as a historical control [24,25]. At one year, the primary composite endpoint of MACCE (death, stroke, non-fatal MI, and TVR) in ARTS II-DES patients was similar to the ARTS I-CABG arm and significantly better than the ARTS I-BMS cohort. CABG surgery continued to afford greater freedom from the need for TVR compared to coronary stenting as a whole [24]. After three years, MACCE rates in non-diabetic patients in ARTS II continued to mirror those of ARTS I-CABG and were vastly superior to ARTS I-PCI patients. Of note, ARTS II patients were at significantly lower risk of death, MI, and stroke when compared to both ARTS I-CABG and ARTS I-PCI individuals. In diabetics, MACCE rates for ARTS II were better than those for ARTS I-BMS, but worse than for ARTS I-CABG, the difference being primarily driven by a substantially greater need for repeat revascularization following PCI in general. The use of DES did, however, result in a 44% decrease in the need for repeat revascularization compared to BMS [26].

Ultimately, however, both ERACI III and ARTS II were non-randomized, prospectively collected registries and as such, all treatment arms were not enrolled concurrently. There was also a time lag between the trials during which both PCI and CABG techniques had been refined and concomitant medical therapy, either given periprocedurally or at discharge, not only varied between trials, but had also improved and were given more rigorously in later years. These limitations led to the initiation of the SYNTAX RCT (see below) which sought to demonstrate non-inferiority of PCI with DES to CABG in patients with triple-vessel or LMCA disease.

The 2-year results from the SYNTAX trial were presented at the European Society of Cardiology Congress in 2009. MACCE rates remained significantly higher in the PCI arm, again primarily driven by a greater need for repeat revascularization. Stroke rates remained higher for CABG, but appeared to be a carryover from the first 12 months. The harder endpoint of death/MI/stroke continued to remain the same between the two modalities.

⊘ **Landmark trial** The Synergy between Percutaneous Coronary Intervention with Taxus and Cardiac Surgery (SYNTAX) trial [27]

- 1,800 patients with triple-vessel or LMCA disease randomized to CABG or PCI with Taxus DES;
- 'All-comers' design with consecutive enrolment of all eligible patients at 85 sites in 17 countries;
- Both a local cardiac surgeon and interventional cardiologist had to agree that an enrolled patient could achieve equivalent anatomical revascularization with either CABG or PCI;
- Utilized the SYNTAX score algorithm to grade the complexity of CAD requiring revascularization [28];
- Primary endpoint was composite of MACCE (i.e. all-cause mortality, stroke, MI, or repeat revascularization);
- At 12 months, significantly lower MACCE for CABG over PCI (12.4% vs 17.8%, p = 0.002);
- Repeat revascularization again as the predominant differentiator (PCI 13.5% vs CABG 5.9%, p < 0.001);
- Stroke rate significantly higher in the CABG group (2.2% vs 0.6%, p = 0.003);
- Combined rates of death, stroke, or MI were similar between the groups;
- Therefore, the non-inferiority of PCI compared to CABG in patients with severe MVD was not proven at 12 months.

Table 1.2 Cumulative event rates to three years from the SYNTAX trial

Cumulative event rate	CABG arm (%)	PCI arm (%)	p value
MACCE	20.2	28.0	<0.001
Death, stroke, MI	12.0	14.1	0.21
All-cause death	6.7	8.6	0.13
Stroke	3.4	2.0	0.07
MI	3.6	7.1	0.002
Repeat revascularization	10.7	19.7	<0.001

The 3-year SYNTAX results were first presented at the European Association of Cardiothoracic Surgery Annual Meeting in 2010. Again, MACCE rates remained lower in the CABG arm, driven predominantly by a persistently higher rate of revascularization procedures in the PCI arm (Table 1.2). Again, however, there was no statistical difference between the two cohorts in terms of the hard composite endpoint of all-cause death/stroke/MI.

The most interesting result to note from SYNTAX at three years was the demarcation of event rates by the baseline SYNTAX score:

- Lowest-risk patients (SYNTAX score 0–22): MACCE rates were very similar between the two treatment modalities.
- Intermediate-risk patients (SYNTAX score 23–32): the 2-year results indicated a trend toward improved outcomes with CABG, but with no statistical significance. The 3-year results have demonstrated a continuing separation of the event curves (DES 27.4% vs CABG 18.9%) such that statistical significance (p=0.02) has been reached.
- Highest-risk patients (SYNTAX score > 33): this cohort represents those individuals with the most complex disease and SYNTAX clearly demonstrates CABG to be the best option.

In conclusion, therefore, the 3-year SYNTAX results suggest PCI or CABG can only be considered a reasonable therapeutic option in those patients at lowest risk by SYNTAX score.

A final word from the expert

In stable angina, patients with multivessel coronary disease, the decision between CABG surgery and PCI is one of the most common, and sometimes most difficult, dilemmas facing interventional cardiologists. There are a number of important points to bear in mind when considering the options:

- Virtually all patients are initially referred to cardiologists rather than cardiac surgeons. As such, we are often seen as the 'gatekeepers' and sometimes subjected to criticism. We must bear this in mind and involve surgeons in the decision-making process, often in a multidisciplinary team (MDT) meeting setting. This allows some objectivity in the process.

- When discussing such patients in an MDT meeting, it is important to not only have full details of the history, examination, non-invasive tests and angiography, but also to have calculated the SYNTAX score (available from: www.Syntaxscore.com). In addition, although the Euroscore (available from: www.euroscore.org) overestimates risk, it nevertheless provides useful information to guide the decision-making process.

continued

- In the vast majority of patients with stable CAD, provided PCI is technically feasible with a high chance of success, but there is no clear difference between the two treatment modalities in terms of the 'hard endpoints' of death or MI. There are, however, certain subsets of patients in whom there may be a prognostic benefit for surgery (e.g. significant left main/3-vessel disease with impaired LV function). From the trials, however, this 'prognostic benefit' is limited and was initially derived from the days when the comparator was suboptimal medical therapy.

- The real difference is in the need for 'repeat revascularization', in other words, the need for a repeat procedure (either PCI or CABG) for recurrent limiting symptoms. Even when using DES, whatever trial or registry you look at, the need for repeat intervention is higher with PCI than with surgery.

- Usually, ISR is a relatively benign phenomenon and can often be treated with repeat angioplasty, albeit with a higher risk of subsequent recurrent restenosis or alternatively, subsequently treated by CABG. Importantly, it must be remembered that the vast majority of patients treated with PCI do not develop restenosis!

In view of this, my opinion is that we can give patients real choice in their treatment as long as the treatment options are clearly explained to the patient as well as the realistic 'risk' of the need to come back for a repeat procedure.

References

1 Antman EM, Cohen M, Bernink PJLM, et al. The TIMI risk score for unstable angina/non-ST-elevation MI. A method for prognostication and therapeutic decision-making. *JAMA* 2000; 284: 835–842.

2 Antman EM, McCabe CH, Gurfinkel EP, et al. Enoxaparin prevents death and cardiac ischaemic events in unstable angina or non-Q wave myocardial infarction: results of the Thrombolysis In Myocardial Infarction (TIMI) IIB trial. *Circulation* 1999; 100: 1593–1601.

3 Cohen M, Demers C, Gurfinkel EP, et al. A comparison of low-molecular-weight heparin with unfractionated heparin for unstable coronary artery disease. *N Engl J Med* 1997; 337: 447–452.

4 Antman EM, Cohen M, Radley D, et al. Assessment of the treatment effect of enoxaparin for unstable angina/non-Q-wave myocardial infarction. *TIMI 11B-ESSENCE meta-analysis. Circulation* 1999; 100: 1602–1608.

5 Granger CB, Goldberg RJ, Dabbous O, et al. Predictors of hospital mortality in the global registry of acute coronary events. *Arch Intern Med* 2003; 163: 2345–2353.

6 Yusuf S, Zhao F, Mehta CR, et al. for the CURE Trial Investigators. Effects of clopidogrel in addition to aspirin in patients with acute coronary syndromes without ST-segment elevation. N *Engl J Med* 2001; 345: 494–502.

7 Peters RJG, Mehta SR, Fox KAA, et al. for the CURE Trial Investigators. Effects of aspirin dose when used alone or in combination with clopidogrel in patients with acute coronary syndromes. Observations from the Clopidogrel in Unstable angina to prevent Recurrent Events (CURE) study. *Circulation* 2003; 108: 1682–1687.

8 British Cardiovascular Intervention Society. BCIS Audit Returns 2008. Available from: http://www.bcis.org.uk/pages/page_box_contents.asp?pageid=705&navcatid=11.

9 Katritis DG, Ioannidis JP. Percutaneous coronary intervention vs conservative therapy in non-acute coronary artery disease: a meta-analysis. *Circulation* 2005; 111: 2906–2912.

10 Yusuf S, Zucker D, Peduzzi P, et al. Effect of coronary artery bypass graft surgery on survival: overview of 10-year results from randomized trials by the Coronary Artery Bypass Graft Surgery Trialists Collaboration. *Lancet* 1994; 344: 563–570.

11 Smith PK, Califf RM, Tuttle RH, et al. Selection of surgical or percutaneous coronary intervention provides differential longevity benefit. *Ann Thorac Surg* 2006; 82: 1420–1428.

12 Soran O, Manchanda A, Schueler S. Percutaneous coronary intervention vs coronary artery bypass surgery in multivessel disease: a current perspective. *Interact CardioVasc Thorac Surg* 2009; 8: 666–671.

13 RITA Trial Participants. Coronary angioplasty vs coronary artery bypass surgery: the Randomized Intervention Treatment of Angina (RITA) trial. *Lancet* 1993; 341: 573–580.

14 Henderson RA, Pocock SJ, Sharp SJ, et al. Long-term results of RITA 1 trial: clinical and cost comparisons of coronary angioplasty and coronary artery bypass grafting. *Lancet* 1998; 352: 1419–1425.

15 The Bypass Angioplasty Revascularization Investigation (BARI) Investigators. Comparison of coronary bypass surgery with angioplasty in patients with multivessel disease. *N Engl J Med* 1996; 335: 217–225.

16 The BARI Investigators. The final 10-year follow-up results from the BARI randomized trial. *J Am Coll Cardiol* 2007; 49: 1600–1606.

17 Hoffman SN, TenBrook Jr JA, Wolf MP, et al. A meta-analysis of randomized controlled trials comparing coronary artery bypass graft with percutaneous transluminal coronary angioplasty: one- to eight-year outcomes. *J Am Coll Cardiol* 2003; 41: 1293–1304.

18 Bravata DM, Glenger AL, McDonald KM, et al. Systematic review: the comparative effectiveness of percutaneous coronary interventions and coronary artery bypass graft surgery. *Ann Intern Med* 2007; 147: 703–716.

19 Kapur A, Hall RJ, Malik IS, et al. Randomized comparison of percutaneous coronary intervention with coronary artery bypass grafting in diabetic patients: 1-year results of the CARDia (Coronary Artery Revascularization in Diabetes) trial. *J Am Coll Cardiol* 2010; 55: 432–440.

20 Hannan EL, Racz MJ, Walford G, et al. Long-term outcomes of coronary artery bypass grafting vs stent implantation. *N Engl J Med* 2005; 352: 2174–2183.

21 Gershlick AH, Thomas M. PCI or CABG: which patients and at what cost? *Heart* 2007; 93: 1188–1190.

22 Rodriguez AE, Maree AO, Mieres J, et al. Late loss of early benefit from drug-eluting stents when compared with bare-metal stents and coronary artery bypass surgery: 3-year follow-up of the ERACI III registry. *Eur Heart J* 2007; 28: 2118–2125.

23 Rodriguez AE, Baldi J, Pereira CF, et al. Five-year follow-up of the Argentine randomized trial of coronary angioplasty with stenting vs coronary bypass surgery in patients with multiple vessel disease (ERACI II). *J Am Coll Cardiol* 2005; 46: 582–588.

24 Serruys PW, Ong ATL, Morice M-C, et al. Arterial Revascularization Therapies Study part II–sirolimus-eluting stents for the treatment of patients with multivessel de novo coronary artery lesions. *EuroIntervention* 2007; 3: 450–459.

25 Serruys PW, Unger F, Sousa JE, et al. Comparison of coronary artery bypass surgery and stenting for the treatment of multivessel disease. *New Engl J Med* 2001; 344: 1117–1124.

26 Daemen J, Kuck KH, Macaya C, et al. Multivessel coronary revascularization in patients with and without diabetes mellitus. 3-year follow-up of the ARTS II trial. *J Am Coll Cardiol* 2008; 52: 1957–1967.

27 Serruys PW, Morice M-C, Kappetein AP, et al. for the SYNTAX Investigators. Percutaneous coronary intervention vs coronary artery bypass grafting for severe coronary artery disease. *N Engl J Med* 2009; 360: 961–972.

28 Sianos G, Morel M-A, Kappetein AP, et al. The SYNTAX Score: an angiographic tool grading the complexity of coronary artery disease. *EuroIntervention* 2005; 1: 219–227.

Can a rash cause stent thrombosis?

Aung Myat

🄖 **Expert commentary** Professor Tony Gershlick

Case history

A 56-year-old Caucasian gentleman presented to his primary care physician with a 10-week history of exertional symptoms typical of angina. There was a previous history of treated hypertension and dyslipidaemia but, by his own admission, the patient was poorly compliant with taking his ramipril and simvastatin. He was a lifelong smoker and had a history of ischaemic heart disease in a first-degree relative. The amount of exertion required to provoke retrosternal chest pain and breathlessness had diminished over this time period to the point where the patient could no longer climb the stairs at work and was forced to use the elevator over the preceding two weeks. On examination, the patient was pain-free and haemodynamically stable. An electrocardiogram (ECG) revealed sinus rhythm and no acute ischaemia. The doctor confirmed the possibility of myocardial ischaemia and referred the patient on to the local Rapid Access Chest Pain clinic (RACPC) for further assessment. The doctor also prescribed aspirin 75 mg once daily (od) and a sublingual glyceryl trinitrate (GTN) spray to help alleviate any recurrent exacerbations of angina.

At the RACPC, a detailed history and examination were conducted prior to the patient performing an exercise tolerance test (ETT). Within five minutes (i.e. stage 2) of a Bruce protocol, the patient became acutely dyspnoeic and complained of mild central chest heaviness. There was a concomitant fall in blood pressure from 150/90 mmHg (pre-exercise) to 110/70 mmHg along with anteroseptal ST-segment depression on the ECG (refer to ETT Learning point in Case 1). The ETT was stopped and deemed to be strongly positive for myocardial ischaemia at low-to-medium workload. In recovery, the patient's symptoms rapidly resolved with rest and two puffs of sublingual GTN. The patient confirmed these symptoms to be identical to those he had had in the last ten weeks. The ECG normalized and the patient was discharged home with a view to an urgent outpatient coronary angiogram within a few days. A beta-blocker (bisoprolol 2.5 mg od) was added to the patient's drug regimen and he was strongly advised to stop smoking and remain compliant with his medication. The patient was also told to either contact the Cardiology department, his primary care physician, or the paramedics should his symptoms recur or fail to settle with GTN spray.

Prior to coronary angiography, the patient was pre-loaded with clopidogrel 600 mg and was consented for percutaneous coronary intervention (PCI) if an appropriate and treatable lesion was found. The procedure was conducted via the right radial artery and revealed a subtotally occluded left anterior descending (LAD) artery secondary to a critical 95% proximal stenosis, but otherwise normal coronary vessels. Left ventricular function was found to be normal. The interventionist relayed the findings and, with the patient's consent, proceeded to PCI of the proximal LAD with unfractionated heparin (UFH)

✚ Clinical tip TIMI grade flow definitions

The TIMI grade flow is an easily accessible and widely adopted scoring system which refers to the degree of coronary blood flow seen during coronary angiography.
- TIMI 0 flow (no perfusion): absence of any antegrade flow beyond a coronary occlusion;
- TIMI 1 flow (penetration without perfusion): faint antegrade coronary flow beyond the occlusion, with incomplete filling of the distal coronary bed;
- TIMI 2 flow (partial reperfusion): delayed or sluggish antegrade flow with complete filling of the distal territory;
- TIMI 3 flow (complete perfusion): normal flow which fills the distal coronary bed completely.

✦ Expert comment

If this initial reaction were due to the clopidogrel, it is starting very early after taking the medication. Even so and in the absence of any other cause, it should have alerted the interventionist to a problem with this drug.

✦ Expert comment

Ticlopidine can be very difficult to get hold of nowadays and in the context of newer agents is probably now obsolete.

cover according to the activated clotting time (ACT). A 3.0 x 18 mm drug-eluting stent (DES) was deployed following pre-dilatation with serial inflations of a 2.5 x 12 mm balloon. Post-procedural balloon dilatation to ensure good stent apposition was undertaken. There were no periprocedural complications and Thrombolysis in Myocardial Infarction (TIMI) myocardial perfusion grade 3 flow was restored to the LAD artery. Residual stenosis was less than 10% of the vessel diameter.

The patient was transferred back to the ward and commenced on regular clopidogrel (75 mg od) alongside his aspirin, bisoprolol, ramipril, simvastatin, and GTN. He was asked to take clopidogrel for 12 months and was advised not to stop it under any circumstances unless prior discussion with his interventionist had taken place.

Within three hours post-procedure, the patient complained of a warm and itchy forehead. The Cardiology Fellow was called at which point an examination revealed nothing untoward. All observations were normal as was a troponin T and repeat ECG that showed no acute ischaemia. The patient was discharged home later that evening.

✪ Learning point The evolution of dual antiplatelet therapy

The central role of platelets in the propagation of intracoronary thrombi has made antiplatelet therapy central to the management of atherothrombotic cardiovascular disease. Over the last two decades, aspirin has become the cornerstone of antiplatelet therapy [1]. Its antithrombotic action is mediated through the irreversible acetylation of cyclooxygenase (COX) enzymes secreted by activated platelets. As such, COX-mediated thromboxane-A$_2$ (TXA$_2$) synthesis from arachidonic acid (AA) release, following phospholipase A$_2$ activation, is inhibited for the entire lifespan of the platelet (approximately 120 days). TXA$_2$ induces platelet aggregation and vasoconstriction. Landmark trials have established the efficacy of aspirin in the prevention of arteriosclerotic vascular disease and have also shown it to reduce the frequency of ischaemic complications after PCI [2,3]. Despite the proven benefits of aspirin, a significant proportion of patients continued to suffer major adverse cardiovascular and cerebrovascular events (MACCE) whilst on therapy. More potent antiplatelet agents, ticlopidine and clopidogrel, which are structurally related thienopyridines with platelet inhibitory properties, were therefore developed.

Both agents are rapidly absorbed prodrugs that require hepatic transformation to an active metabolite by the cytochrome P450 enzyme system to acquire their antiplatelet activity. They exert their action by irreversibly inhibiting adenosine diphosphate (ADP) binding to the P2Y$_{12}$ receptor on the platelet surface. This receptor is central to the amplification of the aggregatory pathways stimulated by all known platelet agonists, including collagen, thrombin, immune complexes, TXA$_2$, adrenaline, and serotonin, and is therefore pivotal in stabilizing and propagating the growth of the platelet-rich intraluminal thrombus. By blocking this receptor, the thienopyridines interfere with platelet activation, degranulation, and aggregation.

Ticlopidine, the first thienopyridine to be developed, given as a twice-daily dose of 250 mg, has been shown to be just as effective as aspirin and significantly superior to placebo for the secondary prevention of ischaemic events in patients at high atherothrombotic risk [4]. There is, however, a clear rationale for combining aspirin with a thienopyridine since they work via complementary mechanisms and have the potential to provide synergistic inhibition of the platelet aggregatory pathway, hence the evolution of dual antiplatelet therapy (DAPT). The association of ticlopidine with hypercholesterolaemia and, more seriously, adverse haematological effects such as neutropaenia, thrombocytopaenia, aplastic anaemia, and thrombotic thrombocytopaenic purpura (TTP) along with its relative expense means that its use is now reserved primarily for those who are found to be allergic to clopidogrel.

Clopidogrel is now well established as the current thienopyridine of choice, used in combination with low-dose aspirin, as DAPT to prevent the deleterious effects of stent thrombosis in the coronary stenting era and for the secondary prevention of ischaemic vascular sequelae in high-risk individuals following an acute coronary syndrome (ACS). It is a prodrug that requires two cytochrome P450-dependent oxidative steps during its hepatic metabolism to produce its active moiety. The superior tolerability of clopidogrel when compared to ticlopidine was first established by the CLASSICS trial [5]. Subsequently, due to its adverse side effect profile and slower onset of action, ticlopidine use fell dramatically and was replaced by the much safer, equally effective and, when a loading dose was given, significantly faster-acting clopidogrel. Since then, landmark trials have established an undoubted benefit of clopidogrel alone or in combination with aspirin in the context of arteriosclerotic vascular disease, ACS, and prolonged DAPT following PCI (see Table 2.1) [6-13].

Table 2.1 Landmark clopidogrel trials in atherothrombotic vascular disease

Study (year)	Patients (n)	Clinical presentation	Treatment arms	Mean follow-up period	Primary endpoint	ER (%) Rx*	ER (%) Ctrl†	RRR (%)	p
CAPRIE (1996)	19,185	Recent MI, CVA, or PAD	Clopidogrel 75 mg od vs ASA 325 mg od	1.9 y	Ischaemic stroke, MI, vascular death	5.32	5.83	8.7	0.043
CURE (2001)	12,562	ACS	Clopidogrel 300 mg bolus, 75 mg od + ASA 75–325 mg od vs placebo + ASA 75–325 mg od	9 mo	CV death, non-fatal MI, CVA	9.3	11.4	20.0	<0.001
PCI-CURE (2001)	2,658	ACS on PCI	Clopidogrel 300 mg bolus, 75 mg od + ASA 75–325 mg od vs placebo + ASA 75–325 mg od	8 mo	CV death, MI, urgent target vessel revascularization	4.5	6.4	30.0	0.03
CREDO (2002)	2,116	Elective PCI or at high likelihood to undergo PCI	Clopidogrel 300 mg bolus, 75 mg od + ASA 325 mg od vs placebo + ASA 325 mg od	1 y	Death, MI, CVA	8.4	11.5	26.9	0.02
CLARITY-TIMI 28 (2005)	3,491	Acute STEMI (<12 h) Thrombolysis ± heparin	Clopidogrel 300 mg bolus, 75 mg od + ASA vs placebo + ASA	3.5 d	Occluded infarct-related artery, death, MI prior to angiography	14.9	21.7	30.9	<0.001
COMMIT/ CCS-2 (2005)	45,852	Suspected acute MI; 54% thrombolyzed + heparin	Clopidogrel 75 mg od + ASA 162 mg od vs placebo + ASA 162 mg od	28 d	Death, reinfarction, CVA	9.2	10.1	9.0	0.002

*Clopidogrel arm; †Aspirin ± placebo arm; ER: event rate; RRR: relative risk reduction; CVA: cerebrovascular accident; PAD: peripheral arterial disease; ASA: aspirin.

> **⊘ Landmark trial** CLASSICS trial [5]
>
> - Confirmed the superior tolerability of clopidogrel (plus aspirin) to that of ticlopidine (plus aspirin);
> - 1,020 patients randomized to three different 28-day antiplatelet regimens following coronary stenting;
> - 300 mg clopidogrel and 325 mg aspirin on day 1, followed by clopidogrel 75 mg od and aspirin 325 mg od; or
> - Clopidogrel 75 mg od and aspirin 325 mg od; or
> - Ticlopidine 250 mg twice daily and aspirin 325 mg od;
> - Primary endpoint of adverse haematological sequelae or early non-cardiac adverse event-related discontinuation of the study drug(s) occurred significantly more often in the ticlopidine group;
> - Overall rates of MACCE were low and comparable between all three groups.

> **✪ Learning point** Current guidelines on DAPT post-coronary stenting
>
> DES can cause bystander endothelial cell inhibition, thus potentially delaying the protective re-endothelialization which would otherwise normally occur within a month or so following bare-metal stent (BMS) deployment. It is widely accepted that DES pose a greater risk of stent thrombosis compared to BMS in the longer term although clinical outcomes between the two stent platforms may be no different.
>
> Furthermore, PCI with stent deployment leads to significant local trauma to the vessel wall increasing the risk of thrombotic and vaso-occlusive complications. Exposure of the stent struts can stimulate further platelet activation, aggregation, and adherence to a non-endothelialized vessel wall. PCI can also potentiate the release of vasoactive agents from the platelet-rich thrombus, thus adding to the pro-thrombotic milieu already present, especially in the context of ACS.
>
> As a result, those individuals receiving DES require a protracted course of DAPT, hence the updated US and European PCI guidelines [14-16]. It is important to note that the length of re-endothelialization delay, in the context of DES, may well vary according to the stent platform, the polymer used to bind and allow a gradual release of the drug over time, and the therapeutic agent used to reduce neointimal proliferation (and hence ameliorate the degree of in-stent restenosis). Guidelines issued by the European Society of Cardiology (ESC) for DAPT post-ACS and coronary stenting are outlined in Table 2.2 (Please note these have since been superceded by the ESC 2010 guidelines on myocardial revascularisation).
>
> According to updated US guidelines (2007), post-PCI patients receiving a BMS should be given clopidogrel for a minimum of one month and **ideally up to 12 months** (unless the patient is at increased risk of bleeding, then it should be given for a minimum of two weeks) [14].
>
> US PCI guidelines (2007) also recommend clopidogrel (75 mg daily) should be given for at least 12 months in all patients receiving DES if they are not at increased risk of bleeding [14].
>
> Of note, the DES-LATE trial, presented at the Annual Scientific Sessions of the American College of Cardiology in March 2010, helped to confirm the generally held belief that 12 months of DAPT following coronary stenting is about right [17]. The trial was an amalgamation of two South Korean trials (REAL-LATE and ZEST-LATE), each of which had slow enrolment, hence the decision to combine their patient cohorts. The single large trial (n = 2,701) compared the continuation or cessation of clopidogrel after 12 months of DAPT in those patients who had received a DES, but had had no MACCE or significant major bleeding event(s) during that time period. Patients were randomized to clopidogrel 75 mg od plus low-dose aspirin (100–200 mg) or just aspirin alone on an open-label basis and followed up at 6-month intervals up to two years. Results revealed no demonstrable benefit of extending DAPT beyond 12 months in terms of reducing the risk of MI or cardiovascular death. Interestingly, prolonged DAPT actually led to a non-significant increase in the composite endpoint of MI, stroke, or death from any cause and MI, stroke and, cardiovascular death. There was insufficient statistical power, however, to make a firm recommendation on the safety of clopidogrel discontinuation following 12 months of DAPT. The much larger American DAPT trial is currently enrolling to answer this question.

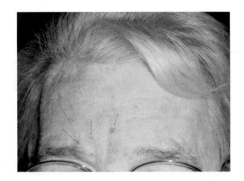

Figure 2.1 Discrete pruritic maculopapular rash following initiation of clopidogrel therapy (arrows).

The next day, the patient was still suffering from pruritus, but now noticed a discrete erythematous maculopapular rash that had erupted over his forehead overnight (Figure 2.1). There was no chest pain or breathlessness, but the patient did not feel well systemically. He was concerned enough to make an appointment to see the family doctor the next day.

The primary care physician later diagnosed a hypersensitivity reaction to clopidogrel. He advised the cessation of clopidogrel therapy and prescribed an antihistamine (chlorpheniramine 4 mg tds) and oral prednisolone (30 mg od) for five days to treat the presumed allergic rash and pruritus. The family doctor arranged to see the patient again after completion of treatment with a view to restarting clopidogrel or to initiate the trial of a different antiplatelet agent. The patient unfortunately failed to mention the strict advice given to him by the Cardiology Fellow upon discharge from hospital only a few days before.

Within two days, the patient's rash had improved markedly and he had returned to work. He was sitting at his desk when suddenly he developed a crushing central chest pain radiating to his neck. He became cold and clammy. He immediately took two puffs of his GTN spray five minutes apart, but this had little effect. In the meantime, his co-workers had called for the paramedics who arrived within eight minutes.

⊕ Clinical tip Clopidogrel hypersensitivity reaction

- A pruritic, maculopapular rash that can occur in up to 15% of individuals;
- Predominantly affects the limbs rather than the trunk;
- Usually occurs by day 3 or 4 post-initiation of therapy (although some reports describe a rash within 20 minutes or after 14 days);
- Can be associated with fever, nausea, vomiting, anaemia, thrombocytopaenia, leucopaenia, and deranged liver function;
- Treated with systemic or topical steroids and antihistamines;
- Management options to prevent STENT THROMBOSIS in PCI patients:
  - Discontinue clopidogrel and commence an alternative thienopyridine (e.g. ticlopidine, prasugrel), bearing in mind the potential risk of cross-sensitivity; or
  - Continue clopidogrel and accept that urticaria/rash will persist; unlikely to be a realistic option for those receiving DES who require a protracted course of DAPT; or
  - Discontinue clopidogrel and initiate an alternative non-thienopyridine antiplatelet agent (e.g. cilostazol, dipyridamole, or more latterly, ticagrelor); or
  - Attempt clopidogrel desensitization once the rash has resolved using incremental doses of the offending drug given over a predetermined time period under close supervision in hospital; again unlikely to be a realistic option in light of the availability of newer oral non-thienopyridine antiplatelet agents such as ticagrelor.

Table 2.2 ESC guidelines on the use of DAPT in patients requiring PCI [15,16]

ESC antiplatelet therapy guideline recommendations for STEMI patients proceeding to PCI	
Aspirin	Patients already on daily aspirin should be given a 75–325 mg stat dose before PCI. Patients not on regular aspirin should be given 500 mg at least 3 h before PCI or 300 mg IV at the time of the procedure. Following PCI, patients should continue on 75–160 mg daily MD indefinitely.
Clopidogrel	Patients should be given a 300 mg LD at least 6 h before PCI; if this is not possible, then a 600 mg LD at least 2 h before the procedure. Following BMS implantation, patients should continue clopidogrel at 75 mg daily MD for four to six weeks. Following DES implantation, patients must continue clopidogrel for at least 12 months.
ESC antiplatelet therapy guideline recommendations for NSTEMI patients proceeding to PCI	
Aspirin	A 160–325 mg LD should be given to all patients presenting with NSTEMI. A long-term MD of 75–100 mg daily should be given indefinitely.
Clopidogrel	All patients undergoing PCI should receive 600 mg LD. Following BMS implantation, patients should continue clopidogrel at 75 mg daily MD for four to six weeks. Following DES implantation, patients must continue clopidogrel for at least 12 months.

⊕ **Clinical tip** Premature discontinuation of clopidogrel after coronary stenting

- Physicians and patients must be made aware that clopidogrel should not be discontinued prematurely, even for minor procedures like dental care, and that the opinion of a cardiologist should be sought if the patient is considering non-emergent, non-cardiac surgery.
- In general, elective non-cardiac surgery should be deferred for one year after DES implantation. Conversely, if it is known that a non-cardiac operation is required prior to PCI, then all efforts should be made to implant a BMS so that clopidogrel need only be continued for four to six weeks as opposed to one year.
- Strict compliance to dual antiplatelet therapy must be maintained.
- The issue of clopidogrel cards to patients that detail the PCI procedure and the recommended length of clopidogrel therapy should be encouraged (Figure 2.2).
- In patients treated with clopidogrel in whom it is decided that coronary artery bypass grafting is more favourable, the surgery should be delayed for five days, if possible, to reduce the risk of bleeding. This may now be of less significance due to the impending introduction of ticagrelor, a reversible (thienopyridines are irreversible) non-thienopyridine oral antiplatelet agent.

❝ **Expert comment**

Acute stent thrombosis is best treated, if possible, with IV glycoprotein IIb/IIIa inhibitor prior to going to the cardiac catheterization laboratory.

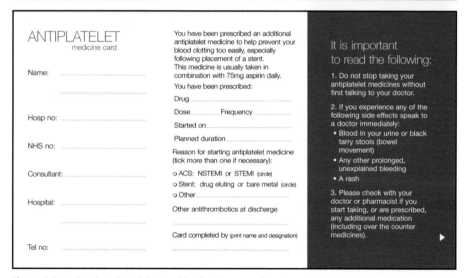

Figure 2.2 A clopidogrel card designed by the Pharmacy department at Barts and The London Heart Centre. With kind permission from Barts and the London NHS Trust. Copyright 2011.

The paramedics took a quick history, gave 300 mg of aspirin to chew, and established intravenous (IV) access. The patient was administered oxygen via a mask and given 10 mg morphine with anti-emetic cover. An ECG was taken which revealed an anterior ST-elevation myocardial infarction (STEMI). The local regional cardiac centre was contacted and asked to prepare for a primary PCI (PPCI).

On arrival to the Emergency department, the patient was met by the same Cardiology Fellow that had been involved in his care previously. The Fellow confirmed an antero-lateral STEMI (Figure 2.3) and also concurred with the primary care physician's diagnosis of clopidogrel hypersensitivity reaction. He did not concur, however, with the premature cessation of clopidogrel therapy without prior referral to the cardiac centre first. The Fellow prescribed a loading dose of prasugrel 60 mg stat. The patient gave verbal consent and was rushed to the cardiac catheterization laboratory for PPCI. Call to needle time was established at 55 minutes.

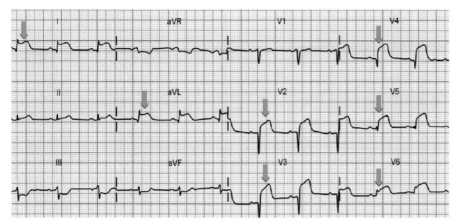

Figure 2.3 ECG on arrival to the Emergency Department demonstrating an anterolateral STEMI (arrows).

Expert comment

Although premature cessation of DAPT was the cause in this case, stent thrombosis is not uncommonly associated with malapposition of the stent to the vessel wall with most 'curves' of timing of stent thrombosis incidence having a steep early phase, so high-pressure balloon dilatation being careful to stay within the stent, is generally indicated. Subsequent intravascular ultrasound (IVUS) examination of the stent, if this is available, should be considered in high-risk lesions (left main stem, large proximal stenting in any of the three main vessels).

Repeat angiography via the right radial artery covered with UFH and IV abciximab (a glycoprotein IIb/IIIa antagonist) demonstrated a total occlusion of the proximal LAD due to stent thrombosis. All other coronary vessels remained patent. A decision to proceed to plain old balloon angioplasty (POBA) of the occluded stent was made by the interventionist on-call. Serial inflations with a 3.0 x 15 mm balloon restored patency to the vessel.

An excellent angiographic result was obtained with TIMI grade 3 flow returning to the LAD artery (Figure 2.4). Anterolateral ST-segment elevation on the ECG also subsided and the patient was pain-free by the end of the procedure with no peri-operative complications. The patient made an uneventful recovery on the ward and was discharged home on the third day of admission. Peak creatine kinase (CK) post-event was measured at 812 U/L and transthoracic echocardiography on the ward revealed hypokinesia of the anterior wall with an estimated ejection fraction by Simpson's biplane method of 45%, suggesting at least a moderate impairment of function. He was prescribed a 12-month course of prasugrel at 10 mg od and asked to contact the Cardiology department directly if there were any adverse reactions to the new therapy. Contact with the cardiac rehabilitation team was established, and a full and thorough discharge summary emphasizing the importance of maintenance of DAPT was relayed to the primary care physician.

Expert comment

The National Institute for Health and Clinical Excellence (NICE) has provided guidance on this matter and has indicated that prasugrel should be used in the setting of stent thrombosis.

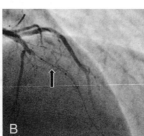
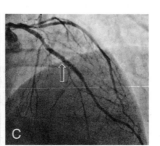

Figure 2.4 Repeat coronary angioplasty. Plate A: proximal LAD artery occlusion (blue arrow) secondary to stent thrombosis (red arrows); plate B: POBA of occluded proximal LAD stent with multiple balloon inflations (red arrow); and plate C: recanalization of the LAD artery with a patent stent and TIMI grade 3 flow (blue arrow).

> ⊕ **Learning point** Definition of stent thrombosis [18]
>
> With the advent of DES, results from a number of trials in the late 1990s/early 2000s had led to the suggestion that DES posed a greater risk of late stent thrombosis, and therefore more death and MI, when compared to BMS. These trials had employed differing definitions of stent thrombosis that made comparisons between them almost impossible. Amid the furore, a group of experts formed the Academic Research Consortium (ARC), their role being to standardize the definition of stent thrombosis and provide consistency in the reporting of future trials involving and comparing both BMS and DES. Definitions are as follows:
>
> - **Definite stent thrombosis** is considered to have occurred by *either* angiographic or pathologic confirmation.
> - **Probable stent thrombosis** is considered to have occurred after intracoronary stenting in the following cases:
>   - Any unexplained death within the first 30 days;
>   - Irrespective of the time after the index procedure, any MI which is related to documented acute ischaemia in the territory of the implanted stent without angiographic confirmation of stent thrombosis and in the absence of any other obvious cause;
> - **Possible stent thrombosis** is considered to have occurred with any unexplained death from 30 days following intracoronary stenting until end of trial follow-up.
>
> **Timing of stent thrombosis**
> - Acute ST: 0–24 h post-implantation;
> - Subacute ST: >24 h to 30 days post-implantation;
> - Late ST: >30 days to 1 year post-implantation;
> - Very late ST: >1 year post-implantation.

Discussion

The case outlined here illustrates how fundamental it is to maintain adequate inhibition of platelet aggregation (IPA) following deployment of intracoronary stents and in particular, for DES in the longer term since delayed re-endothelialization through drug bystander effects may be one mechanism of continued exposure to a risk of stent thrombosis. Adequate prevention of stent thrombosis following PCI requires optimization of four key factors, all of which are intimately interrelated: the patient, the anti-platelet drug therapy, platelet function and reactivity, and the characteristics of the stent along with its correct deployment.

Patient compliance with DAPT is paramount to the success of PCI. In all studies, the greatest hazard ratio for stent thrombosis is 'premature' discontinuation of DAPT and in particular, the thienopyridine portion of it. Without knowledge of the individual's re-endothelialization status, defining what constitutes 'premature discontinuation' is clearly an inexact science. Most will have re-endothelialized within 6–12 months of the DAPT protection period, some as early as three months, whilst some, however, will have not.

To reduce the risk of iatrogenic or patient-driven discontinuation, the use of clopidogrel cards must be encouraged. They are an invaluable source of information both to the patient and to other medical personnel. Presentation of the clopidogrel card to the primary care physician in this case study may well have prevented the adverse sequelae that resulted from premature cessation of clopidogrel. There are also other issues. With an increasingly ageing demographic in the developed world, it is inevitable that the majority of PCI patients will be elderly. It follows that these patients may well require an unplanned non-cardiac procedure in the (1-year) post-stent period, necessitating the consideration of discontinuation of clopidogrel. In these situations, appropriate liaison with a cardiologist is essential. If the stent is large, has been well deployed and is in a distal vessel and the patient requires an important non-surgical procedure four months post-PCI (e.g. biopsy for breast cancer), the clinical decision may well be to stop the clopidogrel five days before the procedure. Alternatively, an ostial LAD stent five weeks post-PCI in a patient requiring a haemorrhoid operation will be a completely different scenario. Each patient has to be considered on his or her individual merits and with it, the surgeon-primary care physician-interventionist communication line is a vital component of this decision-making process. The use of clopidogrel cards can facilitate this communication.

Are the days of aspirin and clopidogrel numbered?

Theoretically, the inhibition of the two main amplification pathways of platelet aggregation should be superior to that of either pathway alone. Despite appropriate DAPT, however, a significant minority of patients continue to suffer MACCE following ACS and coronary stenting. Late stent thrombosis, particularly in the era of DES, can occur in 1–2% of individuals following PCI and is reported to progress at 0.3 to 0.6% each year. In real terms, this can account for 30,000 MACCE per annum worldwide. Death, MI, or stroke occur in 8.5% and 21.4% require revascularization a year after their index PCI procedure [19]. This has led to the postulation that those individuals suffering further events may represent a cohort of patients who are resistant to the platelet inhibitory properties of aspirin and/or clopidogrel.

The term DAPT 'resistance' is controversial in this context since it has been used to encompass both the failure of an agent to prevent the clinical condition for which it is intended and also failure to achieve its full pharmacokinetic and/or pharmacodynamic effect. Since the pathophysiology of atherothrombosis is complex, comprising thrombosis, inflammation, intrinsic vascular biology and haemodynamic variability, no single agent can be expected to abolish ischaemic events completely. Furthermore, a patient may have the appropriate platelet response to a given therapy, but have recurrent events mediated by non-platelet factors. For these reasons, it would seem reasonable to categorize patients suffering recurrent events on therapy as having *treatment failure*, while limiting the term *resistance* to those for whom the antiplatelet drug does not achieve appropriate IPA, i.e. its pharmacological effect. Resistance, in its broadest sense, can be referred to as the continued occurrence of ischaemic events despite adequate duration of antiplatelet therapy, dosing, and compliance alongside optimal stent deployment.

Aspirin resistance

In the purest pharmacological sense, aspirin resistance would suggest a failure to inhibit platelet COX-1-dependent thromboxane formation. The concept of aspirin resistance is made problematic by a lack of definitive evidence to suggest that altering therapy in response to discovering this phenomenon actually improves clinical outcomes. Indeed, although aspirin strongly inhibits the production of TXA_2, it may still fail to inhibit platelet aggregation since there are a number of other potent agonists that will continue to activate platelets. As such, there is no universally accepted definition of aspirin resistance.

Furthermore, selecting an appropriate method for determining aspirin resistance remains a challenge. At present, AA-stimulated platelet aggregation assessed by light transmittance aggregometry (LTA) or platelet mapping by thromboelastography are the most commonly used laboratory assays, but these putative *in vitro* tests

Expert comment

Few regard aspirin resistance as a true clinical entity.

may not be specific or sensitive enough and also suffer from a number of significant limitations:

- Platelets are removed from the circulation and are therefore no longer exposed to the prothrombotic effects of shear stress and contact with the endothelium and neighbouring blood cells;
- Platelet assays tend to use a single agonist whereas *in vivo* multiple agonists act in combination and often synergistically;
- Preactivation may occur and this may be enhanced in already hyper-reactive platelets;
- Essential secretory (autocrine and paracrine) functions of platelet-derived TXA_2 will not be detected by measures of platelet aggregation;
- Anticoagulants may modify platelet aggregation differently [20].

Consequently, no assay standards have been set or widely accepted for determining biochemical aspirin resistance. The cause of aspirin resistance, if it truly exists, remains contentious and is most likely multifactorial. Causes may represent a drug-related or disease-related dichotomy or be divided into clinical, cellular, and genetic factors (Table 2.3).

Currently, the estimated prevalence of aspirin non-responsiveness ranges from 4 to 65%, borne from the heterogeneity of the methodologies used to assess platelet aggregation, the variability of aspirin dosing, the definition of resistance adopted by the particular study, and the population from which trial participants were recruited [22,23]. Interestingly, the ASPECT trial did demonstrate a dose-dependent effect of aspirin on non-responsiveness, which tended to occur less frequently with repeated and increased administration of the drug [24]. At present, however, evidence pointing to the existence of true aspirin resistance remains tenuous at best and a lack of appropriate alternatives means that there is little, if any, justification in withholding the drug when used alone or in conjunction with clopidogrel as DAPT.

Table 2.3 Potential causes of aspirin resistance [20,21]

Clinical factors	• Failure to prescribe appropriately
	• Patient non-compliance
	• Non-absorption/insufficient bioavailability (low-dose enteric-coated preparations)
	• Interaction with NSAIDs (e.g. ibuprofen, indomethacin) preventing access to binding sites inside the COX-1 channel
	• ACS or congestive heart failure
	• Hyperglycaemia
Cellular factors	• Impaired sensitivity of platelet COX-1
	• Insufficient suppression of COX-1
	• Platelet hyper-reactivity ('residual' platelet reactivity)
	• Platelet stimulation by alternative aspirin-insensitive mechanisms (e.g. ADP, shear stress, erythrocyte-induced platelet activation)
	• Platelet sensitizing by isoprostanes (e.g. 8-iso-PGF$_{2\alpha}$)
	• Platelet stimulation by COX-2-dependent TXA_2 formation
Genetic factors	• COX-1 gene polymorphisms (A842G/C50T)
	• Glycoprotein IIb/IIIa receptor polymorphisms
	• von Willebrand factor receptor polymorphisms
	• Collagen receptor polymorphisms

Clopidogrel resistance

In contrast to the phenomenon of aspirin resistance, there is evidence to suggest that clopidogrel resistance is a definite pharmacological entity that can lead to adverse clinical outcomes. There is wide inter-individual variation in clopidogrel response. Like hyporesponsiveness to aspirin, a laboratory definition of true clopidogrel resistance has not been universally accepted. It is agreed that clopidogrel resistance occurs when the drug is unable to achieve appropriate IPA. Since there are a number of different assays available to assess this phenomenon, it follows that there are a number of empiric cut-off values that have been adopted to suggest non-responsiveness. None of these tests have been fully standardized, leading to significant inter-laboratory variation in results. Prevalence figures for non-responders to clopidogrel range from 4 to 34% 24 hours after drug administration, depending on the technique used to measure platelet aggregation and the presence of factors contributing to greater baseline platelet reactivity [25].

Several studies have established clopidogrel resistance as an emerging clinical entity and proposed a link with adverse outcomes. Common to all of them, however, are relatively small sample sizes and short follow-up periods. They have not been sufficiently powered to detect a causal association between clopidogrel resistance and MACCE. One of the largest studies found a normal distribution of clopidogrel responsiveness amongst 544 individuals, consisting of healthy volunteers, patients post-coronary stenting, those with heart failure, and after stroke [26]. The authors subsequently categorized hyporesponders, hyper-responders, and the remaining individuals as standard responders using the mean IPA achieved as a reference point. Another prospectively studied 60 patients who underwent primary PCI following presentation with STEMI to determine whether variability in response to clopidogrel affected clinical outcomes. Patients were stratified into four quartiles according to the percentage reduction of ADP-induced platelet aggregation. Forty per cent of patients in the first quartile, who were considered non-responders, sustained a MACCE during six months of follow-up compared to one patient in the second quartile and none in the third and fourth [27]. The largest study thus far looked at platelet reactivity following clopidogrel administration to 804 patients who had received DES during PCI. They found that patients with over 70% post-clopidogrel platelet aggregation *in vitro* had a nearly four-fold increase in definite or probable stent thrombosis as compared with clopidogrel responders [28]. More recently, Price and colleagues measured post-clopidogrel treatment platelet reactivity with the VerifyNow® $P2Y_{12}$ assay in 380 patients undergoing PCI with sirolimus-eluting stents to determine whether there was an optimal cut-off value for platelet reactivity in predicting 6-month MACCE rates. They found that those patients with high post-treatment platelet reactivity had significantly higher rates of cardiovascular death, stent thrombosis, and overall MACCE [29].

Platelet function tests

Since clopidogrel is specific for the $P2Y_{12}$ receptor, the $P2Y_1$ platelet receptor can still be activated and contribute to platelet aggregation. This can be a confounding factor when using LTA or impedance aggregometry as an *ex vivo* test of clopidogrel response. The vasodilator-stimulated phosphoprotein phosphorylation (VASP-P) assay is more specific to the $P2Y_{12}$ pathway. Levels of VASP-P and dephosphorylation reflect $P2Y_{12}$ inhibition and activation, respectively, and can be measured reliably by quantitative flow cytometry. This is fast becoming the only standardized $P2Y_{12}$-specific assay available. Furthermore, point-of-care assays for platelet aggregation have a promising role in guiding future antiplatelet therapy. The VerifyNow® P2Y$_{12}$ system uses a similar principle to that employed by the VASP-P assay by using a combination of ADP and prostaglandin E$_1$ (PGE$_1$) as agonists to specifically evaluate inhibition of the P2Y$_{12}$ pathway. PGE$_1$ increases VASP-P by stimulation of adenylate cyclase. Binding of ADP to P2Y$_{12}$ leads to inhibition of adenylate cyclase, thereby reducing PGE$_1$-induced VASP-P levels. If, however, P2Y$_{12}$ receptors are successfully blocked by clopidogrel, the addition of ADP will have no theoretical effect on PGE$_1$-stimulated VASP-P levels. The VerifyNow® P2Y$_{12}$ system has recently been approved by the Food and Drug Administration (FDA) in the United States, but remains primarily a research tool and is yet to be used widely in the clinical forum.

The POPULAR study, which was first reported at the American Heart Association (AHA) meeting in November 2009, sought to identify the platelet function test that best predicted clinical outcomes in 1,069 consecutive patients on DAPT undergoing elective PCI with coronary stenting between December 2005 and December 2007 in a single Dutch centre [30]. The study performed a parallel head-to-head comparison of seven platelet function tests:

- LTA (laboratory-based, requiring trained technicians and labour-intensive; using platelet-rich plasma);
- VerifyNow® P2Y$_{12}$ (bedside assay, whole blood, aggregation-based);
- Plateletworks (bedside assay, whole blood, ADP stimulation, must be performed within ten minutes or results can become unstable);
- IMPACT-R (adhesion and shear stress-based, whole blood);
- IMPACT-R ADP (stimulation with ADP, whole blood);
- PFA-100 COL/ADP (i.e. collagen/ADP, whole blood, shear stress-based);
- INNOVANCE® PFA P2Y (shear stress-based, whole blood).

The primary efficacy endpoint was the composite of death, non-fatal MI, stent thrombosis, and stroke at one year. The primary safety endpoint was set at TIMI major and minor bleeding in the same time period. The study found that the platelet aggregation tests, LTA, VerifyNow® P2Y$_{12}$, and Plateletworks, were all able to predict adverse events. In essence, the primary ischaemic endpoint occurred more frequently in patients with high on-treatment platelet reactivity (HPR) as identified by these three tests. In contrast, the remaining four platelet adhesion and/or shear stress-based tests were unable to predict MACCE. None of the tests, however, were able to discriminate those patients at increased risk of TIMI major and minor bleeding. Overall, the ability of these tests to predict atherothrombotic outcomes in this relatively low-risk, non-ACS population was described as 'modest' by the authors. Perhaps more pertinently, this study served to highlight the importance of HPR as opposed to pharmacological clopidogrel resistance. Also of note, the Multiplate analyzer, the thromboelastograph, and the VASP-P assay were not available at the time when the POPULAR study was recruiting. Ongoing trials (e.g. TRIGGER PCI and GRAVITAS) in higher-risk ACS populations will help to determine which platelet test best serves those individuals with clopidogrel resistance and/or HPR.

Mechanisms of clopidogrel resistance

Several mechanisms of clopidogrel resistance have been postulated and encompass genetic, cellular, and clinical factors, either acting alone or in conjunction (Table 2.4). Again, a common thread of small sample sizes, empirical definitions for responsiveness, a lack of robust clinical outcome data, differing methods of assessing platelet

Expert comment

The GRAVITAS trial will be an important study since it will direct therapy based on near-patient platelet function testing. However, one should stress that the most important factor in limiting stent thrombosis, other than ensuring continuance of DAPT, is still optimal stent deployment with IVUS, if necessary.

aggregation, and contradictory findings exists in studies aiming to identify a cause-and-effect relationship.

No one mechanism has been accepted as the true cause of clopidogrel resistance. Particular interest has, however, focused recently on several functional polymorphisms found in genes encoding cytochrome P450 isoenzymes involved in the hepatic biotransformation of clopidogrel to its active form. Abnormal functional variants of the CYP2C9 and CYP2C19 genotypes have been associated with a decreased pharmacodynamic response to clopidogrel, resulting in less exposure to the active metabolite [31]. Collet and colleagues have shown that a cohort of patients aged under 45 years taking clopidogrel, who were carriers of the loss-of-function CYP2C19 681 > G (*2) allele, had a greater propensity to stent thrombosis and the composite of death, MI, and urgent coronary revascularization when compared with non-carriers [32]. These findings were further substantiated by the TIMI group who examined the association between functional variants of the CYP genes in 1,477 individuals who had been enrolled into the clopidogrel arm of the TRITON-TIMI 38 trial [33,34]. They were able to demonstrate a significant relative increase in the risk of CV death, MI, stent thrombosis, and stroke in those carriers of the CYP2C19 reduced-function allele compared with non-carriers. Carriers were also shown to produce lower levels of the active thiol clopidogrel metabolite and demonstrated diminished IPA.

The CHARISMA Genomics substudy has also shown that those patients homozygous for the CYP2C19*2 allele are at increased risk of ischaemic events [35]. This prospective, placebo-controlled study genotyped for CYP2C19*2, *3, and *17 alleles in 4,862 of the 15,603 patients consented for the CHARISMA trial [36] and randomized them to aspirin with clopidogrel or aspirin with placebo to evaluate whether this polymorphism had any effect on both ischaemic and bleeding outcomes. Homozygotes for the reduced-function allele were found to suffer more ischaemic events, but less

Table 2.4 Proposed mechanisms of clopidogrel resistance

Genetic factors	• Polymorphisms of hepatic CYP3A4, CYP2C9, CYP2C19 and 1A2 • Polymorphisms of glycoprotein Ia • Polymorphisms of P2Y$_{12}$ • Polymorphisms of glycoprotein IIIa
Cellular factors	• HPR • Reduced CYP3A4/CYP3A5 metabolic activity • Increased ADP exposure • Upregulation of the P2Y$_{12}$ pathway • Upregulation of the P2Y$_1$ pathway • Upregulation of P2Y-independent pathways • (collagen, adrenaline, TXA$_2$, thrombin)
Clinical factors	• Failure to prescribe or under-dosing • Poor compliance • Poor absorption • Suboptimal stent deployment • Drug-drug interactions • (e.g. lipophilic statins such as atorvastatin and simvastatin, omeprazole, calcium channel blockers) • Increased baseline platelet reactivity • (e.g. ACS, increased body mass index, diabetes mellitus, and insulin resistance) • Clopidogrel side effects such as thrombotic thrombocytopaenic purpura (i.e. creation of a pro-thrombotic state)

GUSTO-defined bleeding when compared with wild type (WT) alleles. This trend was also seen in patients taking placebo although this finding did not reach significance. Patients with the WT alleles experienced more GUSTO bleeding with DAPT. In contrast to the findings from TRITON-TIMI 38, heterozygotes did not display the same effects on outcomes. This study was the first of its kind to indicate a potential relationship between bleeding and genotype. Homozygotes for CYP2C19*2 may have relatively less conversion to the active metabolite of clopidogrel, thereby conferring a reduced chance of bleeding, but an increased risk of MACCE.

Although further large-scale prospective studies are required to definitively outline the clinical relevance of CYP2C19 polymorphisms, the clear weight of evidence accumulated thus far has led the FDA to issue a requirement for the makers of clopidogrel to add a 'boxed warning' to their product from March 2010. The warning states that those with poor clopidogrel metabolism may not receive its full benefits. The warning also states that there are tests available to determine the genetic make-up of the individual's CYP 450 enzymes and advises clinicians to consider using alternative antiplatelet therapies or augmented dosing strategies for clopidogrel in non-responders.

Optimizing the dose of clopidogrel

The potential clinical validity of clopidogrel resistance has led to the construction of several studies designed to elucidate the optimal loading and maintenance doses for clopidogrel that can potentially overcome hyporesponsiveness and yet remain safe in terms of bleeding rates. The ARMYDA-2 study indicated the benefit of pre-treatment with a loading dose (LD) of 600 mg when compared with 300 mg in reducing periprocedural MI in patients with stable angina or NSTEMI undergoing planned PCI without any increase in bleeding hazards [37].

The ALBION and ISAR-CHOICE studies looked at increasing the LD further to 900 mg [38,39]. A higher LD did display a greater degree of platelet inhibition, more rapid onset of action (approximately two hours although maximal IPA may not be achieved until three to four hours after ingestion), and a lower percentage of non-responders compared to the standard 300 mg strategy, but the differences observed between the 600 mg and 900 mg regimens were less remarkable and not significant. These studies confirm the dose-dependent inhibitory effects of clopidogrel, but also show there is a threshold for the platelet inhibitory function achieved which may be linked to the saturation of intestinal absorption as opposed to a limit on hepatic metabolism.

To establish further the mechanistic aspects of clopidogrel resistance, Bonello and colleagues undertook a prospective, randomized, multicentre study of 162 patients due to undergo coronary stenting. Clopidogrel resistance was defined as a VASP-P index of greater than 50% after a 600 mg LD. Patients who were non-responsive to clopidogrel were randomized to a control group or to a VASP-guided group; the latter received additional boluses of clopidogrel to reduce the VASP-P index to below 50% as measured by the VerifyNow® P2Y$_{12}$ assay. Although the study sample was small, there was a significantly lower MACCE rate in the VASP-guided group, suggesting that adjusting the LD according to clopidogrel response was appropriate, safe (i.e. there was no difference in bleeding between the two groups), and could potentially improve clinical outcome [40].

The standard 75 mg/day maintenance dose (MD) of clopidogrel requires three to seven days to achieve maximal IPA. The ISAR-CHOICE-2 study revealed the advantage of a 150 mg clopidogrel MD over standard dosing in patients one month after low-risk PCI [41]. Additionally, the OPTIMUS study showed that a 150 mg MD of clopidogrel resulted in pronounced platelet inhibition of numerous platelet function measures compared to the standard 75 mg daily in patients with diabetes mellitus, although a significant number of patients continued to display HPR [42].

More definitive data on the optimal dosing of clopidogrel has come from the CURRENT-OASIS 7 trial, the results of which were first reported at the ESC Annual Congress in September 2009. Over 25,000 patients presenting with stent thrombosis and non-ST-elevation ACS intended for early (≤72 hours) revascularization were enrolled into a 2 x 2 factorial trial and randomized to either 600 mg LD followed by 150 mg/day for one week, then 75 mg/day MD of clopidogrel or a 300 mg LD followed by 75 mg/day MD [43]. Individuals were also randomized to receive either high-dose (300–325 mg) or low-dose (75–100 mg) aspirin in an open-label manner.

Of the 17,232 patients who did receive early intervention, the primary composite endpoint of CV death, MI, and stroke at 30 days occurred in 4.5% of those on the 'standard' clopidogrel regimen and 3.9% on the 'augmented' regimen (p=0.036), the benefit primarily driven by a reduction in MI. There was no significant difference in the primary endpoint in those 7,855 patients who did not proceed to PCI because of no significant CAD identified on angiography or those scheduled for CABG. Overall, the rate of stent thrombosis was significantly higher in the standard group compared to the double clopidogrel therapy (1.2% vs 0.7%, p=0.001). There was no significant difference in the primary endpoint between a high- or low-dose aspirin strategy although, conversely, there was also no difference in bleeding indices between the two strategies either. Data from CURRENT-OASIS 7 suggest that those patients scheduled to undergo PCI following an ACS should receive a 600 mg LD of clopidogrel which is already advocated in Europe and is current practice. A MD of 150 mg for one week following PCI would be simple enough to institute thereafter and then patients could return to the 75 mg MD that we are all familiar with. Whether this practice will become commonplace in the 'real world' is yet to be seen.

What is clear from the evidence accumulated so far is that further work is needed to establish the role of genotyping vs platelet function measurements (i.e. complementary or alternative) and how they can be transferred from the laboratory to the bedside. The idea of tailoring antiplatelet therapy for those patients found to have a suboptimal response to current standard DAPT after coronary stenting and ACS may soon become reality.

⚙ Expert comment

The 'augmented regimen' used in CURRENT-OASIS 7 is certainly worth considering in contemporary ACS intervention.

💬 A final word from the expert

Stent thrombosis can clearly result in serious adverse clinical outcomes. Careful stenting is the key and all patients should be discharged with a DAPT treatment card indicating which therapies they are on and most importantly, how long they should remain on them. From the development and evidence-based perspective, it is still unclear how long any particular patient treated with any particular DES and with any particular antiplatelet agent should be treated for. Consensus remains that 12 months is the minimum period, but second and third generation stents are more conformable (and so there is less stent-to-vessel wall space for thrombus to form) and have more bioneutral polymers, so arterial healing is better. Some suggest that patients with such stents need treatment for only three or six months and there are studies from the ISAR group addressing this. Others believe that events occurring late (beyond 12 months), irrespective of whether they are due to delayed arterial healing or to new events, need continued antiplatelet protection. As such, the DAPT trial of 20,000 patients will address the use of clopidogrel for 12 vs 30 months.

Newer agents have also become available. Prasugrel, a third generation thienopyridine which requires a single metabolic step to produce the active moiety (compared with two steps for clopidogrel),

continued

generally attenuates the variable response in individual patients to clopidogrel. Following the issue of NICE guidance in October 2009, it is currently the recommended first-line therapy in diabetics and those undergoing primary PCI [44]. Providing prescribing care is taken to exclude those high-risk groups (age greater than 75 years, weight less than 60 kg, previous minor/major stroke), then prasugrel is a useful addition to our pharmacological armamentarium. It should not be used beyond 12 months since many of the bleeding events occurred in patients treated out to a mean of 450 days in the TRITON-TIMI 38 trial as opposed to the recommended 360 days [34].

Ticagrelor, a non-thienopyridine $P2Y_{12}$ receptor antagonist, will add yet another dimension to our therapies. It appears to be more potent than clopidogrel to reduce mortality and is reversible. This may thus have significant advantages when patients need a non-cardiac operation or those who may ultimately require cardiac bypass surgery during their index ACS admission [46]. In the ONSET/OFFSET study, Gurbel and colleagues demonstrated the greater and faster onset of action of ticagrelor compared with clopidogrel in patients with stable CAD. On discontinuation, platelets regained function within two to three days in the ticagrelor group compared with five days in the clopidogrel cohort [46].

It is likely that despite all these advances, DAPT will continue to play a fundamental role in post-PCI care. Which combination of agents and for how long and whether this will be tailored to individual patient's needs and/or the stent are research questions still to be resolved.

References

1 Selwyn AP. Prothrombotic and antithrombotic pathways in acute coronary syndromes. *Am J Cardiol* 2003; 91: 3H–11H.
2 Antithrombotic Trialists' Collaboration. Collaborative meta-analysis of randomized trials of antiplatelet therapy for prevention of death, myocardial infarction, and stroke in high-risk patients. *BMJ* 2002; 324: 71–86.
3 ISIS-2 (Second International Study of Infarct Survival) Collaborative Group. Randomized trial of intravenous streptokinase, oral aspirin, both, or neither among 17,187 cases of suspected acute myocardial infarction: ISIS-2. *Lancet* 1988; 332: 349–360.
4 Patrono C, Coller B, Fitzgerald GA, et al. Platelet-active drugs: the relationships among dose, effectiveness, and side effects: The Seventh ACCP Conference on Antithrombotic and Thrombolytic Therapy. *Chest* 2004; 126: 234–264.
5 Bertrand M, Rupprecht HJ, Urban P, et al. for the CLASSICS Investigators. Double-blind study of the safety of clopidogrel with and without a loading dose in combination with aspirin compared with ticlopidine in combination with aspirin after coronary stenting: the clopidogrel aspirin stent international cooperative study (CLASSICS). *Circulation* 2000; 102: 624–629.
6 CAPRIE Steering Committee. A randomized, blinded trial of clopidogrel versus aspirin in patients at risk of ischaemic events (CAPRIE). *Lancet* 1996; 348: 1329–1339.
7 CURE Study Investigators. Effects of clopidogrel in addition to aspirin in patients with acute coronary syndromes without ST-segment elevation. *N Engl J Med* 2001; 345: 494–502.
8 Mehta SR, Yusuf S, Peters RJG, et al. Effects of pre-treatment with clopidogrel and aspirin followed by long-term therapy in patients undergoing percutaneous coronary intervention: the PCI-CURE study. *Lancet* 2001; 358: 527–533.
9 Steinhubl SR, Berger PB, Mann JT III, et al. Early and sustained dual oral antiplatelet therapy following percutaneous coronary intervention: a randomized controlled trial. *JAMA* 2002; 288: 2411–2420.
10 Chen ZM, Jiang LX, Chen YP, et al. Addition of clopidogrel to aspirin in 45,852 patients with acute myocardial infarction: randomized placebo-controlled trial. *Lancet* 2005; 366: 1607–1621.
11 Sabatine MS, Cannon CP, Gibson CM, et al. for the CLARITY-TIMI 28 Investigators. Addition of clopidogrel to aspirin and fibrinolytic therapy for myocardial infarction with ST-segment elevation. *N Engl J Med* 2005; 352: 1179–1189.

12 Sabatine MS, Cannon CP, Gibson CM, et al. for the Clopidogrel as Adjunctive Reperfusion Therapy (CLARITY)–Thrombolysis in Myocardial Infarction (TIMI) 28 Investigators. Effect of clopidogrel pre-treatment before percutaneous coronary intervention in patients with ST-elevation myocardial infarction treated with fibrinolytics: the PCI-CLARITY study. *JAMA* 2005; 294: 1224–1232.

13 Maree AO, Fitzgerald DJ. Variable platelet response to aspirin and clopidogrel in atherothrombotic disease. *Circulation* 2007; 115: 2196–2207.

14 King SB, Smith SC, Hirshfeld JW, et al. 2007 focused update of the ACC/AHA/SCAI 2005 Guideline update for percutaneous coronary intervention: a report of the American College of Cardiology/American Heart Association Task Force on practice guidelines: (2007 Writing Group to review new evidence and update the 2005 ACC/AHA/SCAI guideline update for percutaneous coronary intervention). *Circulation* 2008; 117: 261–295.

15 Silber S, Albertsson P, Aviles FF, et al. Guidelines for percutaneous coronary interventions. *Eur Heart J* 2005; 26: 804–847.

16 Bassand JP, Hamm CW, Ardissino D, et al. Guidelines for the treatment of non-ST-segment elevation acute coronary syndromes. *Eur Heart J* 2007; 28: 2–63.

17 Park S-J, Park D-W, Kim Y-H, et al. Duration of dual antiplatelet therapy after implantation of drug-eluting stents. *N Engl J Med* 2010; 362: 1374–1382.

18 Cutlip DE, Windecker S, Mehran R, et al. Clinical endpoints in coronary stent trials: a case for standardized definitions. *Circulation* 2007; 115: 2344–2351.

19 Steinhubl SR, Berger PB, Mann JT III, et al. Early and sustained dual oral antiplatelet therapy following percutaneous coronary intervention: a randomized controlled trial. *JAMA* 2002; 288: 2411–2420.

20 Schror K. What is aspirin resistance? *Br J Cardiol* 2009; 17(Suppl 1): S5–S7.

21 Bhatt DL. Aspirin resistance: more than just a laboratory curiosity. *J Am Coll Cardiol* 2005; 43: 1128.

22 Lordkipanidze M, Pharand C, Schampaert E, et al. A comparison of six major platelet function tests to determine the prevalence of aspirin resistance in patients with stable coronary artery disease. *Eur Heart J* 2007; 28: 1702–1708.

23 Snoep JD, Hovens MMC, Eikenboom JCJ, et al. Association of laboratory-defined aspirin resistance with a higher risk of recurrent cardiovascular events: a systematic review and meta-analysis. *Arch Intern Med* 2007; 167: 1593–1599.

24 Gurbel PA, Bliden KP, DiChiara J, et al. Evaluation of dose-related effects of aspirin on platelet function: results from the Aspirin-Induced Platelet Effect (ASPECT) study. *Circulation* 2007; 115: 3156–3164.

25 O'Donoghue M, Wiviott SD. Clopidogrel response variability and future therapies. Clopidogrel: does one size fit all? *Circulation* 2006; 114: e600–e606.

26 Serebruany VL, Steinhubl SR, Berger PB, et al. Variability in platelet responsiveness to clopidogrel among 544 individuals. *J Am Coll Cardiol* 2005; 45: 246–251.

27 Matetzky S, Shenkman B, Guetta V, et al. Clopidogrel resistance is associated with increased risk of recurrent atherothrombotic events in patients with acute myocardial infarction. *Circulation* 2004; 109: 3171–3175.

28 Buonamici P, Marcucci R, Migliorini A, et al. Impact of platelet reactivity after clopidogrel administration on drug-eluting stent thrombosis. *J Am Coll Cardiol* 2007; 49: 2312–2317.

29 Price MJ, Endemann S, Raghava G, et al. Prognostic significance of post-clopidogrel platelet reactivity assessed by a point-of-care assay on thrombotic events after drug-eluting stent implantation. *Eur Heart J* 2008; 29: 992–1000.

30 Breet NJ, van Werkum JW, Bouman HJ, et al. Comparison of platelet function tests in predicting clinical outcome in patients undergoing coronary stent implantation. *JAMA* 2010; 303: 754–762.

31 Brandt JT, Close SL, Iturria SJ, et al. Common polymorphisms of CYP2C19 and CYP2C9 affect the pharmacokinetic and pharmacodynamic response to clopidogrel but not prasugrel. *J Thromb Haemost* 2007; 5: 2429–2436.

32 Collet JP, Hulot JS, Pena A, et al. Cytochrome P450 2C19 polymorphism in young patients treated with clopidogrel after myocardial infarction: a cohort study. *Lancet* 2009; 373: 309–317.

33 Mega JL, Close SL, Wiviott SD, et al. Cytochrome P450 polymorphisms and response to clopidogrel. *New Engl J Med* 2009; 360: 354–362.

34 Wiviott SD, Braunwald E, McCabe CH, et al. Prasugrel versus clopidogrel in patients with acute coronary syndromes. *N Engl J Med* 2007; 357: 2001–2015.

35 Bhatt DL. Plenary Session XII. LBCT II. Presented at: Transcatheter Cardiovascular Therapeutics, 21–25 September, 2009, San Francisco.

36 Bhatt DL, Fox KAA, Hacke W, et al. for the CHARISMA Investigators. Clopidogrel and aspirin versus aspirin alone for the prevention of atherothrombotic events. *New Engl J Med* 2006; 354: 1706–1717.

37 Patti G, Colonna G, Pasceri V, et al. Randomized trial of high loading dose of clopidogrel for reduction of periprocedural myocardial infarction in patients undergoing coronary intervention: results from the ARMYDA-2 (Antiplatelet therapy for Reduction of MYocardial Damage during Angioplasty) study. *Circulation* 2005; 111: 2099–2106.

38 Montalescot G, Sideris G, Meuleman C, et al. A randomized comparison of high clopidogrel loading doses in patients with non-ST-elevation acute coronary syndromes: the ALBION trial. *J Am Coll Cardiol* 2006; 48: 931–938.

39 von Beckerath N, Taubert D, Pogatsa-Murray G, et al. Absorption, metabolization, and antiplatelet effects of 300, 600, and 900 mg loading doses of clopidogrel: results of the ISAR-CHOICE (Intra-coronary Stenting and Antithrombotic Regimen: Choose between 3 High Oral doses for Immediate Clopidogrel Effect) trial. *Circulation* 2005; 112: 2946–2950.

40 Bonello L, Camoin-Jau L, Arques S, et al. Adjusted clopidogrel loading doses according to vasodilator-stimulated phosphoprotein phosphorylation index decrease rate of major adverse cardiovascular events in patients with clopidogrel resistance. *J Am Coll Cardiol* 2008; 51: 1404–1411.

41 von Beckerath N, Kastrati A, Wieczorek A, et al. A double-blind randomized study on platelet aggregation in patients treated with a daily dose of 150 or 75 mg of clopidogrel for 30 days (ISAR-CHOICE-2 trial). *Eur Heart J* 2007; 28: 1814–1819.

42 Angiolillo DJ, Shoemaker SB, Desai B, et al. Randomized comparison of a high clopidogrel maintenance dose in patients with diabetes mellitus and coronary artery disease: results of the optimising antiplatelet therapy in diabetes mellitus (OPTIMUS) study. *Circulation* 2007; 115: 708–716.

43 Mehta SR, Bassand JP, Chrolavicius S, et al. Design and rationale of CURRENT-OASIS 7: a randomized 2x2 factorial trial evaluating optimal dosing strategies for clopidogrel and aspirin in patients with ST and non-ST-elevation acute coronary syndromes managed with an early invasive strategy. *Am Heart J* 2008; 156: 1080–1088.

44 National Institute for Health and Clinical Excellence. Prasugrel for the treatment of acute coronary syndromes with percutaneous coronary intervention. NICE Technology Appraisal Guidance 182 [issued October 2009]. Available from: http://www.nice.org.uk/nicemedia/live/12324/45849/45849.pdf.

45 Wallentin L, Becker RC, Budaj A, et al. Ticagrelor versus clopidogrel in patients with acute coronary syndromes. *N Engl J Med* 2009; 361: 1045–1057.

46 Gurbel PA, Bliden KP, Butler K, et al. Randomized double-blind assessment of the ONSET and OFFSET of the antiplatelet effects of ticagrelor versus clopidogrel in patients with stable coronary artery disease. The ONSET/OFFSET study. *Circulation* 2009; 120: 2577–2585.

Triple antithrombotic therapy after coronary stenting for chronically anticoagulated patients: too much of a good thing?

Aung Myat

Expert commentary Professor Gregory YH Lip

Case history

A 68-year-old lady was directly referred by her family physician to the Medical Admissions Unit (MAU) with a 2-week history of exertional angina which had, in the last few days, deteriorated to central chest pain occurring both at rest and on minimal activity. Each episode had been relieved with a sublingual application of glyceryl trinitrate (GTN) spray. There was an extensive medical history, including rheumatic fever in childhood, systemic lupus erythematosus (requiring long-term steroid therapy), type II diabetes mellitus (necessitating both oral antidiabetic therapy and regular subcutaneous insulin), paroxysmal atrial fibrillation (PAF), a 29 mm Bjork–Shiley mitral valve replacement (MVR) for mixed mitral valve disease in 1990, an 18 mm Carbomedics aortic valve replacement (AVR) for critical aortic stenosis (AS) plus two coronary artery bypass grafts (CABG-saphenous vein graft (SVG) to an obtuse marginal (OM) artery and a left internal mammary artery (LIMA) graft to the left anterior descending (LAD) artery) in 1998, and a cerebrovascular accident (CVA) of ischaemic origin in 2004. She had been taking warfarin since the MVR operation in 1990, along with insulin, bumetanide, atorvastatin, metformin, ramipril, lansoprazole, and isosorbide mononitrate. There was a longstanding intolerance of beta-blockers and a lifelong non-smoking history.

> **Learning point** Indications for chronic oral anticoagulation (OAC) therapy
>
> Warfarin and other synthetic coumadin derivatives represent a family of vitamin K antagonists (VKA) that have now become standard therapy for patients at moderate to high risk of thromboembolism. Warfarin was first developed as a rodenticide in 1948 and approved for medicinal use in humans in 1954. Its anticoagulant property derives from its ability to inhibit vitamin K epoxide reductase which is fundamental to the γ-carboxylation of the vitamin K-dependent coagulation factors II, VII, IX, and X. Warfarin also inhibits the carboxylation of the regulatory anticoagulant proteins C and S [1].
>
> Indications for warfarin use include: moderate- and high-risk AF, prevention and treatment of venous thromboembolism (VTE), prosthetic heart valves, cerebrovascular disease and cryptogenic stroke, left ventricular aneurysm and mural thrombus, thrombophilia, individuals who have suffered one or more episodes of systemic thromboembolism, and hypertension associated with any of the above [1].
>
> *continued*

For the majority of conditions, moderate anticoagulant intensity (international normalized ratio [INR] 2.0 to 3.0) is sufficient. In the case of VTE, dosing to produce only moderate intensity anticoagulation is just as effective as a more intense regime (target INR 3.0 to 4.5) and leads to less bleeding complications [2]. Furthermore, four randomized studies have indicated that a reduction in the target INR range from 3.0–4.5 to 2.0–3.0 leads to a significant lowering of haemorrhagic risk, both in the context of tissue and mechanical prosthetic heart valves and VTE [3-6].

On arrival, the patient was pain-free and haemodynamically stable. An electrocardiogram (ECG) confirmed sinus rhythm with significant first degree heart block (PR interval 310 ms), left ventricular hypertrophy by voltage criteria with fixed inferolateral ST-segment depression (when compared to old traces), and no acute ischaemia (Figure 3.1). In light of the history and extensive cardiac background, the patient was given stat bolus doses of aspirin 300 mg and clopidogrel 300 mg, but no low molecular weight heparin (LMWH) in view of her chronic OAC. She was transferred to the Coronary Care Unit (CCU), at which point her OAC was stopped temporarily and eventually proceeded to an inpatient left heart catheterization via the right femoral artery on an unfractionated heparin (UFH) infusion once her INR had fallen below 2.0. A 12-hour troponin T was normal.

⭐ Learning point Radial vs femoral access for coronary angiography

- The right radial artery is now the preferred method of vascular access for both diagnostic coronary angiography and percutaneous coronary intervention (PCI) since it is associated with less access site complications.
- A meta-analysis published in 2009 revealed that radial artery access reduced major bleeding by 73% when compared with femoral access and also indicated a trend toward reductions in death, myocardial infarction (MI) and stroke [8].
- A transradial approach also obviates the need to interrupt OAC prior to coronary angiography ± PCI and therefore avoids the potential hazard of using additional heparin bridging (with UFH or LMWH) periprocedure and also post-procedure when OAC is recommended to achieve adequate INR levels.
- In the setting of previous CABG surgery, however, and in particular LIMA grafts, it is advisable to use the right femoral artery approach.
- A left radial artery approach may be considered for a graft study if the patient is known to have significant peripheral vascular disease or previous vascular surgery for the lower extremities.

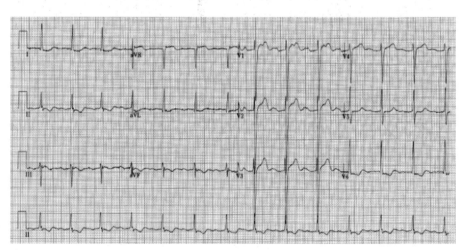

Figure 3.1 ECG on admission showing fixed inferolateral ST-segment depression.

Coronary angiography revealed a patent SVG to an OM branch and LIMA graft to the LAD artery. There was a critical ostial left main stem (LMS) stenosis which fed a widely patent first diagonal (D1) branch of the LAD artery which was itself occluded distal to the origin of D1. There was a tight proximal lesion in the native left circumflex (LCx) artery and the right coronary artery (RCA) was dominant and had a normal anatomy (Figure 3.2). At this stage, it was thought prudent to stop the procedure there and discuss the findings at a multidisciplinary team (MDT) meeting later in the week. Haemostasis of the puncture site was achieved with manual pressure to safely allow for the possibility of PCI at a later date.

An MDT meeting was convened with both interventional and non-interventional cardiologists and cardiac surgeons in attendance. It was felt the patient's symptoms could well have been emanating from the ungrafted D1 artery which appeared to cover a relatively large myocardial territory and was being fed by an LMS which had a critical stenosis at its ostium. However, the risks of PCI to the LMS were considered too high

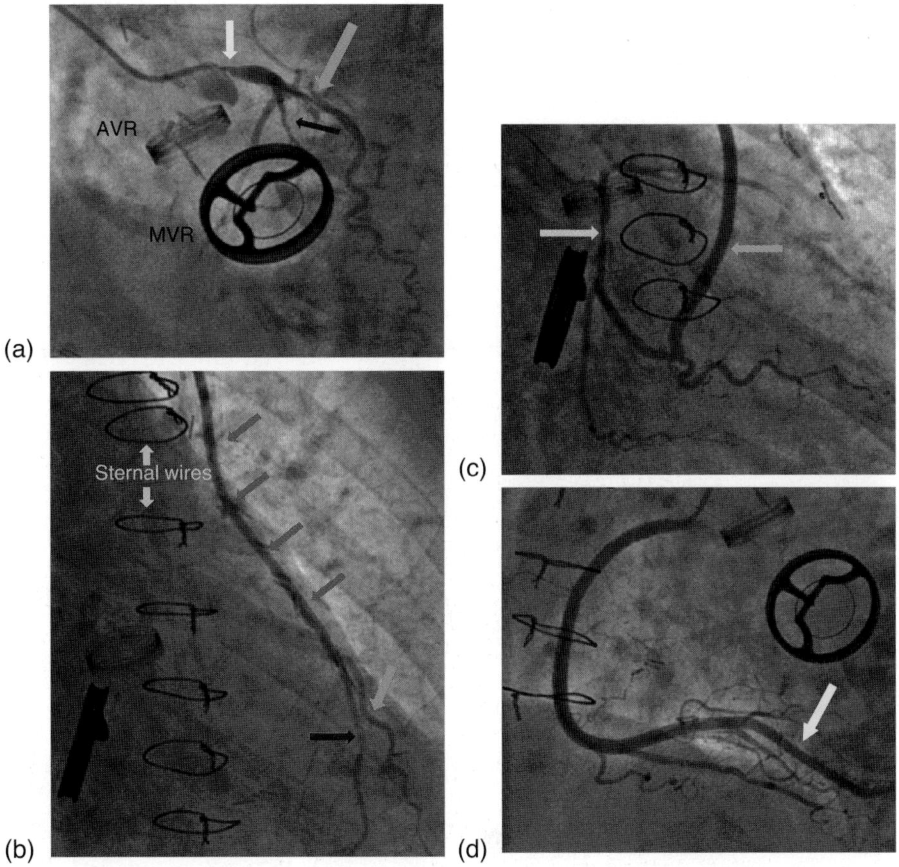

Expert comment

A recent European Society of Cardiology (ESC) Working Group on Thrombosis Consensus document [9], endorsed by the European Heart Rhythm Association (EHRA) and European Association of Percutaneous Coronary Interventions (EAPCI) recommends an uninterrupted anticoagulation strategy where possible, based on case series (but no randomized trials) that an uninterrupted anticoagulation strategy was associated with less thromboembolic and bleeding complications. A radial approach is recommended where possible and in this particular case, a femoral approach was necessary due to her previous grafts.

Clinical tip Coronary artery dominance

The artery supplying the posterior descending artery (PDA) or posterior interventricular artery determines the coronary dominance.
- If the PDA is supplied by the RCA, then the coronary circulation is classified as 'right-dominant'.
- If the PDA is supplied by the LCx artery, then the coronary circulation is classified as 'left-dominant'.
- If the PDA is supplied by both the RCA and LCx, then the coronary circulation is classified as 'co-dominant'.

Approximately 70% of the general population are right-dominant, 20% are co-dominant, and 10% are left-dominant.

Figure 3.2 Coronary angiography images. (a) Left anterior oblique (LAO) cranial view on diagnostic coronary angiography. Critical LMS ostial stenosis (yellow arrow) feeding a large and widely patent, but ungrafted, D1 branch with moderate proximal disease (green arrow) and a proximally occluded LAD (red arrow); (b) Patent LIMA graft (blue arrows) to LAD artery (red arrow) and a relatively large D1 artery (green arrow); (c) Widely patent SVG (orange arrow) to OM and a 90% lesion of the proximal LCx artery (blue arrow); (d) A normal dominant RCA. The posterior descending artery (PDA) branch (yellow arrow) indicates 'dominant' anatomy.

at this juncture and the consensus decision was to trial the patient on optimized anti-anginal therapy to improve her symptom burden, especially in light of a negative troponin T. The patient was recommenced on warfarin with a target INR of 2.5–3.5; her long-acting nitrate was uptitrated from 60 to 90 mg and nicorandil, a potassium channel activator, was started at 10 mg twice daily with a view to her family physician uptitrating the dose according to patient response and angina severity/frequency. At her consultant's discretion, both aspirin and clopidogrel (dual antiplatelet therapy (DAPT)) were stopped since the bleeding risk from triple therapy (TT), i.e. OAC and DAPT, was considered to be too high and far outweighed the presumed benefits.

A month later, the patient was re-admitted with a similar episode of unstable angina despite the enhanced medical therapy. There were no changes on the ECG and troponin T was again found to be normal. The decision, however, was made to proceed to PCI of the LMS stenosis on the basis of recurrent symptoms. The procedure was conducted via the right radial artery on this occasion so that OAC did not have to be stopped. The lesion was directly stented with a 4 x 16 mm drug-eluting stent (DES), and post-dilated with 4 x 15 mm and then 4.5 x 15 mm non-compliant balloons which achieved a good angiographic result (Figure 3.3). There were no peri-procedural complications and the patient made an uneventful recovery. In light of DES deployment, the patient was discharged on TT (i.e. long-term OAC, aspirin, and clopidogrel) for six weeks until outpatient clinic review at which point the plan would be to stop aspirin if the patient remained well and warfarin and clopidogrel would be continued lifelong.

⊕ **Learning point** OAC after coronary stenting

Contemporary guidelines advocate the use of DAPT after coronary stenting. OAC plus aspirin, however, was the precursor to DAPT until four landmark trials were published (ISAR [11], STARS [12], FANTASTIC [13], and MATTIS [14]). In total, these studies clearly demonstrated the superiority of DAPT over OAC and aspirin in the prevention of stent thrombosis and other major adverse cardiovascular and cerebrovascular events (MACCE) following PCI and further significantly reduced the risk of bleeding complications. All four trials used a combination of ticlopidine (the precursor of clopidogrel) and aspirin and compared them to OAC and aspirin. Although patients were randomized to either treatment arm, each study had an open-label design. Different patient populations were studied with variation in disease severity. Differences in peri-procedural anticoagulation and definitions of safety endpoints were also potential confounders. Despite this, all four studies came to the same conclusion: DAPT was superior to OAC plus aspirin in terms of reducing the incidence of adverse events and haemorrhagic/vascular complications following coronary stent deployment. A subsequent meta-analysis of the trials confirmed the net clinical benefit of DAPT over OAC and aspirin [15]. This advantage was essentially driven by significant reductions in non-fatal MI and the need for repeat target lesion revascularization (TLR). Interestingly, there was no significant difference in mortality between the two treatment strategies.

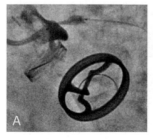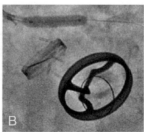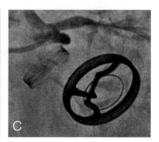

Figure 3.3 Left main stem PCI with coronary stenting of the critical LMS stenosis. A: placement of stent across critical ostial LMS stenosis; B: stent deployment; C: final result following post-stent dilatation.

⊙ Learning point OAC and thromboembolic risk

To date, the decision to continue or withdraw OAC following PCI has largely been empiric and generally based on the 'guesstimated' risk made by the attending physician of thromboembolic and atherothrombotic (i.e. stent thrombosis) complications balanced against the perceived increased risk of bleeding. General consensus might suggest that there are very few instances in which OAC can be stopped safely and a complete switch to DAPT be made after coronary stenting, low thromboembolic-risk atrial fibrillation (AF) and low-risk VTE being the only potential likely scenarios.

By far, the most common indication for OAC is AF. The prevalence of AF has risen dramatically in line with the current trend towards an ageing population. It affects 5% of those aged over 65 years and almost 10% of people above the age of 80 [16]. This is set to double over the next two generations. Various schema such as CHADS$_2$ have been postulated to stratify AF patients for thromboembolic risk and the subsequent need for OAC or aspirin [17]. None are ideal with marked variability between individuals categorized as having low, moderate, and high risk factors. Current National Institute for Health and Clinical Excellence (NICE) guidelines on AF favour a more pragmatic and algorithm-based approach to stroke prevention based on the Birmingham risk stratification schema [16,18]. The NICE schema has been compared to the CHADS$_2$ scoring system and was found to be comparable for predicting stroke and other vascular events [19]. Such schema can be used to stratify the potential risk of discontinuing warfarin.

Since AF commonly coexists with vascular disease, it follows that the incidence of patients in AF on warfarin therapy presenting with an acute coronary syndrome (ACS) or requiring scheduled PCI is set to rise exponentially over the coming years. Currently, given that the prevalence of AF is approximately 1–2% of the population, it follows that one to two million Europeans on chronic OAC will be candidates for coronary revascularization, often through PCI with stent deployment [20]. It is also important to remember that PAF carries the same thromboembolic risk as persistent and permanent AF [16].

ⓘ Expert comment

Given the increasing prevalence of AF in the general population and the common association of AF with vascular disease (including CAD), we are likely to see even more anticoagulated AF patients who present with an ACS and/or require PCI/stenting. Stroke risk is closely correlated to bleeding risk and the commonly used CHADS$_2$ score is a modest predictor of thromboembolic risk, but a good predictor of bleeding risk!

The CHADS$_2$ stroke risk scheme was recently refined to create the CHA$_2$DS$_2$-VASc score (Table 3.1). CHA$_2$DS$_2$-VASc includes all of the risk factors from the CHADS$_2$ index, but age between 65 and 74 years, female sex, and the presence of vascular disease are additional risk factors, each scoring one point. This schema improves on the CHADS$_2$ score for predicting stroke, but more importantly, those it categorizes as 'low risk' are truly low risk and only a small proportion are classified into the 'moderate risk' category, thus minimizing clinical uncertainty over whether to use VKA or aspirin in those patients [21].

Table 3.1 The CHA$_2$DS$_2$-VAS$_c$ schema for predicting stroke risk in patients with non-valvular AF (based on an initial validation cohort reported by Lip et al.; actual rates of stroke in contemporary cohorts may vary from these estimates) [21]

CHA$_2$DS$_2$-VAS$_c$ criteria	Score	CHA$_2$DS$_2$-VAS$_c$ total score	Rate of stroke/ other TE, %/year (95% CI)*
Congestive heart failure/LV dysfunction	1	0	0 (0–0)
Hypertension	1	1	0.6 (0–3.4)
Age ≥75 years	2	2	1.6 (0.3–4.7)
Diabetes mellitus	1	3	3.9 (1.7–7.6)
Stroke/TIA/TE	2	4	1.9 (0.5–4.9)
Vascular disease (prior MI, plaque, or aortic plaque)	1	5	3.2 (0.7–9.0)
Age 65–74 years	1	6	3.6 (0.4–12.3)
Sex category female	1	7	8.0 (1.0–26.0)
		8	11.1 (0.3–48.3)
		9	100 (2.5–100.0)

* Assuming aspirin not taken.

The patient was re-admitted to the MAU six weeks later, just before her planned cardiology review, complaining of epigastric pain, dyspnoea and dark offensive stool, but no angina. Urgent blood tests were ordered and revealed a hypochromic microcytic anaemia (Table 3.2). Blood pressure (BP) was measured at 98/60 mmHg with a heart rate of 110 beats per minute in sinus rhythm. There was no evidence of pulmonary congestion and prosthetic first and second heart sounds were audible. Two large-bore

Table 3.2 Urgent blood test results on admission

Haematology		Biochemistry	
Hb	**6.4 g/dL** (11.5–16.0)	Na	139 mmol/L (133–146)
Hypochromic RBC	**19.6%** (0.0–8.0)	K	3.8 mmol/L (3.5–5.3)
MCV	**75.2 fL** (80.0–100.0)	Urea	**16.1 mmol/L** (2.5–7.8)
WCC	**12.15 x 10⁹/L** (4.0–11.0)	Creatinine	111 micromol/L (50–110)
Platelet count	433 × 10⁹/L (150–400)		
		Creatine kinase	74 U/L (<130)
INR	**3.2** (0.9–1.2)	Troponin T	<0.01 ng/mL (0.00–0.01)
		Iron	**<5.0 micromol/L** (14.0–29.0)
		Total iron binding capacity	61 micromol/L (45–72)
		Serum ferritin	29 ng/mL (13–150)
		LFTs	Normal

Clinical tip Rapid reversal of OAC using PCC (Octaplex®)

- Used for the reversal of warfarin therapy or vitamin K deficiency in those patients who are either exhibiting major bleeding manifestations or those who require an urgent (less than six hours) surgical procedure;
- Should only be used following specialist haematological consultation;
- A more rapid and complete reversal of the effects of warfarin are achieved with PCC when compared with fresh frozen plasma (FFP) and as such, PCC is recommended by the British Committee for Standards in Haematology (BCSH) in preference to FFP for major bleeding [22];
- PCC is given intravenously along with 5–10 mg vitamin K.

Expert comment

The difficulty here is balancing the need for prevention of stent thrombosis and recurrent cardiac ischaemia against the potential for bleeding. In this particular case, the cause of anaemia was eventually thought to be as a result of a low-grade haemolytic process, but the marked drop in haemoglobin levels (alongside a microcytic picture) clearly necessitates the aggressive investigations described to identify a source of potential bleeding.

venous cannulae were inserted in each arm and six units of blood were cross-matched. Specialist cardiology and haematology opinions were sought by the admitting general medical team whilst the patient was receiving an immediate 2-unit blood transfusion. The cardiologist advised cessation of aspirin and warfarin for the meantime and conversion to heparin, but the clopidogrel was to be continued in order to prevent, as much as possible, any adverse atherothrombotic sequelae. The haematologist concurred and further advised the use of both intravenous (IV) vitamin K and prothrombin complex concentrate (PCC) to rapidly reverse the oral anticoagulation. Both prosthetic valves were to be covered with LMWH in the acute period before haemodynamic stability and a source of bleeding could both be attained.

A per rectum examination was conducted which demonstrated no evidence of melaena. The patient proceeded to urgent oesophagogastroduodenoscopy (OGD) which revealed nothing more than a small sliding hiatus hernia. Both the stomach and duodenum were normal and no fresh or old blood were seen in the upper gastrointestinal (GI) tract. The patient was stabilized haemodynamically on the ward and a general surgical consult was obtained. They advised a computed tomography (CT) mesenteric angiogram to search for a source of the bleeding. This scan demonstrated no signs of significant GI blood loss. As such, the decision was made by the GI team, in collaboration with the cardiologists, to discharge the patient on the same TT as before: warfarin, aspirin, and clopidogrel as there was no evidence of GI blood loss. The haemoglobin (Hb) was 9.0 g/dL and the patient was sent home with ferrous sulphate (200 mg three times a day).

Unfortunately, the patient returned to hospital as an emergency a fortnight later with melaena and generalized abdominal pain. The Hb had fallen to 5.2 g/dL on this occasion and therefore required several units of blood to maintain haemodynamic stability. An urgent repeat OGD demonstrated only two very superficial abrasions to the gastric mucosa which were deemed unlikely to have given rise to such a significant GI bleed. A colonoscopy was also found to be normal. Despite the normal investigations, it was thought prudent to stop the patient's aspirin completely and leave her on OAC and clopidogrel. The patient remained well thereafter and made a full recovery. No definite cause of haemorrhage was found although it was postulated that the blood loss could have been the result of a low-grade haemolytic anaemia caused by the prosthetic AVR and/or MVR.

⊕ **Learning point** Prosthetic heart valves and their complications

- Replacement of a diseased heart valve exchanges the haemodynamic instability and with it, the adverse cardiac remodelling and the morbidity and mortality caused by native valve disease, with the inherent complications associated with the implanted prosthetic device.
- The nature, frequency, and severity of complications experienced depend on the valve type and position and several other clinical risk factors. In general, the incidence of complications, despite appropriate management, is approximately 3% per year [23].
- Complications associated with prosthetic heart valves are as follows:
  1 Primary structural failure, e.g. paravalvular leaks, strut fracture and subsequent embolization, and peri-prosthetic valve regurgitation;
  2 Valve obstruction and thromboembolism, e.g. with pannus formation (i.e. fibrous tissue in-growth), prosthetic valve thrombosis, or vegetations;
  3 Infection, e.g. infective endocarditis and paravalvular abscesses;
  4 Mechanical haemolytic anaemia; and
  5 Anticoagulant-related haemorrhage.

⊕ **Learning point** Mechanical haemolytic anaemia

- This phenomenon is usually seen with mechanical heart valves. Ordinarily, it is at most mild and subclinical, but can be severe in up to 15% of patients with specific prostheses such as a ball-and-cage device or bileaflet valves or those suffering perivalvular regurgitation.
- Although uncommon, it can occur with tissue valves and may be the initial presentation of porcine valve failure.
- Clinical presentation may manifest as:
  1 Anaemia;
  2 Jaundice with dark urine and pale stool;
  3 Cardiac decompensation;
  4 Increasing serum lactate dehydrogenase (LDH); and
  5 A new or changed regurgitant murmur;
- The 'Waring blender' syndrome refers to the appearance of peripheral blood smears, demonstrating marked red cell fragmentation and small fragmented cells with multiple sharp edges which can be a direct result of the shear forces from a defective prosthetic valve, effectively cleaving red blood cells as they pass through the device.
- Oral iron therapy is usually adequate although blood transfusion and even redoing cardiac surgery may be necessary in the most severe cases, especially if there is associated regurgitation from a perivalvular leak or valve failure.

⊕ **Clinical tip** Anticoagulant-related haemorrhage

The overriding concern with OAC is the risk of bleeding which correlates with the INR level. Other factors include the underlying disease pathology, concomitant administration of gastro-toxic drugs such as aspirin and other non-steroidal anti-inflammatory drugs (NSAIDs) or other agents that impair platelet function, cause gastric erosions, and in escalated doses, impair the hepatic production of vitamin K-dependent clotting factors. The risk of haemorrhagic complications are also dependent on demographic factors such as age greater than 65 years, low body mass index, a previous history of stroke or previous GI bleeding, and comorbid conditions such as renal failure, anaemia, and diabetes.

Discussion

This case clearly demonstrates an altogether increasingly common clinical dilemma faced by cardiologists and general medical physicians alike, i.e. what the optimal antithrombotic therapy that provides net clinical benefit to those patients on chronic OAC following an ACS and, in particular, those who proceed to subsequent PCI and coronary stenting is.

When managing such individuals, we must first decide whether long-term OAC is indeed appropriate. In this particular patient's case, OAC was absolutely essential. Not withstanding the obvious need to prevent thrombotic complications arising from both mechanical valve prostheses, this individual was also over the age of 65, had had a previous cerebral infarct, a history of PAF, ischaemic heart disease, and type II diabetes mellitus. Her CHADS$_2$ score is 3 which equates to a 5.9% risk of stroke per annum without treatment [17]. Similarly, she also lies in the high-risk category of the NICE guidelines for thromboprophylaxis in AF, giving an annual stroke risk lying somewhere between 3 and 15% [16,18] (Table 3.3).

Table 3.3 Risk of thromboembolic events occurring per annum without oral anticoagulation
(adapted from Rubboli A et al. and the NICE guidelines for thromboprophylaxis in AF [18,24])

Clinical scenario	Thromboembolic risk (per annum) (%)
Low-risk AF (NICE guidelines)	1
• Age <65 with no history of embolism or other high/moderate risk factors	
• **Aspirin 75–300 mg/day if no contraindications**	
Moderate-risk AF (NICE guidelines)	3–7
• Age ≥65 not in the high risk category or	
• All patients <75 with diabetes, hypertension, or vascular disease (i.e. PAD or CAD) not identified in the high-risk category	
• **Consider OAC or aspirin**	
High-risk AF (NICE guidelines)	12–15
• Previous transient ischaemic attack or ischaemic cerebrovascular accident or thromboembolism	
• Age ≥75 with diabetes or vascular disease or hypertension	
• Clinical evidence of valve disease, heart failure, or impaired LV function on echocardiography	
• **Anticoagulation with warfarin**	
Bileaflet mechanical aortic prostheses (St Jude, Carbomedics)	10–12
Tilting-disc mechanical aortic prostheses (Bjork–Shiley, Medtronic–Hall, Omnicarbon)	23
Bileaflet mechanical mitral prostheses (St Jude, Carbomedics)	22
Multiple bileaflet mechanical prostheses (St Jude, Carbomedics)	91
Low-risk VTE	2–5
• VTE >6 months ago	
• Reversible risk factors	
High-risk VTE	10–27
• Recent VTE <3 weeks ago	
• Neoplasm	
• Persistent risk factors	
• Antiphospholipid syndrome	
• Homozygous for factor V Leiden	
• Protein C and S deficiency	
• Chronic heart or lung disease	

As mentioned previously, there are very few clinical scenarios that exist in which long-term OAC can potentially be stopped without exposing the patient to an unacceptably high risk of thromboembolic phenomena (Table 3.4). Results from the ACTIVE W trial also demonstrated the superiority of warfarin over aspirin and clopidogrel in AF patients with one or more thromboembolic risk factors for the primary prevention of stroke, non-central nervous system embolism, MI, and vascular death. OAC demonstrated such a clear morbidity and mortality advantage over DAPT that the Data and Safety Monitoring Board was forced to stop the trial early. Interestingly, there were also similar major bleeding rates between the two treatment arms [25]. It follows, therefore, that DAPT should not be used as a substitute for OAC in those at moderate to high thromboembolic risk.

Table 3.4 Which patients potentially can and cannot stop oral anticoagulation

Can potentially stop OAC	Cannot safely or should not stop OAC
Low-risk AF, i.e. low risk according to NICE guidelines or CHADS$_2$ score 0–1	Moderate-risk AF, i.e. moderate risk according to NICE guidelines or CHADS$_2$ score 2–3
Mitral stenosis and no AF (whether paroxysmal, persistent, or permanent)	High-risk AF, i.e. high risk according to NICE guidelines or CHADS$_2$ score 4–6
Biological heart valve and no AF (whether paroxysmal, persistent, or permanent)	Mechanical heart valve in the aortic or mitral positions
LV systolic dysfunction, but no AF (whether paroxysmal, persistent, or permanent) or intracardiac thrombus	LV mural thrombus/apical aneurysm
Non-cardioembolic ischaemic stroke, i.e. cryptogenic or secondary to patent foramen ovale	One or more episodes of systemic/arterial thromboembolism
Low-risk VTE	High-risk VTE

With the appropriate need for long-term OAC established, other factors come into play when selecting the best antithrombotic combination for patients proceeding to PCI with coronary stenting. The following must all be considered:

- What type of stent platform to use (bare-metal or drug-eluting);
- Lesion type, length, and diameter;
- Duration of adjunctive antiplatelet mono- or dual therapy;
- Which vascular access site to use (radial vs femoral);
- Should OAC be interrupted with heparin bridging prior to PCI or remain uninterrupted;
- INR range, control within that range, and frequency of monitoring; and
- The overall haemorrhagic risk of the patient (Table 3.5).

Table 3.5 The HAS-BLED bleeding risk score [27]

Letter	Clinical characteristic	Points awarded (max 9 points)
H	Hypertension, defined as systolic BP >160 mmHg	1
A	Abnormal kidney function, i.e. chronic dialysis/renal transplantation/serum creatinine ≥200 micromol/L Abnormal liver function, i.e. chronic hepatic disease (e.g. cirrhosis) or biochemical evidence of hepatic derangement: • Bilirubin >2 x upper limit of normal (ULN) in association with • AST/ALT/ALP >3 x ULN	1 or 2
S	Stroke	1
B	Bleeding (previous bleeding history and/or predisposition to bleeding, e.g. bleeding diathesis, anaemia)	1
L	Labile INR unstable/high INR or insufficient time in therapeutic range (<60%)	1
E	Elderly (age >65 years)	1
D	Drugs (e.g. antiplatelet agents, NSAIDs) or alcohol abuse	1 or 2

This simple bleeding risk score was derived from a 'real world' cohort of 3,978 European subjects with AF from the Euro Heart Survey and has now been incorporated into the new ESC guidelines for the management of AF issued in 2010 [26]. A score of ≥3 indicates 'high risk' and therefore, caution and regular review of the patient is advised following the initiation of antithrombotic treatment, whether it be aspirin or VKA (adapted from Pisters et al. [27]).

There are currently no large-scale, prospective, multicentre, randomized clinical trials published in the medical literature that address this issue. To date, 21 studies have been published, but they represent only single-centre registries, small case-controlled series or post hoc analyses of prospective studies and have tended to focus on safety endpoints such as bleeding risk. Significantly less emphasis has been dedicated to elucidating the most suitable therapeutic strategy that is able to provide net clinical benefit (i.e. the sum of bleeding vs atherothrombotic and thromboembolic sequelae). Furthermore, the frequency and severity of bleeding events vary substantially between these studies as a consequence of differing bleeding definitions recorded, varying doses of aspirin, sample size inequalities, intensity of the anticoagulant regimen,

Table 3.6 Recommended antithrombotic strategies following coronary artery stenting in patients with AF at moderate-to-high thromboembolic risk (in whom oral anticoagulation therapy is required) [9,26]

Haemorrhagic risk	Clinical setting	Stent implanted	Anticoagulation regimen
Low or intermediate (e.g. HAS-BLED score 0–2)	Elective	Bare-metal	**1 month:** triple therapy of VKA (INR 2.0–2.5) + aspirin ≤100 mg/day + clopidogrel 75 mg/day **Up to 12th month:** combination of VKA (INR 2.0–2.5) + clopidogrel 75 mg/day[b] (or aspirin 100 mg/day) **Lifelong:** VKA (INR 2.0–3.0) alone
	Elective	Drug-eluting	**3 (-olimus[a] group) to 6 (paclitaxel) months:** triple therapy of VKA (INR 2.0–2.5) + aspirin ≤100 mg/day + clopidogrel 75 mg/day **Up to 12th month:** combination of VKA (INR 2.0–2.5) + clopidogrel 75 mg /day[b] (or aspirin 100 mg/day) **Lifelong:** VKA (INR 2.0–3.0) alone
	ACS	Bare-metal/ drug-eluting	**6 months:** triple therapy of VKA (INR 2.0–2.5) + aspirin ≤100 mg/day + clopidogrel 75 mg/day **Up to 12th month:** combination of VKA (INR 2.0–2.5) + clopidogrel 75 mg /day[b] (or aspirin 100 mg/day) **Lifelong:** VKA (INR 2.0–3.0) alone
High (e.g. HAS-BLED score ≥3)	Elective	Bare-metal[c]	**2–4 weeks:** triple therapy of VKA (INR 2.0–2.5) + aspirin ≤100 mg/day + clopidogrel 75 mg/day **Lifelong:** VKA (2.0–3.0) alone
	ACS	Bare-metal[c]	**4 weeks:** triple therapy of VKA (INR 2.0–2.5) + aspirin ≤100 mg/day + clopidogrel 75 mg/day **Up to 12th month:** combination of VKA (INR 2.0–2.5) + clopidogrel 75 mg /day[b] (or aspirin 100 mg/day) **Lifelong:** VKA (INR 2.0–3.0 alone)

[a] Sirolimus, everolimus, and tacrolimus; [b] Combination of VKA (INR 2.0–3.0) + aspirin ≤100 mg/day (with proton pump inhibitor, if indicated) may be considered as an alternative; [c] Drug-eluting stents should be avoided as far as possible, but if used, consideration of more prolonged (3– 6 months) triple antithrombotic therapy is necessary.
Reproduced with permission from European Heart Rhythm Association; European Association for Cardio-Thoracic Surgery, Camm AJ, Kirchhof P, Lip GY, et al. Guidelines for the management of atrial fibrillation: the Task Force for the Management of Atrial Fibrillation of the European Society of Cardiology (ESC). *Eur Heart J* 2010; 31: 2369–2429. Epub 2010 Aug 29 with permission and copyright of Oxford University Press.

and the clinical characteristics of the patient populations under investigation [28]. It has also been difficult to differentiate those patients actually taking TT and those only receiving OAC plus a single antiplatelet agent.

In an era of evidence-based medicine, large randomized controlled trials (RCTs) and guideline-driven therapeutics, robust prospective randomized data on the best anti-thrombotic regimen for this subset of patients on chronic OAC requiring PCI are currently undefined. Many of the recommendations available are anecdotal and centre on the need to strike the perfect balance between avoiding stent thrombosis and thromboembolic complications against minimizing the risk of bleeding. The need for RCT data is all the more pressing since it is evident this subset of patients is expanding fast alongside the growth of an elderly population.

> **⊕ A final word from the expert**
>
> This case neatly illustrates the dilemma over how best to manage such patients. Given the lack of prospective blinded RCT data, following an evidence-based expert consensus approach would be prudent. Table 3.6 illustrates recommendations issued by the ESC in its new AF guidelines for this patient cohort [9,26]. Bleeding risk assessment is also problematic and current published scores have not been adequately validated in AF populations nor are user-friendly or practical, hence the emergence of the HAS-BLED risk score and its incorporation into the new ESC AF guidelines.

References

1 Hirsh J, Fuster V, Ansell J, et al. American Heart Association/American College of Cardiology foundation guide to warfarin therapy. *Circulation* 2003; 107: 1692–1711.

2 Landefeld CS, Rosenblatt MW. Bleeding in outpatients treated with warfarin: relation to the prothrombin time and important remediable lesions. *Am J Med* 1989; 87: 153–159.

3 Hull R, Hirsh J, Jay R, et al. Different intensities of oral anticoagulant therapy in the treatment of proximal vein thrombosis. *N Engl J Med* 1982; 307: 1676–1681.

4 Turpie AGG, Gunstensen J, Hirsh J, et al. Randomized comparison of two intensities of oral anticoagulant therapy after tissue heart valve replacement. *Lancet* 1988; 1: 1242–1245.

5 Saour JN, Sieck JO, Mamo LAR, et al. Trial of different intensities of anticoagulation in patients with prosthetic heart valves. *N Engl J Med* 1990; 322: 428–432.

6 Altman R, Rouvier J, Gurfinkel E, et al. Comparison of two levels of anticoagulant therapy in patients with substitute heart valves. *J Thorac Cardiovasc Surg* 1991; 101: 427–431.

7 Bassand J, Hamm C, Ardissino D, et al. Guidelines for the diagnosis and treatment of non-ST-segment elevation acute coronary syndromes. *Eur Heart J* 2007; 28: 1598–1660.

8 Jolly SS, Amlani S, Hamon M, et al. Radial versus femoral access for coronary angiography or intervention and the impact on major bleeding and ischaemic events: a systematic review and meta-analysis of randomized trials. *Am Heart J* 2009; 157: 132–140.

9 Lip GYH, Huber K, Andreotti F, et al. Management of antithrombotic therapy in atrial fibrillation patients presenting with acute coronary syndrome and/or undergoing percutaneous coronary intervention/stenting. *Thromb Haemost* 2010; 103: 13–28.

10 Rubboli A, Colletta M, Sangiorgio P, et al. Antithrombotic treatment after coronary artery stenting in patients on chronic oral anticoagulation: an international survey of current clinical practice. *Ital Heart J* 2004; 5: 851–856.

11 Schomig A, Neumann FJ, Kastrati A, et al. A randomized comparison of antiplatelet and anticoagulant therapy after the placement of coronary artery stents. *N Engl J Med* 1996; 334: 1084–1089.

12 Leon MB, Baim DS, Popma JJ, et al. A clinical trial comparing three antithrombotic drug regimens after coronary artery stenting. *N Engl J Med* 1998; 339: 1665–1671.

13 Bertrand ME, Legrand V, Boland J, et al. Randomized multicentre comparison of conventional anticoagulation versus antiplatelet therapy in unplanned and elective coronary stenting. The Full Anticoagulation Versus Aspirin and Ticlopidine (FANTASTIC) study. *Circulation* 1996; 98: 1597–1603.

14 Urban P, Macaya C, Rupprecht HJ, et al. Randomized evaluation of anticoagulation versus antiplatelet therapy after coronary stent implantation in high-risk patients. The Multicentre Aspirin and Ticlopidine Trial after Intracoronary Stenting (MATTIS). *Circulation* 1998; 98: 2126–2132.

15 Rubboli A, Milandri M, Castelvetri C, et al. Meta-analysis of trials comparing oral anticoagulation and aspirin versus dual antiplatelet therapy after coronary stenting. Clues for the management of patients with an indication for long-term anticoagulation undergoing coronary stenting. *Cardiology* 2005; 104: 101–106.

16 Lip GYH, Boos CJ. Antithrombotic treatment in atrial fibrillation. *Heart* 2006; 92: 155–161.

17 Gage BF, Waterman AD, Shannon W, et al. Validation of clinical classification schemes for predicting stroke: results from the National Registry of atrial fibrillation. *JAMA* 2001; 285: 2864–2870.

18 National Institute for Health and Clinical Excellence. Atrial fibrillation: the management of atrial fibrillation. NICE guideline CG36 [issued June 2006]. Available from: http://www.nice.org.uk/CG36.

19 Lip GY, Edwards SJ. Stroke prevention with aspirin, warfarin and ximelgatran in patients with atrial fibrillation: a systematic review and meta-analysis. *Thromb Res* 2006; 118: 321–333.

20 Stewart S, Hart CL, Hole DJ, et al. Population, prevalence, incidence, and predictors of atrial fibrillation in the Renfrew/Paisley study. *Heart* 2001; 86: 516–521.

21 Lip GY, Nieuwlaat R, Pisters R, et al. Refining clinical risk stratification for predicting stroke and thromboembolism in atrial fibrillation using a novel risk factor-based approach: the Euro Heart survey on atrial fibrillation. *Chest.* 2010; 137: 263–272.

22 British Committee for Standards in Haematology Guidelines on oral anticoagulation (warfarin): third edition, 2005 update. *Br J Haematol* 2006; 132: 277–285.

23 Vongpatanasin W, Hillis D, Lange RA. Prosthetic heart valves. *N Engl J Med* 1996; 335: 407–416.

24 Rubboli A, Verheugt FWA. Antithrombotic treatment for patients on oral anticoagulation undergoing coronary stenting. A review of the available evidence and practical suggestions for the clinician. *Intl J Cardiol* 2008; 123: 234–239.

25 The ACTIVE Writing Group on behalf of the Active Investigators. Clopidogrel plus aspirin versus oral anticoagulation for atrial fibrillation in the Atrial Fibrillation Clopidogrel Trial with Irbesartan for prevention of Vascular Events (Active W): a randomized controlled trial. *Lancet* 2006; 367: 1903–1912.

26 European Heart Rhythm Association; European Association for Cardiothoracic Surgery, Camm AJ, Kirchhof P, Lip GY, et al. Guidelines for the management of atrial fibrillation: the Task Force for the Management of Atrial Fibrillation of the European Society of Cardiology (ESC). *Eur Heart J* 2010; 31: 2369–2429.

27 Pisters R, Lane DA, Nieuwlaat R, et al. A novel user-friendly score (HAS-BLED) to assess 1-year risk of major bleeding in patients with atrial fibrillation: the Euro Heart Survey. *Chest* 2010; 138: 1093–1100.

28 Holmes DR, Kereiakes DJ, Kleiman NS, et al. Combining antiplatelet and anticoagulant therapies. *J Am Coll Cardiol* 2009; 54: 95–109.

4 A closer look at lipid management following an acute coronary syndrome

William Moody and Aung Myat

Expert commentary Dr Anthony Wierzbicki

Case history

A 40-year-old company director presented to A&E with a 4-hour history of crushing central chest pain. His admission electrocardiogram (ECG) revealed deep T wave inversion in leads V1–V6. He was obese with a body mass index (BMI) of 35 kg/m² and xanthelasmata were noted around his eyes. His untreated non-fasting lipid profile on admission was: total cholesterol (TC) 9.5 mmol/L, triglycerides (TG) 3.9 mmol/L, high-density lipoprotein cholesterol (HDL-C) 0.9 mmol/L, and calculated low-density lipoprotein cholesterol (LDL-C) 6.5 mmol/L. Troponin T at 12 hours was elevated at 1.2 ng/mL (0.00–0.01 ng/mL), confirming the diagnosis of anterior non-ST-elevation myocardial infarction (NSTEMI). Deemed high risk, he was started on atorvastatin 80 mg once daily (od) as part of the acute coronary syndrome (ACS) treatment regime. He underwent percutaneous coronary intervention (PCI) to his left anterior descending (LAD) artery the following day and a successful angiographic outcome was achieved. He was discharged home on day 4 after being given lifestyle advice from the cardiac rehabilitation nurse specialist.

He was followed up eight weeks later by his general practitioner at which point his repeat lipid profile was: TC 4.3, HDL-C 1.2, and TG 1.3. His calculated LDL-C fraction was 2.5 mmol/L. Despite high-dose statin therapy, he had not met optimal TC and LDL-C goals (TC 4 mmol/L and LDL-C 2 mmol/L) now approved by NICE [1].

> **Learning point** Calculating LDL-C using the Friedewald formula [3]
>
> LDL-C is most commonly estimated from quantitative measurements of TC, HDL-C, and plasma TG using the empirical relationship first described by Friedewald et al.: $[LDL-C] = [TC - HDL-C] - [TG/2.19]$, where all concentrations are given in mmol/L. The ultracentrifugal reference method of measuring LDL-C is time-consuming, expensive, and requires specialist equipment. Newer assays that measure LDL-C directly on automated systems are available in some centres.
>
> The quotient [TG/2.19] is used as an estimate of very low density lipoprotein cholesterol (VLDL-C) concentration. It assumes that virtually all of the plasma TG is carried on VLDL-C and that the TG:TC ratio of VLDL is constant at about 5:1.
>
> The Friedewald equation should not be used under the following circumstances:
> - When chylomicrons are present (i.e. non-fasting samples);
> - When plasma TG concentration exceeds 4.52 mmol/L and underestimates TG from levels >2.5 mmol/L with significant bias from TG >3.5 mmol/L;
> - In patients with dysbetalipoproteinaemia (type III hyperlipoproteinaemia); and
> - In patients with diabetes.

> **Clinical tip** Higher vs lower intensity statins
>
> - Troponins are good indices of the extent of myocardial necrosis and are of prognostic benefit in ACS. Additional prognostic information can be obtained with B-type natriuretic peptide (BNP) and high sensitivity C reactive protein (hsCRP) levels.
> - Higher intensity statins such as atorvastatin 80 mg, rosuvastatin 20/40 mg are now recommended in those patients with ACS in order to achieve the increasingly stringent TC and LDL-C targets approved by the National Institute of Health and Clinical Excellence (NICE) [1].
> - Though some guidelines recommend simvastatin 80 mg, data from the SEARCH study showed only a 7% non-significant reduction in cardiovascular events with incremental simvastatin therapy (80 vs 20 mg) and a large increase in myopathic events [2].
> - Simvastatin came off patent in 2003 and is therefore ten-fold cheaper than alternative statins. Atorvastatin is due to come off patent in late 2011.

The patient made no complaints of gastrointestinal side effects, but was concerned about muscle aches and pains, particularly in his calves. He had recently read a newspaper article about statins and now feared he may have developed a dangerous myositis. Despite this, he had maintained strict adherence to his treatment plan.

Serum creatine kinase (CK) was measured and found to be only mildly elevated at 165 U/L (< 130 U/L). Despite this reassuring result, he was not keen to continue on the atorvastatin even at a lower dose. He was switched to low-dose pravastatin, initially at 10 mg daily which was subsequently uptitrated to 80 mg nocte over a 6-month period. Given his difficulties with tolerating higher intensity statin therapy, a further review in a specialist lipid clinic was arranged.

Learning point North American lipid targets

Since the publication of Acute Treatment Panel III (ATP III) in 2004, the National Cholesterol Education Programme (NCEP) in the United States cite five major clinical trials of statin therapy that have addressed clinical endpoints not adequately covered in previous studies [5]. They have highlighted the Heart Protection Study (HPS), the Prospective Study of Pravastatin in the Elderly at Risk (PROSPER) study, the Antihypertensive and Lipid-Lowering Treatment to Prevent Heart Attack Trial-Lipid-Lowering Trial (ALLHAT-LLT), the Anglo-Scandinavian Cardiac Outcomes Trial-Lipid-Lowering Arm (ASCOT-LLA), and the Pravastatin or Atorvastatin Evaluation and Infection Therapy (PROVE-IT) trial as having important implications for the management of those with lipid disorders, especially high-risk patients [6-10]. They suggest an additional benefit in **aggressively** treating those in the very high-risk subset (i.e. those with established coronary heart disease (CHD) who also have multiple risk factors, including diabetes and metabolic syndrome) to LDL levels <1.8 mmol/L. This new guidance supports the use of adding in alternative lipid-lowering agents to baseline statin therapy to achieve these goals [4].

Landmark trial HPS trial [6]

- Huge combined primary and secondary prevention trial;
- A randomized 2 by 2 factorial design assessing statin as well as vitamin E therapy;
- 20,536 patients, including males and females aged 40–80 years, 13,379 of whom had pre-existing CHD;
- High-risk patients with a wide range of TC ≥3.5 mmol/L;
- Simvastatin 40 mg daily vs placebo with mean follow-up at five years;
- Primary endpoints were all-cause mortality, CHD mortality, and all mortality from causes other than CHD;
- A 12% relative reduction in all-cause mortality, p < 0.001; 17% reduction in vascular mortality, p < 0.0002;
- A 24% relative reduction in major vascular events (total of CHD, stroke, and revascularizations), p < 0.00001;
- **Conclusion:** Patients at high risk, particularly those with existing CHD, should receive statin treatment, irrespective of LDL-C.

Landmark trial PROSPER trial [7]

- Combined primary and secondary prevention trial in the elderly;
- 5,804 men and women, aged 70–82 years from Scotland, Ireland, and the Netherlands with plasma TC of 4–9 mmol/L and TG levels <6 mmol/L;
- Enrolled patients included those with pre-existing vascular disease (coronary, cerebral, or peripheral) or those at increased risk for vascular disease due to such factors as smoking, hypertension, or diabetes;
- Pravastatin 40 mg daily vs placebo; follow-up at 3.2 years;
- A 15% relative reduction in primary outcome (a composite of definite or suspected death from CHD, non-fatal MI, and fatal or non-fatal stroke), p = 0.014;
- No measured impact on cognitive function;
- **Conclusion:** There is a need to expand statin therapy to include this elderly patient population in order to reduce the incidence of vascular-related events.

○ **Landmark trial** ALLHAT-LLT trial [8]

- Combined primary and secondary prevention trial in 10,355 patients aged ≥55 years with moderate hypercholesterolaemia;
- Fasting LDL-C of 3–5 mmol/L with no known CHD or LDL-C of 2.5–3.5 mmol/L with known CV disease;
- Pravastatin 40 mg daily vs placebo with mean follow-up at 4.8 years;
- A 28% reduction in LDL-C from baseline;
- No benefit in either the primary outcome (all-cause mortality) or the key secondary outcome (combined non-fatal and fatal MI);
- **Conclusion:** Insufficient statistical power to demonstrate a clinical benefit resulting in an apparent null result.

○ **Landmark trial** ASCOT-LLA trial [9]

- Randomized, double-blind, placebo-controlled, 2 by 2 factorial primary prevention trial of blood pressure lowering and lipid lowering;
- 10,297 European patients with hypertension and non-fasting TC concentrations of ≤6.5 mmol/L;
- Atorvastatin 10 mg daily vs placebo;
- Atorvastatin reduced LDL-C by 35% and TC by 24% after one year of follow-up;
- The trial was originally planned for five years, but was stopped after a median follow-up of 3.3 years because of a significant 36% reduction in the primary outcome of CHD events (p = 0.0005);
- A 27% reduction in the secondary outcome of fatal and non-fatal stroke (p = 0.0236), 21% reduction in total cardiovascular events, including revascularization procedures (p = 0.0005), and a 29% reduction in total coronary events (p = 0.0005);
- **Conclusion:** Clear benefit of statin therapy in at-risk hypertensive patients with average or lower-than-average cholesterol concentrations.

Three months later, he was reviewed in the specialist lipid clinic. His fasting profile now measured TC 5.3, HDL-C 2.0, and TG 1.3, giving an estimated LDL-C of 2.7. A secondary cause for his dyslipidaemia was excluded. Thyroid, liver and renal function, fasting glucose, and a urine dipstick for protein were all within normal limits. There was no family history of premature cardiac death and the patient denied the consumption of any alcohol since his heart attack. His lipid profile history was reviewed and a diagnosis of mixed dyslipidaemia was made. After discussion with the patient, a decision was made to add in ezetimibe 10 mg daily. A repeat fasting profile eight weeks later showed the patient had achieved the lipid targets approved by NICE guidance 067 and no side effects had been reported.

○ **Learning point** Mixed dyslipdaemia and the metabolic syndrome

This gentleman suffers from mixed dyslipidaemia as characterized by high TG, low HDL-C, and elevated LDL-C which almost certainly relates to his underlying obesity and the presence of the metabolic syndrome. This syndrome is closely linked to insulin resistance and is defined by a constellation of lipid and non-lipid risk factors of metabolic origin. The NCEP ATP III recognizes mixed dyslipidaemia (atherogenic dyslipidaemia) as the most common dyslipidaemia associated with metabolic syndrome and diabetes [5].

In the JUPITER trial, a primary prevention study (n = 17,802) evaluating the effect of rosuvastatin compared with placebo in low-risk patients with LDL <3.4 and hsCRP ≥2 mg/L, the prevalence of metabolic syndrome at baseline in both treatment and placebo groups was as high as 41%. ATP III recognizes low HDL-C as a major risk factor and elevated TG and small LDL-C particles as the emerging risk factors for CV disease [16]. The higher CV disease risk in patients with diabetes and metabolic syndrome who are at target LDL-C levels with statin treatment may be explained, in part,

continued

⊕ **Clinical tip** Statins and associated myopathy

- If levels of CK exceed ten times the upper limit of normal (ULN), the statin should be stopped.
- In patients with a normal CK, but persistent muscle pain, halving the dose of statin or switching to an alternative preparation like pravastatin are both reasonable strategies.
- In patients taking statins, a form of subclinical myositis is now recognized (through elevations in transaminases and CK from baseline levels) where persistent muscle pain may reflect structural muscle damage on a microscopic level, even in the absence of CK levels outside the reference range [11].
- In the large, placebo-controlled, randomized controlled trials (RCTs), there was no significant difference in the frequency of muscle symptoms between those on statin therapy and those on placebo [12].
- Even in those patients on higher intensity statins, in three out of four large RCTs reviewed by NICE, the incidence of myopathy is no greater than in those on lower intensity statins. The same is true for rhabdomyolysis [10,13-15].
- Statins are generally well tolerated drugs although reports exist that some are better tolerated than others. Atorvastatin, simvastatin, and lovastatin are all oxidized by the cytochrome P450 (CYP450) 3A4. Pravastatin and rosuvastatin are not metabolized by the P450 system and fluvastatin is metabolized by the CYP450 2C9 isoenzyme. This difference in pharmacokinetics is thought to reflect the lower incidence of associated rhabdomyolysis in patients on fluvastatin and pravastatin compared with those on atorvastatin, simvastatin, and lovastatin (0 vs 4.2 cases per 100,000 person years). These figures are drawn from large cohort studies [12].

by mixed dyslipidaemia in this group of patients. This is shown in a substudy of the PROVE-IT trial that for each 10 mg/dL (0.11 mmol/L) reduction in on-treatment TG, the incidence of death, MI, and recurrent ACS was lowered by 1.6% or 1.4% after adjustment for LDL-C or non-HDL-C and other covariates (p < 0.001 and p = 0.01, respectively) [17]. There is a need for further treatment of mixed dyslipidaemia in patients on appropriate statin treatment and the addition of fibrates, niacin, and omega-3 fatty acids can improve the TG and HDL-C profiles.

✪ Learning point Unified clinical criteria for the identification of the metabolic syndrome (2010) [18]

	Risk factor	Defining level
PRIMARY		
Abdominal obesity[†] (waist circumference)[‡]	Men (Caucasian)	≥102 cm (>40 inches)
	Women (Caucasian)	≥88 cm (> 35 inches) and 2 of the following:
SECONDARY (requires 2 from 4 factors)		
Fasting TG		≥1.7 mmol (150 mg/dL)
HDL-C	Men	≥1.04 mmol/L (40 mg/dL)
	Women	≥1.3 mmol/L (50 mg/dL)
BP		≥130/85 mmHg
Fasting glucose		≥5.6 mmol/L (90 mg/dL)

† The presence of abdominal obesity is more highly correlated with metabolic risk factors than is an elevated BMI;
‡ Some males can develop multiple risk factors with only a slight increase in waist circumference (94–102 cm, 37–40 inches). Such patients are likely to have a strong genetic predisposition to insulin resistance and should be identified for intensive therapeutic lifestyle changes.

Discussion

Higher vs lower intensity statins

To date, there have been five RCTs comparing higher and lower intensity statins in patients with CHD: PROVE-IT TIMI 22 and A-Z (in patients post-ACS), IDEAL (in patients with previous MI), TNT (in patients with previous MI and/or angina/revascularization), and SEARCH (in patients with previous CHD) [2,10,13-15]. None of these trials treated to a pre-specified target TC or LDL-C, although the achieved levels were lower in each of the higher intensity statin groups compared with the corresponding lower intensity statins.

PROVE-IT TIMI 22 recruited patients within ten days of an ACS (29% had unstable angina (UA), 36% NSTEMI, and 35% STEMI). Two thirds of trial participants were revascularized for treatment of the index event. At recruitment, patients had to have a TC of ≥6.21 mmol/L. Patients were randomized to receive either higher intensity atorvastatin therapy (80 mg od) or lower intensity pravastatin therapy (40 mg od). At follow-up, patients in the atorvastatin group achieved lower levels of LDL-C compared with the pravastatin group (1.60 vs 2.46) and patients in the pravastatin group achieved higher HDL-C levels. During a mean follow-up of 24 months, there was no significant reduction in death from any cause or reinfarction with the higher intensity therapy. There was, however, a 28% risk reduction in the primary outcome (a composite of all-cause mortality, MI, documented UA requiring rehospitalization, revascularization, or stroke) with higher intensity therapy. Similarly, higher intensity therapy was associated with a 14% reduction in the secondary outcome which was a composite of CV death, non-fatal MI, or revascularization [10].

A to Z (Aggrastat to Zocor) was the first large RCT to compare early intensive statin therapy with delayed lower intensity statin therapy. This trial consisted of two overlapping phases. The first phase was an open-labelled trial comparing enoxaparin with unfractionated heparin in patients with non-ST-elevation ACS who were treated with tirofiban and aspirin. The second phase recruited patients from the first phase who had initially stabilized (for at least 12 consecutive hours within five days of symptom onset). In addition, recruits had at least one of the following characteristics: age over 70 years, diabetes mellitus, prior history of coronary artery disease, peripheral arterial disease, or stroke. Subsequently, the protocol was amended to allow patients with non-ST-elevation ACS who were not enrolled in the first phase and also patients with STEMI to enter into the second phase directly (overall 60% NSTEMI and 40% STEMI). This trial of patients compared receiving 40 mg/day of simvastatin for one month followed by 80 mg/day thereafter (n=2,265) with placebo for four months followed by 20 mg/day of simvastatin (n=2,232). Early high intensity statin therapy decreased LDL levels by 39% compared with baseline levels during the first month of therapy and then by a further 6% following an increase in simvastatin dosage to 80 mg. For the delayed conservative treatment group, LDL levels increased by 11% during the 4-month placebo period, then decreased from baseline by 31% after four months of therapy with simvastatin 20 mg od. The placebo/low-dose simvastatin group achieved an LDL-C of 3.20 mmol/L at one month and 2.0 mmol/L at eight months with 20 mg simvastatin. The simvastatin only group achieved an LDL-C of 1.8 mmol/L at one month and 1.6 mmol/L at eight months on 80 mg simvastatin. For the primary endpoint (combination of CV death, non-fatal MI, readmission for ACS or stroke), early higher intensity statin therapy did not confer benefit compared with delayed lower intensity therapy. No difference was evident during the first four months between the groups for the primary endpoint, but from four months in the primary endpoint, it was significantly reduced in the simvastatin only group (hazard ratio 0.75, 95% CI, 0.60–0.95, p=0.02). Myopathy (CK greater than ten times the ULN associated with myalgia) occurred in nine patients (0.4%) receiving simvastatin 80 mg. There was a reduction in the incidence of new onset congestive heart failure in the early intensive treatment group, but the trend in reduced incidence of CV-related death did not quite reach significance [15].

IDEAL was an open-labelled, randomized trial in patients with prior MI (median time since last MI was 22 months). Most trial participants were taking aspirin and beta-blockers, but almost two thirds were not taking angiotensin-converting enzyme (ACE) inhibitors or angiotensin receptor blockers (ARBs). Patients were assigned to atorvastatin 80 mg od or simvastatin 20 mg od. Further drug titration could be undertaken at 24 weeks within the study protocol, based on achieved TC levels. At the end of the study, 23% were treated with simvastatin 40 mg daily and 13% with atorvastatin 40 mg daily. Mean LDL-C levels were 2.7 mmol/L for those taking simvastatin and 2.1 mmol/L in the atorvastatin group. During a median follow-up of 4.8 years, there were no differences in CV or all-cause mortality or in the primary endpoint of major coronary events (defined as CV death, hospitalization for non-fatal acute MI or cardiac arrest with resuscitation) between the two treatment groups. There was a reduction in the non-fatal MI component of this primary endpoint with atorvastatin therapy. Atorvastatin was associated with a reduction in the secondary endpoint of any CHD event and also a reduction in any major CV event compared with simvastatin [13].

TNT recruited patients with clinically evident stable CHD (59% had a prior MI, 82% angina). To ensure that at baseline, all patients had LDL-C levels consistent with

ⓔ Expert comment

Obesity is often forgotten as a contributory cause for hyperlipidaemia and weight reduction remains the first-line therapy, not only improving lipid profiles but also improving blood pressure control.

ⓔ Expert comment

Patients with the metabolic syndrome, including increased visceral adiposity (waist circumference) and atherogenic dyslipidaemia (elevated fasting triglycerides (>1.7 mmol/L), HDL-C <1.0 mmol/L in men or <1.2 mmol/L in women), raised blood pressure (>130/80 mmHg), and dysglycaemia (>5.5 mmol/L) have increased CV disease risk due to small dense LDL particles (measured by increased apolipoprotein B levels) [18].

the then current guidelines for the treatment of stable CHD, patients with LDL-C levels between 3.4 and 6.5 entered an 8-week run-in period of open-labelled treatment with 10 mg of atorvastatin od. At the end of the run-in phase, those patients with a mean LDL-C of less than 3.4 were randomized. Patients were assigned to either high intensity atorvastatin (80 mg od) or lower intensity atorvastatin (10 mg od). The trial follow-up was for a median of 4.9 years. Mean LDL-C levels during the study were 2.0 in the higher intensity group and 2.6 in the lower intensity arm. There was a 22% reduction in the primary endpoint (defined as the combination of CV death, non-fatal non-procedural MI, resuscitation after cardiac arrest, and fatal or non-fatal stroke) in patients treated with high-dose atorvastatin. Higher intensity treatment was also associated with a lower incidence of the following secondary outcomes: major coronary or cerebrovascular event, hospitalization for congestive heart failure, and any CV or coronary event. There was no difference in all-cause mortality between the two cohorts [14].

The SEARCH study is the largest randomized trial to assess directly the efficacy and safety of lowering LDL-C using simvastatin. It recruited 12,064 men and women with a history of MI: 6,031 were randomized to 80 mg simvastatin daily, and 6,033 were given 20 mg simvastatin daily. During an average of 6.7 years of treatment, the 80 mg simvastatin regimen lowered LDL-C by an average of 0.35 mmol/L more than the 20 mg simvastatin regimen. This additional reduction in LDL-C was associated with a non-significant 6% reduction in CV events [2].

A meta-analysis of the early studies concluded that higher intensity statin therapy did not confer any significant benefit over lower intensity statin therapy for the outcomes of all-cause mortality and CV or non-CV mortality. Higher intensity statin therapy was associated with a reduction in the combination of coronary death or MI, stroke and coronary death or any CV event [19,20]. An updated meta-analysis of low vs high dose statin trials by the Cholesterol Treatment Trialists' (CTT) collaboration has shown that these are consistent with the results previously published for the statin vs placebo studies implying a 11% extra reduction in events for the extra 0.5 mmol/L achieved in these studies (available at: www.ctsu.ox.ac.uk/projects/ctt).

Are targets such a good thing?

There has been considerable debate as to whether treating patients to a specified target should be our objective. Supporters of targets quote the log linear hypothesis from the CTT collaboration that confirmed 'lower is better' for LDL-C [21]. This study showed a proportional reduction in the CV event rate of 23% per 1 mmol/L reduction in LDL-C. This was largely independent of the presenting cholesterol level. It is worth appreciating that although the relative risk reduction remains constant, at lower cholesterol levels, there is a smaller absolute reduction in events and it is the absolute reduction in events that determines cost-effectiveness.

There are also concerns that patients may be left under-treated if targets are not set in stone. Opponents of setting targets argue that none of the major trials treated to a pre-specified target TC or LDL-C, but rather used specific drugs to treat patients. The greatest LDL-C reduction is made with the first dose of statin with an average of 6% further LDL-C reduction when the dose is doubled [1]. Thus lower cholesterol levels for individual patients may be achieved by using higher intensity statins, but for each doubling of dose, there is a smaller absolute reduction in events. Following the Heart Protection Study, a strong argument was made that all CHD patients should receive statin therapy irrespective of lipid profile [6]. Indeed, some proposed that lipid measurements were no longer required; after all, platelet function is not routinely measured with aspirin or clopidogrel therapy.

When to start and at what dose?

A to Z (Aggrastat to Zocor) was the first large RCT to compare early intensive statin therapy with delayed lower intensity statin therapy. This trial, though negative in its primary endpoint, suggested that early statin-based therapy might be better in reducing future events than delayed treatment with a standard dose [15].

In those high-risk patients undergoing intervention, the argument for initiating early higher intensity statin therapy was recently strengthened by the ARMYDA-ACS (Atorvastatin for Reduction of Myocardial Damage During Angioplasty) trial [22]. Patients with UA/NSTEMI were randomized to receive 80 mg atorvastatin at 12 hours and 40 mg atorvastatin at two hours before intervention or placebo. This demonstrated that short-term pre-treatment with atorvastatin improved outcomes in patients with ACS undergoing an early invasive strategy. Pre-treatment with high-dose atorvastatin conferred an 88% risk reduction in 30-day major adverse cardiac events (MACE) compared with placebo supporting the routine use of high-dose statins before intervention. This benefit was essentially driven by a reduction in periprocedural MI as defined by biomarkers. After PCI, the proportion of patients with elevated levels of CK-MB and troponin I was significantly lower in the treatment arm (CK-MB 7% vs 27%, $p < 0.001$; troponin I 41% vs 58%, $p < 0.039$).

The ARMYDA trial in patients with stable angina, which preceded ARMYDA-ACS, showed that 7-day pre-treatment with atorvastatin was associated with an 81% risk reduction of periprocedural MI in those undergoing elective PCI [23]. Similarly the Novel Approaches for Preventing or Limiting Events (NAPLES) II trial has shown that in patients undergoing elective PCI, a single dose of 80 mg atorvastatin reduced the incidence of peri-procedural MI [24]. The possible mechanisms underlying the early protective effect of atorvastatin are unclear, but are unlikely to be due to cholesterol-lowering effects, which would intuitively require a longer duration of treatment. This phenomenon has been largely attributed to the so called 'pleiotropic' effects of statins.

> ⊕ **Learning point** Pleiotropic effects of statins
>
> • Statins have an ability to affect the stability of atherosclerotic plaques as well as improving endothelial function, decreasing oxidative stress and inflammation, and inhibiting the thrombogenic response.
> • Many of these effects are supposedly mediated by inhibition of isoprenoids which serve as lipid attachments for intracellular signalling molecules. In particular, the inhibition of small GTP-binding proteins, Rho, Ras and Rac, whose proper membrane localization and function are dependent on isoprenylation, may play an important role in mediating the pleiotropic effects of statins [25].

Conclusion

In patients presenting with ACS, there is now considerable evidence to support the early use of higher intensity statins as supported by the latest NICE guidance. In those undergoing PCI, there is increasing data to support even an 'upstream' use of such agents. The primary goal of lipid therapy is to reduce TC and LDL-C to pre-defined targets. Ezetimibe remains an attractive addition to achieve LDL-C goals when statin monotherapy is inadequate or associated with side effects such as myopathy.

In patients with metabolic syndrome as reflected by mixed dyslipidaemia, even if NICE targets of '4 and 2' are achieved, a residual risk of CV disease remains secondary to low HDL-C and elevated TG levels. Statins have little effect on the HDL-C side of the risk equation and are only slightly better at addressing adverse TG profiles. Where this situation arises, combination therapy with fibrates, niacin, or omega-3-fatty acids warrants careful consideration.

💬 **A final word from the expert**

This case is typical of high-risk populations presenting with acute chest pain. Lipids should be measured immediately on admission as cytokine-induced reductions in LDL-C and HDL-C occur within 24 hours and persist for at least one month post-angioplasty and up to three months for coronary bypass grafting. A number of biochemical markers, including troponin levels, CRP, and BNP levels predict prognosis at one year. The introduction of ultrasensitive troponin assays will probably result in a further reclassification of ACS, especially for UA with a recognition that prognosis will relate to the peak troponin level achieved.

After initial stabilization and intervention (if appropriate), patients should be discharged on high-dose statin as only 30% of patients will achieve an LDL-C of 2 mmol/L on simvastatin 40 mg so most will require 80 mg atorvastatin (or 20–40 mg rosuvastatin). The reduction of 0.4–0.5 mmol/L in LDL-C produced with high-dose modern statins is likely to reduce subsequent events by 11%. Simvastatin 80 mg, though recommended in the NICE guidelines of 2008, has been superseded following the presentation of the results of the SEARCH trial where increased therapy with 80 mg compared with 20 mg (let alone 40 mg) was ineffective and resulted in a large increase in myositis events. Patients sensitized to statins by the presence of myositis may require a statin-free treatment period of up to two years before they can be successfully rechallenged.

If patients do not reach LDL-C targets, then there is no evidence as yet to support any of the additional lipid-lowering drugs. Ezetimibe reduces LDL-C by 23%, but has not shown benefits on surrogate markers of atherosclerosis (carotid intima media thickness, ENHANCE trial) or events (in combination with simvastatin) in patients with aortic stenosis (SEAS study) [26,27]. However, these studies may have either been confounded (ENHANCE) or underpowered (SEAS) so it will require the IMPROVE-IT study to show the benefits of ezetimibe in ACS in 2015 [28]. Some fibrates (fenofibrate, bezafibrate) can reduce LDL-C and there is evidence that fibrates can reduce non-fatal myocardial events, but as yet no evidence exists for endpoint benefit in fibrate-statin combination therapy and there is an increased risk of rhabdomyolysis with all combinations involving gemfibrozil [29]. Niacin reduced CV events as monotherapy in the Coronary Drug Project and improved both coronary mean lumen diameter (HATS) and carotid intima media thickness (cIMT) (ARBITER-2 and -3) when added to statin therapy. Niacin-statin therapy was superior to ezetimibe-statin combination therapy in reducing cIMT in the ARBITER-6 trial [30]. Endpoint trials with niacin in dyslipidaemic post-MI patients (AIM-HIGH) and patients with CV disease (HPS-2/THRIVE) with optimized LDL-C are underway.

This patient has severely elevated cholesterol levels and elevated TGs. The potential diagnoses once secondary causes have been excluded include familial hypercholesterolaemia (FH) allied with metabolic syndrome, a secondary hypertriglyceridaemia or a remnant hyperlipidaemia (assessed by apolipoprotein E genotype) or familial combined hyperlipidaemia (FCH) [31]. Familial hypercholesterolaemia needs to be diagnosed if present, in line with NICE guidance CG71 [32]. The patient's family (including children) should have both cholesterol and TG levels checked. The patient should be examined for the presence of tendon xanthomata to assess whether he meets the Simon Broome criteria for FH. In any case, treatment should be considered in line with the NICE FH guidelines with the aim of reducing LDL-C by 50% from baseline in line with evidence from the ASAP trial. If FH is suspected, then a genetic test for LDL receptor (LDLR), apolipoprotein B LDLR binding domain, and PCSK-9 mutations should be carried out. If a mutation is found, then lipid levels and genotypes need to be checked in all blood relatives after systematic family (cascade) testing and treatment instituted. If no FH mutation is found, then the diagnosis by exclusion is FCH which carries a similar risk of premature CHD, but the lipid phenotypes in relatives tend to be diverse and dependent on other factors, including age, gender, and insulin resistance-related risk factors.

> ⊙ **Learning point** Diagnostic criteria for definite familial hypercholesterolaemia using the Simon Broome register
>
> - If aged <16 years: TC >6.7 mmol/L or LDL-C >4.0 mmol/L; or
> - In an adult: TC >7.5 mmol/L or LDL-C >4.9 mmol/L;
>
> Plus
> - Tendon xanthomas in the patient or in a first-degree relative (parent, sibling, child) or in a second-degree relative (grandparent, uncle, aunt); or
> - DNA-based evidence of an LDLR mutation or a familial defective apo B-100.

References

1 National Institute for Health and Clinical Excellence. Lipid modification: cardiovascular risk assessment and the modification of blood lipids for the primary and secondary prevention of cardiovascular disease. NICE guideline CG67 [issued May 2008]. Available from: http://guidance.nice.org.uk/CG67.

2 The SEARCH Collaborative Group. SLCO1B1 variants and statin-induced myopathy–a genomewide study. *N Engl J Med* 2008; 359: 789–799.

3 Friedewald WT, Levy R, Frederickson DS. Estimation of the concentration of low density lipoprotein cholesterol in plasma without the use of the preparative ultracentrifuge. *Clin Chem* 1972; 18: 499–502.

4 Penning-van Beest FJA, Termorshuizen F, Goettsch WG, et al. Adherence to evidence-based statin guidelines reduces the risk of hospitalization for acute myocardial infarction by 40%: a cohort study. *Eur Heart J* 2007; 28: 154–159.

5 Grundy SM, Cleeman JI, Merz CN, et al. Implications of recent clinical trials for the National Cholesterol Education Program Adult Treatment Panel III guidelines. *Circulation* 2004; 110: 227–239.

6 Heart Protection Study Collaborative Group. MRC/BHF Heart Protection Study of cholesterol lowering with simvastatin in 20,536 high-risk individuals: a randomized placebo-controlled trial. *Lancet* 2002; 360: 7–22.

7 Shepherd J, Blauw GJ, Murphy MB, et al. PROSPER study group. Pravastatin in elderly individuals at risk of vascular disease (PROSPER): a randomized controlled trial. *Lancet* 2002; 360: 1623–1630.

8 The ALLHAT Officers and Coordinators for the ALLHAT Collaborative Research Group. Major outcomes in moderately hypercholesterolaemic, hypertensive patients randomized to pravastatin vs usual care: The Antihypertensive and Lipid-Lowering Treatment to Prevent Heart Attack Trial (ALLHAT-LLT). *JAMA* 2002; 288: 2998–3007.

9 Sever PS, Dhalof B, Poulter NR, et al. ASCOT investigators. Prevention of coronary and stroke events with atorvastatin in hypertensive patients who have average or lower-than-average cholesterol concentrations, in the Anglo-Scandinavian Cardiac Outcomes trial–Lipid Lowering Arm (ASCOT-LLA): a multicentre randomized controlled trial. *Lancet* 2003; 361: 1149–1158.

10 Cannon CP, Braunwald E, McCabe CH, et al. PROVE-IT TIMI 22 trial. Intensive vs moderate lipid lowering with statins after acute coronary syndromes. *N Engl J Med* 2004; 350: 1495–1504.

11 Mohaupt MG, Karas RH, Babiychuk EB, et al. Association between statin-associated myopathy and skeletal muscle damage. *CMAJ* 2009; 181: E11–E18.

12 Law M, Rudnicka AR. Statin safety: a systematic review. *Am J Cardiol* 2006; 97: 52C–60C.

13 Pedersen TR, Faergeman O, Kastelein JJ, et al. High dose atorvastatin vs usual dose simvastatin for secondary prevention after myocardial infarction, the IDEAL study: a randomized controlled trial. *JAMA* 2005; 294: 2437–2445.

14 LaRosa JC, Grundy SM, Waters DD, et al. Intensive lipid lowering with atorvastatin in patients with stable coronary disease. *N Engl J Med* 2005; 352: 1425–1435.

15 de Lemos JA, Blazing MA, Wiviott SD, et al. Early intensive vs a delayed conservative simvastatin strategy in patients with acute coronary syndromes: phase Z of the A to Z trial. *JAMA* 2004; 292: 1307–1316.

16 Ridker M, Danielson E, Fonseca FA, et al. Rosuvastatin to prevent vascular events in men and women with elevated C reactive protein. *N Engl J Med* 2008; 359: 2195–2207.

17 Miller M, Cannon CP, Murphy SA, Qin J, Ray KK, Braunwald E. Impact of triglyceride levels beyond low-density lipoprotein cholesterol after acute coronary syndrome in the PROVE-IT TIMI 22 trial. *J Am Coll Cardiol* 2008; 51: 724–730.

18 Eckel RH, Alberti KG, Grundy SM, et al. The metabolic syndrome. *Lancet* 2010; 375: 181–183.

19 Cannon CP, Steinberg BA, Murphy SA, et al. Meta-analysis of cardiovascular outcomes trials comparing intensive vs moderate statin therapy. *J Am Coll Cardiol* 2006; 48: 438–445.

20 Armitage J. The safety of statins in clinical practice. *Lancet* 2007; 370: 1781–1790.

21 Baigent C, Keech A, Kearney PM, et al. Efficacy and safety of cholesterol-lowering treatment: prospective meta-analysis of data from 90,056 participants in 14 randomized trials of statins. *Lancet* 2005; 366: 1267–1278.

22 Patti G, Pasceri V, Colonna G, et al. Atorvastatin pre-treatment improves outcomes in patients with acute coronary syndromes undergoing early percutaneous coronary intervention: results of the ARMYDA-ACS randomized trial. *J Am Coll Cardiol* 2007; 49: 1272–1278.

23 Pasceri V, Patti G, Nusca A, et al. Randomized trial of atorvastatin for reduction of myocardial damage during coronary intervention: results from the ARMYDA study. *Circulation* 2004; 110: 674–678.

24 Briguori C, Visconti G, Focaccio A, et al. Novel Approaches for Preventing or Limiting Events (NAPLES) II trial: impact of a single high loading dose of atorvastatin on periprocedural
myocardial infarction. *J Am Coll Cardiol* 2009; 54: 2157–2163.

25 Liao JK, Laufs U. Pleiotropic effects of statins. *Ann Rev Pharm Toxicol* 2005; 45: 89–118.

26 Kastelein JJP, Akdim F, Stroes ESG, et al. Simvastatin with or without ezetimibe in familial hypercholesterolaemia. *N Engl J Med* 2008; 358: 1431–1443.

27 Rossebo AB, Pedersen TR, Boman K, et al. Intensive lipid lowering with simvastatin and ezetimibe in aortic stenosis. *N Engl J Med* 2008; 359: 1343–1356.

28 IMPROVE-IT: examining outcomes in subjects with acute coronary syndrome: Vytorin (ezetimibe/simvastatin) vs simvastatin (study P04103AM3). Available from: http://clinicaltrials.
gov/ct2/show/NCT00202878.

29 Saha SA, Kizhakepunnur LG, Bahekar A, et al. The role of fibrates in the prevention of cardiovascular disease: a pooled meta-analysis of long-term randomized placebo-controlled clinical trials. *Am Heart J* 2007; 154: 943–953.

30 Taylor AJ, Villines TC, Stanek EJ, et al. Extended-release niacin or ezetimibe and carotid intima-media thickness. *N Engl J Med*. 2009; 361: 2113–2122.

31 Wierzbicki AS, Graham CA, Young IS, et al. Familial combined hyperlipidaemia: under-defined and under-diagnosed? *Curr Vasc Pharmacol* 2008; 6: 13–22.

32 National Institute for Health and Clinical Excellence. Identification and management of familial hypercholesterolaemia. NICE guideline CG71 [issued August 2008]. Available from: http://guidance.nice.org.uk/CG71.

5 Management of prosthetic heart valves in pregnancy

Kate von Klemperer and Shouvik Haldar

⬤ **Expert commentary** Dr Fiona Walker

Case history

An 18-year-old woman with a mechanical mitral valve (St Jude 31 mm) was referred to a high-risk obstetric service having had an unplanned pregnancy of six weeks' gestation. There was a background history of a primum atrial septal defect which had been surgically repaired at the age of 4 years. By the age of 12, she had developed significant mitral regurgitation which required valve replacement. At 13 years of age, she had infective endocarditis (IE) which was successfully treated with intravenous antibiotics. More recently, she had had episodes of persistent atrial flutter with one failed attempt at DC cardioversion.

⭐ **Learning point** Selection of valve prosthesis in young women

It is important to consider several factors when choosing the type of valve prosthesis in young women of childbearing age. In general, women with well-functioning bioprosthetic heart valves (Table 5.1) are more likely to have uncomplicated pregnancies because these valves are less thrombogenic than their mechanical counterparts, eliminating the need for anticoagulation during pregnancy. The principal disadvantage for this choice of valve implant in a young patient is limited durability, which means that women with bioprosthetic valves will require 're-do' valve replacement surgery at a later stage. Tissue valve degeneration in young patients can occur as early as two to three years after surgery, and is as high as 50% at ten years, and 90% at 15 years [1,2]. Whether pregnancy accelerates tissue valve degeneration remains an unresolved issue with a number of studies reporting conflicting data [3-7]. There is still limited evidence with regards to the effects of pregnancy on valve durability for the newer xenograft and autograft valves, which have improved haemodynamic profiles compared with their older counterparts. Despite a lack of clear evidence that pregnancy has a detrimental impact on valve function long-term, all tissue valves will require replacement at some point and the risk of re-do surgery must be given careful consideration.

Conversely, mechanical heart valves have excellent durability, but are highly thrombogenic and require lifelong anticoagulation with warfarin. In pregnancy, they are associated with a high number of maternal, obstetric, and fetal complications.

Table 5.1 Bioprosthetic valve options

Valve type	Source
Autograft	Valves harvested from the patient themselves, e.g. in the Ross procedure where the pulmonary autograft is transplanted into the aortic position
Homograft	Valve from another human donor
Xenograft	Valves from another species, e.g. bovine or porcine (currently the most commonly used)

⬤ **Expert comment**

The dilemma over which type of valve prosthesis to implant in a young woman arises because there is no ideal anticoagulant for a mechanical valve in pregnancy. In light of this, one is balancing the **potential** risk of a mechanical valve thrombosis during pregnancy with the **definite** risk of re-do cardiac surgery in the future in those who choose a tissue valve. This balance of risk must be considered carefully. If there is a coordinated high-risk maternal cardiology team in place, which includes input from a haematology specialist, the risk of mechanical valve thrombosis should be low because patients are assessed fully for thrombotic risk and anticoagulation is meticulously monitored. The risk of mechanical aortic valve thrombosis is less than that of mechanical mitral valve thrombosis and this needs to be borne in mind. Ultimately, the choice of valve implant must be made by the patient after a full discussion of the advantages and disadvantages of tissue vs mechanical valve replacement as any risks are hers to accept.

Expert comment

Although many cardiologists in the UK are adhering to the NICE Guidance on endocarditis prophylaxis, there is some flexibility in the recommendations, allowing clinicians to manage their patients on an individual basis. Many cardiologists consider those with mechanical valves and/or a past history of IE to be at significant risk of subsequent IE and therefore, would advise endocarditis prophylaxis for vaginal or operative delivery.

At the point of referral, the patient was eight weeks' pregnant. She was in permanent atrial flutter. Her medications included aspirin, warfarin, and amiodarone. At this point, the amiodarone was stopped due to its feto-toxicity and replaced with metoprolol 50 mg twice daily (bd) to maintain effective rate control. The plan was to continue with medical therapy during pregnancy unless the arrhythmia became poorly tolerated. The long-term plan was to refer to an electrophysiologist for curative treatment postpartum. She received counselling on anticoagulation and opted for low molecular weight heparin (LMWH).

Learning point Mechanical heart valves in pregnancy

Women with mechanical heart valves are at high risk during pregnancy, predominantly due to valve thrombosis (Figure 5.1), with reported maternal mortality rates of up to 4% [10]. Pregnancy is a hypercoagulable state due to increased levels of fibrinogen, factors VII, VIII and X, decreased levels of protein S activity, and venous hypertension and stasis [11]. In the non-pregnant state, risk factors for valve thrombosis include subtherapeutic anticoagulation, type of valve prosthesis (size and position), presence of arrhythmias, left atrial size, and a prior history of thrombosis (Table 5.2). Pregnancy increases these predefined risks and hence it is paramount that anticoagulation is therapeutic at all times in order to avoid thromboembolic complications. At present, there is a lack of consensus between the American and European guidelines regarding the optimum choice of anticoagulant in these patients (Tables 5.3 and 5.4). The European guidelines consider warfarin the anticoagulant of choice and feel that there is insufficient evidence to support the use of LMWH, whilst the American Heart Association consider both warfarin and LMWH as acceptable treatment options [12-14].

Table 5.2 Factors that convey a greater risk of valve thrombosis

- Certain prosthetic valves such as the single tilting and ball-and-cage valves convey a higher risk than others:
- Suboptimal anticoagulation
- Position (mitral and tricuspid valves have higher thrombotic risk)
- Past arrhythmias
- Past history of thromboembolism

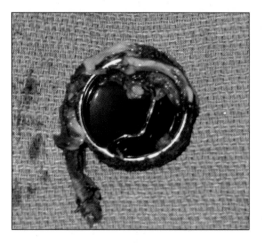

Figure 5.1 Pathological specimen of a thrombosed mitral valve prosthesis.

Due to poor compliance with LMWH, her medication was changed back to warfarin in the second trimester. At twenty weeks, the fetus suffered a fatal intracerebral bleed. During this period, she was receiving 8 mg of warfarin daily and her INR at the time of the event was optimal at 3.3.

Table 5.3 ACC/AHA (class I) recommendations for anticoagulation during pregnancy in patients with mechanical prosthetic valves

All pregnant patients with mechanical prosthetic valves must receive continuous therapeutic anticoagulation with frequent monitoring.

For women requiring long-term warfarin therapy who are attempting pregnancy, pregnancy tests should be monitored with discussions about subsequent anticoagulation therapy so that anticoagulation can be continued uninterrupted when pregnancy is achieved.

Pregnant patients with mechanical prosthetic valves who elect to stop warfarin between weeks 6 and 12 of gestation should receive continuous intravenous UFH, dose-adjusted UFH, or dose-adjusted subcutaneous LMWH.

For pregnant patients with mechanical prosthetic valves up to 36 weeks of gestation, the therapeutic choice of continuous intravenous or dose-adjusted subcutaneous UFH, dose-adjusted LMWH, or warfarin should be discussed fully. If continuous intravenous UFH is used, the fetal risk is lower, but the maternal risks of prosthetic valve thrombosis, systemic embolization, infection, osteoporosis, and heparin-induced thrombocytopaenia are relatively higher.

In pregnant patients with mechanical prosthetic valves who receive dose-adjusted LMWH, the LMWH should be administered twice daily subcutaneously to maintain the anti-Xa level between 0.7 and 1.2 U/mL four hours after administration.

In pregnant patients with mechanical prosthetic valves who receive warfarin, the INR goal should be 3.0 (range 2.5–3.5).

In pregnant patients with mechanical prosthetic valves, warfarin should be discontinued and continuous intravenous UFH given starting two to three weeks before planned delivery.

Bonow RO, Carabello BA, Chatterjee K, et al. ACC/AHA 2006 guidelines for the management of patients with valvular heart disease. *J Am Coll Cardiol* 2006;48:e1–148.

Table 5.4 ESC recommendations for anticoagulation during pregnancy in patients with mechanical prosthetic valves

As LMWH is not approved for use in prosthetic heart valve patients in pregnancy due to the high risk of thrombosis and as subcutaneous UFH carries a similar high risk, the strategies which should be discussed with the patient are:

* Heparin during the first trimester (to avoid warfarin embryopathy) followed by oral anticoagulation up to week 36 with subsequent replacement by heparin until delivery; or
* Oral anticoagulation throughout pregnancy until week 36, followed by heparin until delivery.

Because of the high rate of maternal complications with heparin therapy, particularly when given throughout pregnancy, the committee strongly recommends strategy (b).

Vahanian A, Baumgartner H, Bax J, et al. Guidelines on the management of valvular heart disease: the Task Force on the Management of Valvular Heart Disease of the European Society of Cardiology. *Eur Heart J* 2007;28:230–6.

⭐ Learning point Warfarin in pregnancy: can it be used?

Warfarin crosses the placenta and confers a significant risk to the fetus. Its use in the first trimester is associated with a risk of embryopathy (chondrodysplasia punctata and nasal hypoplasia) to the order of 5–12% [4]. Studies have also shown that when used for the duration of pregnancy, there is an association with fetal central nervous system abnormalities and an increased incidence of low IQ in older children [15,16]. A study by Vitale et al. found extremely low fetal anomaly rates in those pregnant women taking less than 5 mg warfarin daily. However, nearly half of their study population required larger doses and in those taking over 5 mg warfarin daily, only 25% of infants survived, 50% of whom had fetal anomalies [17].

It is important to remember that fetal liver enzyme function is also immature and this can potentiate the anticoagulant effect of warfarin. As a result, the fetus is often excessively anticoagulated, which may lead to spontaneous fetal intracranial haemorrhage, particularly in the peripartum period [18]. If warfarin is used in pregnancy, it should be stopped and converted to heparin (LMWH or unfractionated heparin (UFH)) at 36 weeks' gestation in preparation for delivery. The shorter half-life of these agents allows delivery to be planned with the aim of reducing maternal and fetal haemorrhagic complications. Warfarin is not secreted in significant amounts in breast milk and hence is safe for use in breastfeeding mothers.

ⓘ Expert comment

LMWH anticoagulation can only be used in pregnancy if the patient is compliant with administering the injections, and the monitoring of the anti-Xa levels is meticulous. Any lack of patient compliance can have catastrophic consequences (e.g. valve thrombosis, stroke, death), which is why in this case, the patient was converted back to warfarin.

Data to support the use of LMWH anticoagulation for mechanical valves in pregnancy is accumulating, but remains limited. The optimal anti-Xa for mechanical aortic and mitral valves is not known and in some centres, mitral valve thrombosis has occurred with anti-Xa levels between 0.8 and 1.0 U/mL. In our unit, the anti-Xa is kept between 1.0 and 1.2 U/mL for mitral valve replacement (MVR) and between 0.8 and 1.0 U/mL for aortic valve replacement (AVR), with good outcomes thus far. We also give concomitant aspirin to patients with MVR.

⊙ Learning point Heparin in pregnancy explained

UFH and LMWH do not cross the placenta and so are not associated with embryopathy. Of course, intravenous UFH is not practical for the duration of pregnancy and in most studies, it has been given subcutaneously twice daily. Subcutaneous UFH requires mid-interval APTT monitoring, with current recommendations stating that the APTT should be >2.0 times the normal range. Thus far, UFH has not been shown to provide consistent therapeutic anticoagulation during pregnancy, which may explain the high incidence of valve thrombosis if UFH is used [19].

A comprehensive meta-analysis of 1,234 pregnancies in 976 women by Chan et al. demonstrated a 25% incidence of maternal thromboembolism if adjusted dose UFH was used for the duration of pregnancy [1]. UFH has been shown to carry a 2.2% risk of heparin-induced osteoporotic fractures and a 2–3% risk of heparin-induced thrombocytopaenia (HIT), an immune reaction associated with venous thrombosis. This has led to the use of LMWH as an alternative agent. It is already accepted as the anticoagulant of choice to prevent and treat venous thromboembolism in pregnancy, but there is little information with respect to its efficacy and safety for anticoagulating patients with mechanical valves in pregnancy.

LMWH, a derivative of UFH, can be administered as a twice-daily subcutaneous injection. LMWH has improved bioavailability (85%) and a longer half-life, which provides a more consistent anticoagulant effect over 24 hours when compared with UFH. It also has a low incidence of HIT (<1%) and osteoporosis [20].

In pregnant women, the clearance and volume of distribution of LMWH are increased due to weight gain and increases in plasma volume and glomerular filtration rate [21]. The most recent meta-analysis of its use for mechanical valves in pregnancy reported an 8.64% incidence of valve thrombosis [22]. This is worryingly high; however, 90% of the valve (mitral) thromboses occurred in patients on a fixed dose treatment regime. In the 51 cases where anti-Xa levels were monitored regularly with appropriate dose adjustment, there was only one thromboembolic event. It is now recommended that LMWH is given twice daily and the dose adjusted to maintain a target anti-Xa of between 0.8 and 1.2 U/mL four hours after administration. In order to adjust the dose of LMWH to maintain these levels during the physiological changes in pregnancy, anti-Xa levels should be monitored regularly (at least every two weeks) [23].

A year later, at the age of 19, she became pregnant again. She had not attended her electrophysiology appointment and thus remained in rate-controlled atrial flutter. In view of her previous fetal loss whilst on warfarin, she opted for LMWH anticoagulation in combination with aspirin for the duration of her pregnancy. Her anti-Xa level was monitored every two weeks, with LMWH dose adjustment to maintain anti-Xa levels at 1.0–1.2 (four hours post-dose). Her starting dose was 8,000 IU bd and in her third trimester, she required 13,000 IU bd.

⊙ Learning point Aspirin in pregnancy

Aspirin has been commonly used in pregnancy and hence there is a better understanding of its safety compared with other drugs [24]. Low doses such as 75 mg daily appear to have beneficial effects in pregnancies complicated by systemic lupus erythematosus and antiphospholipid antibodies [25]. These benefits extend to the prevention of pregnancy-induced hypertension and pre-eclampsia as well as in those women deemed to be at high risk of thromboembolism [26,27]. Although higher doses of aspirin and other non-steroidal anti-inflammatory drugs (NSAIDs) can be toxic to the fetus, low doses have been shown to be safe throughout pregnancy [28]. In addition to warfarin or heparin in pregnancy, current guidelines recommend concomitant use of aspirin in women who are at high risk of thromboembolism. In this case, the arrhythmia and mitral position of her mechanical valve placed her in this high-risk category [12,13].

During this pregnancy, she developed intra-chorionic bleeding and intrauterine growth retardation (IUGR). Her case was therefore discussed at a high-risk multidisciplinary team (MDT) meeting and plans were made to deliver the baby at 35 weeks' gestation by elective Caesarean section. The LMWH was stopped 12 hours prior to delivery. She had an uncomplicated procedure under general anaesthetic and was given a prophylactic dose of LMWH six hours post-operatively (5,000 IU). The baby weighed 1.5 kg and was admitted to the special care baby unit for 48 hours. The baby was healthy and had no congenital anomalies. The day after delivery, the mother restarted full-dose therapeutic LMWH bd and on day 5, she restarted warfarin. Once she had achieved a therapeutic INR, LMWH was stopped on day 7 and mother and baby were discharged home.

⊙ **Learning point** Valve thrombosis in pregnancy

The diagnosis of valve thrombosis should always be considered in patients who present with progressive dyspnoea, orthopnoea, dry cough, or worsening peripheral oedema. Some will present acutely in pulmonary oedema. Cerebral, coronary, and peripheral embolization have been noted in up to 25% of cases of valve thrombosis [28]. Echocardiography may demonstrate thrombus on the valve and Doppler studies will show an increased flow gradient across the valve (Figures 5.2 and 5.3). The management of this complication is challenging and is dependent on the clinical status of the patient and the gestational age of the fetus. If the mother presents acutely in pulmonary oedema and the fetus is viable, emergency delivery should be undertaken followed by emergency valve replacement. If, however, the patient is clinically stable, other treatments such as intravenous UFH or thrombolytic therapy can be considered. The success rate of thrombolysis in this context is between 85 and 93% with lower mortality rates when compared with surgery [29-31]. Recombinant tissue plasminogen activator does not cross the placenta and a recent review of 28 case reports of its use in pregnancy found an 8% rate of fetal loss [32]. Cardiopulmonary bypass during pregnancy is high-risk with maternal mortality rates of 3-15% and fetal mortality rates of 20-33% reported [33]. Therefore, thrombolytic therapy should be used as first-line therapy when managing valve thrombosis in pregnancy unless the patient is haemodynamically unstable and requires urgent surgical intervention.

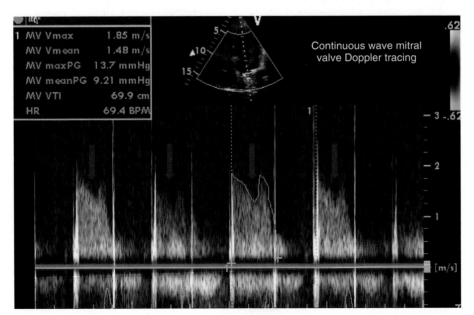

Figure 5.2 Continuous wave Doppler across a thrombosed prosthetic mitral valve showing increased flow gradients (arrows).

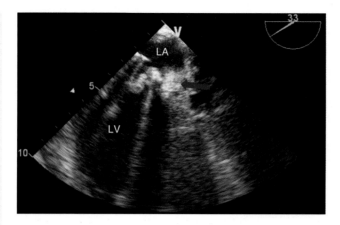

Figure 5.3 Transoesophageal echocardiogram demonstrating thrombus material on a mitral valve prosthesis (arrow). LA = left atrium, LV = left ventricle.

Discussion

Pregnancy in women with prosthetic heart valves is high-risk. The increased maternal mortality in these patients is mainly due to valve thrombosis, which in turn is due to the lack of an ideal anticoagulant for mechanical valves in pregnancy. Drenthen et al. recently identified mechanical valve prosthesis as a strong predictor of maternal and foetal risk in pregnancy [34].

It is crucial that young women with mechanical valve replacements are made aware of the risks when embarking on pregnancy. More importantly, all young women requiring valve surgery should be thoroughly counselled before undergoing the procedure. This should enable them to make an informed decision regarding their choice of valve implantation. Counselling must cover potential issues with the valves themselves and the risks of anticoagulation and future pregnancies. All women with mechanical valves should be cared for by an MDT during pregnancy (cardiologist, haematologist, obstetrician, and anaesthetist) with meticulous monitoring of their anticoagulation, irrespective of whether warfarin or heparin is used.

References

1 Yum KL, Miller DC, Moore KA, et al. Durability of the Hancock MO bioprostheses compared with the standard aortic valve bioprostheses. *Ann Thorac Surg* 1995; 60(2 Suppl): S221–228.

2 North RA, Sadler L, White HD, et al. Long-term survival and valve-related complications in young women with cardiac valve replacement. *Circulation* 1999; 99: 2669–2676.

3 Born D, Martinez EE, Almeida PAM, et al. Pregnancy in patients with prosthetic heart valves: the effects of anticoagulation on mother, fetus, and neonate. *Am Heart J* 1992; 124: 413–417.

4 Ginsberg JS, Barron WM. Pregnancy and prosthetic heart valves. *Lancet* 1994; 344: 1170–1172.

5 Bartolloti U, Milano A, Massucco A, et al. Pregnancy in patients with a porcine valve bioprosthesis. *Am J Cardiol* 1982; 50: 1051–1054.

6 Dore A, Sommerville J. Pregnancy in patients with pulmonary autograft valve replacement. *Eur Heart J* 1997; 18: 1659–1662.

7 Jamieson WRE, Miller DC, Akins CW, et al. Pregnancy and bioprosthesis: influence on structural valve deterioration. *Ann Thorac Surg* 1995; 60: S282–287.

8 Dajani AS Jr, Taubert KA, Zuccaro G, et al. Prevention of bacterial endocarditis. Recommendations by the American Heart Association. *JAMA* 1997; 277: 1794–1801.

9 National Institute for Health and Clinical Excellence. Prophylaxis against infective endocarditis. NICE Guidance CG64 [issued March 2008]. Available from: http://guidance.nice.org.uk/CG64

10 Chan WS, Anand S, Ginsberg JS. Anticoagulation of pregnant women with mechanical heart valves: a systematic review of the literature. *Arch Intern Med* 2000; 160: 191–196.

11 David GL. Haemostatic changes associated with normal and abnormal pregnancies. *Clin Lab Science* 2000; 13: 223–228.

12 ACC/AHA guidelines for the management of patients with valvular heart disease: a report of the American College of Cardiology/American Heart Association Task Force on practice guidelines (Committee on management of patients with valvular heart disease). J Am Coll Cardiol 1998; 32: 1486–1588.

13 Bonow RO, Carabello BA, Riegel B. ACC/AHA 2006 guidelines for the management of patients with valvular heart disease: a report of the American College of Cardiology/American Heart Association Task Force on practice guidelines (writing committee to revise the 1998 guidelines for the management of patients with valvular heart disease): developed in collaboration with the Society of Cardiovascular Anaesthesiologists: endorsed by the Society for Cardiovascular Angiography and Interventions and the Society of Thoracic Surgeons. *Circulation* 2006; 114: e84–e231.

14 Butchart EG, Gohlke–Bärwolf C, Vahanian A, et al. Working Groups on valvular heart disease, thrombosis and cardiac rehabilitation and exercise physiology, European Society of Cardiology. Recommendations for the management of patients after heart valve surgery. *Eur Heart J* 2005; 26: 2463–2471.

15 Stevenson RE, Burton M, Ferlauto GJ, et al. Hazards of oral anticoagulants during pregnancy. *JAMA* 1980; 243: 1549–1551.

16 Wesseling J, Van Driel D, Heymans HS, et al. Coumarins during pregnancy: long term effects on growth and development of school age children. *Thromb Haemost* 2001; 85: 609–613.

17 Vitale N, De Feo M, Contrufo M, et al. Dose-dependent fetal complications of warfarin in pregnant women with mechanical heart valves. *J Am Coll Cardiol* 1999; 33: 1637–1641.

18 Thorpe JA, Poskin MF, Heimes B, et al. Perinatal factors predicting severe intracranial haemorrhage. *Am J Perinatol* 1997; 27: 1704–1706.

19 Brill-Edwards, Ginsberg JS, Hirsh J, et al. Establishing a therapeutic range for heparin therapy. *Ann Intern Med* 1993; 119: 104–105.

20 Monreal M, Lafoz E, Olive A, et al. Comparison of subcutaneous unfractionated heparin with a low molecular weight heparin (Fragmin) in patients with venous thromboembolism and contraindications to coumarin. *Thromb Haemost* 1994: 71: 7–11.

21 Casele HL, Laifer SA, Venkataramanan R, et al. Changes in the pharmacokinetics of the low molecular weight heparin enoxaparin sodium during pregnancy. *Am J Obstet Gynecol* 1999); 181: 1113–1117.

22 Oran B, Lee–Parritz A, Ansell J. Low molecular weight heparin for the prophylaxis of thromboembolism in women with prosthetic mechanical heart valves during pregnancy. *Thromb Haemst* 2004; 92: 747–751.

23 Barbour LA, Oja JA, Schultz LK, et al. A prospective trial that demonstrates that dalteparin requirements increase in pregnancy to maintain therapeutic levels of anticoagulation. *Am J Obstet Gynecol* 2004; 191: 1024–1029.

24 Corby DG. Aspirin in pregnancy: maternal and fetal effects. *Pediatrics* 1978; 62(Suppl): 9307.

25 Rai R, Cohen H, Dave M, et al. Randomized controlled trial of aspirin and aspirin plus heparin in pregnant women with recurrent miscarriage associated with phospholipid antibodies (or antiphospholipid antibodies). *BMJ* 1997; 314: 253–257.

26 CLASP (Collaborative Low-dose Aspirin Study in Pregnancy) Collaborative Group. CLASP: a randomized trial of low-dose aspirin for the prevention and treatment of pre-eclampsia among 9,364 women. *Lancet* 1992; 343: 619–629.

27 Cartis S, Sibai B, Thom E, et al. Low-dose aspirin to prevent pre-eclampsia in women at high risk. *N Engl J Med* 1998; 338: 701–705.

28 Kozer E, Nikfar S, Costei A, et al. Aspirin consumption during the first trimester of pregnancy and congenital anomalies: a meta-analysis. *Am J Obstet Gynecol* 2002; 187: 1623–1630.

29 Bates SM, Greer IA, Ginsberg JS, et al. Use of antithrombotic agents during pregnancy: the seventh ACCP conference on antithrombotic and thrombolytic therapy. *Chest* 2004; 126: S627–644.

30 Lengyel M. Management of prosthetic valve thrombosis. *J Heart Valve Dis* 2004; 13: 329–344.

31 Lengyel M. Thrombolysis should be regarded as first-line therapy for prosthetic valve thrombosis in the absence of contraindications. *J Am Coll Cardiol* 2005; 45: 325.

32 Leonhardt G, Gaul C, Schleusser E, et al. Thrombolytic therapy in pregnancy. *J Thromb Thrombolysis* 2006; 21: 271–276.

33 Chambers CE, Clark SL. Cardiac surgery during pregnancy. *Clin Obstet Gynecol* 1994; 37: 316–323.

34 Drenthen W, Roos–Hesselink JW, Van Der Tuuk K, et al. Predictors of pregnancy-related cardiac, obstetric and neonatal complications in women with congenital heart disease. European Society of Cardiology Congress 2007; September 1–5, 2007, Vienna, Austria.

6 Symptomatic aortic stenosis: new horizons in management

Shouvik Haldar

Expert commentary Dr Martyn Thomas

Case history

A 71-year-old gentleman attended his local cardiology clinic for routine surveillance of his aortic stenosis (AS). A transthoracic echocardiogram (TTE) conducted a year earlier had revealed a tricuspid aortic valve (AV) with a mean AV gradient of 32 mmHg, peak gradient of 52 mmHg, and a valve area of 1.3 cm². Left ventricular (LV) systolic function was preserved with an ejection fraction estimated at 55%. The right heart was dilated with good systolic function and pulmonary artery systolic pressure was elevated at 50 mmHg. The echocardiographic parameters were consistent with moderate AS, and had deteriorated significantly compared with the previous year's scan.

He now complained of a recurrence of angina and marked breathlessness on exertion, limiting him to a walking distance of fifty yards. He denied syncope, pre-syncope, or palpitations. A review of his history revealed extensive comorbidities, including previous percutaneous coronary intervention (PCI) to the right coronary artery (RCA) and left anterior descending artery (LAD), paroxysmal atrial fibrillation (PAF), hypertension, hypercholesterolaemia, type II diabetes mellitus, symptomatic peripheral vascular disease, and chronic renal impairment (baseline creatinine of 205 micromol/L). He drank very little alcohol and had never smoked. His medical therapy included aspirin, atorvastatin, amlodipine, ramipril, furosemide, doxazosin, lanzoprazole, and insulin.

Clinical examination revealed an ejection systolic murmur radiating throughout the precordium with a soft aortic component to the second heart sound. There was no evidence of cardiac failure. A repeat TTE during the consultation now confirmed severe AS (Table 6.1) with a mean gradient of 50 mmHg, peak gradient of 90 mmHg, a valve area of 0.7 cm², and preserved LV systolic function. His pulmonary artery systolic pressure was estimated at 65 mmHg. As this represented a significant deterioration in symptoms and exercise tolerance, he was admitted to hospital for further investigations.

The patient had rapidly progressed to severe symptomatic AS and required consideration for aortic valve replacement (AVR). He was not keen on surgical intervention, but having been counselled on a very poor prognosis without surgery (Figure 6.4), he

Expert comment

In some patients with AS, teasing out the presence of symptoms can be difficult. Symptoms can be subtle and patients tend to adapt their lives to cope. Exercise testing and stress echocardiography can be useful in more objectively assessing the patient's exercise capacity and the full haemodynamic significance of the AS.

Expert comment

Appropriate and timely follow-up in patients with moderate AS is very important. In this case, given the deterioration in the previous two years, annual follow-up may have been too infrequent. It is reasonable to wait for symptoms, but only if follow-up can be very diligent and reactive. Once symptoms develop, the event rate is rapid with increasing mortality. The 'system' of any institution needs to be able to react quickly and appropriately at this point to changes in the patient's condition.

Table 6.1 How to grade the severity of AS (adapted from ACC guidelines 2006) [1]

	Mild	Moderate	Severe
Peak velocity (m/s)	2.0–3.0	3.0–4.0	>4.0
Peak gradient (mmHg)	16–35	36–65	>65
Mean gradient (mmHg)	<25	25–40	>40
Valve area (cm²)	>1.5	1.0–1.5	<1.0

Learning point Calculating the severity of AS

- The peak transvalvular pressure gradient can be calculated from the aortic peak velocity via the simplified Bernoulli equation, provided that LV systolic function is normal:
Pressure gradient = 4 x peak velocity^2
- The longer form of the Bernoulli equation should ideally be used if the peak velocity is <3.0 m/s to avoid inaccuracies:
Pressure gradient = $4 \times (v2^2 - v1^2)$
(where v2 = peak aortic velocity and v1 = peak LV outflow tract velocity)
- Mean aortic pressure gradients can be obtained by tracing the envelope of the continuous wave Doppler signal through the AV. Echo machines will automatically calculate the velocity time integral (VTI) and mean transaortic pressure gradient from this information.
- An AV area of <1.0 cm^2 and mean transvalvular gradient >40 mmHg are markers of severe AS [1].

Learning point Calculating the effective valve area–the continuity equation explained

- If LV function is impaired or hyperdynamic, the generated peak velocities will be either underestimated or overestimated, respectively. This will subsequently lead to errors in peak transvalvular gradients when using the simplified Bernoulli equation.
- In these circumstances, the severity of AS is best assessed by valve area using the continuity equation.
- The continuity equation is based on the principle that the volume of blood passing through the LV outflow tract (LVOT) in 1 second is the same as the volume of blood crossing the AV in 1 second.
- To calculate the volume of blood crossing a particular structure requires knowledge of the VTI and the cross-sectional area (CSA) of that structure. The VTI is the product of velocity and time and takes into account the pulsatile nature of blood flow within the heart.
Volume of blood flow = VTI x CSA
- Therefore, if the volume of blood flow at the LVOT = LVOT VTI x LVOT CSA, then this must equal the volume of blood flow at the AV = AV VTI x AV CSA.
Hence, AV area = LVOT area x LVOT VTI/AV VTI.
- In practice, you need three measurements for the continuity equation which can be obtained from two views (Figures 6.1, 6.2, and 6.3).

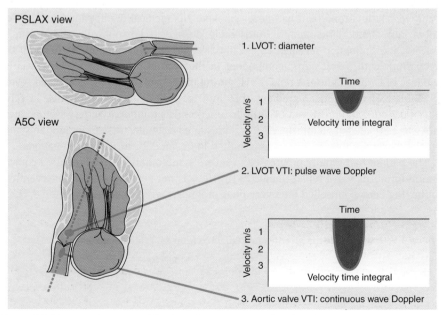

Figure 6.1 Measurements required for the continuity equation (this figure was published in Essential Echocardiography, 1st edition, A. Ryding, p. 89, copyright Elsevier 2008).

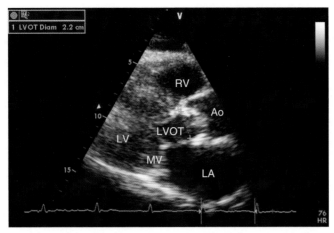

Figure 6.2 Parasternal long axis (PSLAX) view: 2D measurement of the left ventricular outflow tract (LVOT) diameter for the continuity equation beneath a heavily calcified aortic valve. RV = right ventricle; Ao = aorta; LA = left atrium; MV = mitral valve; LV = left ventricle.

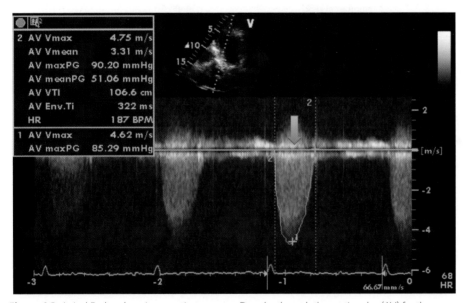

Figure 6.3 Apical 5-chamber view: continuous wave Doppler through the aortic valve (AV) for the velocity time integral (VTI) measurement. Taking a trace of the Doppler signal (arrow) allows for calculation of the maximum and mean gradients across the AV.

> **⊕ Expert comment**
>
> Echocardiographic assessment of AS can be difficult. In the presence of good LV function, the peak and mean Doppler gradients provide adequate information. However, once LV function is reduced, the aortic valve area must be calculated. This must be done carefully as there is significant potential for error, particularly when measuring the LV outflow tract, and should also be interpreted in keeping with the clinical and radiographic findings. There is also a developing concept of low-flow aortic stenosis in the setting of preserved LV function, but this is relatively unusual.

agreed to proceed with further investigations. A repeat coronary angiogram revealed diffusely calcified coronary arteries with patent stents in the LAD and RCA and no new flow-limiting disease.

Given the extent of this gentleman's comorbidities, the case was subsequently presented at a multidisciplinary team (MDT) meeting attended by interventional cardiologists, cardiothoracic surgeons, and cardiac anaesthetists. The patient's predicted mortality was calculated from cardiac surgery scoring systems and ranged from > 20% (Logistic Euroscore) to 9.6% (Society of Thoracic Surgeons). The surgical opinion deemed the risks of conventional AVR to be unacceptably high, and trans-catheter

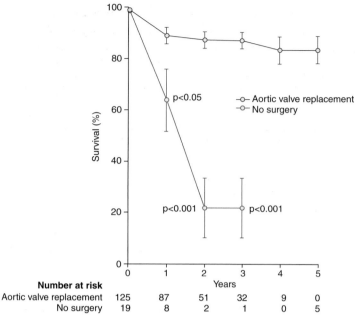

Figure 6.4 Mean survival of patients with symptomatic aortic stenosis. Reprinted with permission from Carabello and Paulus [2].

> ⭐ **Learning point** When to operate in AS?
>
> Once patients with severe AS become symptomatic, their prognosis is poor (Figure 6.4). They require a prompt mechanical solution to the outflow obstruction via AVR.
>
> Asymptomatic patients with severe stenosis are more difficult to manage. Generally, this group of patients have an excellent prognosis without valve replacement. The caveat is that approximately 1% of asymptomatic patients will die unexpectedly or will deteriorate rapidly enough to become symptomatic and die suddenly before seeking medical attention [2,3].
>
> Some experts advocate risk stratification of this high-risk subset of asymptomatic patients although this can prove to be very challenging. Exercise testing may unmask a limited exercise capacity, show abnormal blood pressure responses, or even exercise-induced symptoms [4,5,6]. If these ominous features are shown, then these patients should probably undergo AVR although at present, there are no definitive data to show that this high-risk group would prognostically benefit from such an intervention. Ultimately, asymptomatic patients should be followed up closely to allow prompt surgical referral should symptoms develop.

aortic valve implantation (TAVI) was thought to be the better option. The patient was quoted a 10% risk of mortality with TAVI and was subsequently transferred to a tertiary referral centre for evaluation of his suitability for the procedure.

The patient's TAVI work-up included transoesophageal echocardiography (TOE). This confirmed severe AS with preserved biventricular function. The mitral valve (MV) was calcified with mixed mild stenosis and regurgitation and in addition, pulmonary hypertension was noted. Accurate assessment of the AV annulus was difficult due to some shadow artefacts from the calcified valve, but was measured at 29 mm. A subsequent computed tomography (CT) aortogram confirmed this as the annulus size, but also demonstrated significant peripheral vascular disease with eccentric areas of calcification involving the ilio-femoral vessels. The minimum diameter of these vessels at certain points was less than 7 mm. He was discharged home to await the decision regarding his suitability for TAVI.

⊗ **Learning point** Preoperative risk evaluation for valvular heart surgery

Multivariate scoring systems such as the European Euroscore [7] (available from: www.euroscore.org) and the US-based Society of Thoracic Surgeons (STS) score [8] (available from: www.sts.org/sections/stsnationaldatabase/riskcalculator/) are based on cardiac and non-cardiac risk factors. They have been well validated in cardiac surgery, but have limitations in their predictive accuracy when assessing valvular heart disease in the elderly. This may be, in part, due to the fact that these high-risk groups were under-repres ented in the populations from which the scores were derived. At present, an expected mortality of >20% on the logistic Euroscore and >10% with the STS score is deemed high-risk for surgery [9]. The current and most logical approach to risk evaluation is to use a combination of these scoring systems in conjunction with sound clinical judgement.

⊗ **Learning point** What is TAVI?

TAVI is a procedure designed and reserved for patients who are deemed too high a risk for conventional surgery. The procedure eliminates the need for a traditional midline sternotomy and cardiopulmonary bypass. It also does not involve excision of the diseased valve or associated annular tissue. Cribier reported the first human procedure in 2002 [10]. Since then, two devices have been 'CE marked' and are being used and investigated in a limited number of centres worldwide.

Current indications for TAVI include a logistic Euroscore of >20%, an STS score of >10% or a patient being turned down for surgery by two consecutive cardiothoracic surgeons. It is not, however, indicated for those patients who have been offered, but then declined, conventional AVR [9].

The procedure is usually performed under general anaesthetic with fluoroscopic and transoesophageal echocardiographic guidance. It involves initial balloon aortic valvuloplasty (BAV) to dilate the native valve. This is followed by simultaneous rapid right ventricular pacing to decrease cardiac output transiently, allowing the deployment of a stented bioprosthesis into the aortic annulus. If successfully placed, the mean pressure gradient across the valve can be reduced to near normal with an immediate improvement in haemodynamics.

Currently approved devices include the Edwards SAPIEN™ valve, Edwards SAPIEN XT™ valve (Figure 6.5), and the CoreValve® (Figure 6.6). The Edwards valve is a bovine pericardial valve mounted within a balloon-expandable stent which can be delivered transapically or transfemorally. The Corevalve® is a self-expanding porcine pericardial valve which can be delivered via the transfemoral or transaxillary route, with a transapical device soon to follow.

Current technology limits TAVI to those with an aortic annulus size ≤27 mm and if a transfemoral approach is planned, then a minimum calibre of 6 mm (if using the Edwards Sapien XT™) for the peripheral vessels is required [11]. Other contraindications include bicuspid valves (due to a significant risk of incomplete valve deployment), close proximity of coronary arteries that may be compromised during the procedure, and the presence of LV thrombus [9].

Potential complications for TAVI include paravalvular aortic regurgitation (AR), stroke, need for pacemaker implantation (secondary to compression of the adjacent atrioventricular node and conduction tissue during stent deployment), and vascular problems. Complication rates vary according to which route is taken, but in general, have declined significantly as centres ascend the learning curve of early procedures alongside numerous technical refinements. Mild to moderate AR post-procedurally is not uncommon, but meticulous attention to valve positioning and sizing the prosthesis dimensions to the aortic annulus has reduced the incidence of severe AR down to less than 5%. Reported stroke rates are less than 6% whilst the rate of pacemaker implantation is between 5–10%. Vascular complications have remained high until recently, with reports showing a decline from 10–15% to 5–10% [12].

⊕ **Expert comment**

Risk assessment for aortic valve surgery is difficult. The logistic Euroscore has traditionally been used, but is widely believed to overestimate risk, especially at the higher values. Nonetheless, a logistic Euroscore of >20% is considered to be high-risk and is one of the criteria which allows patients to be considered for 'on label' TAVI. Over and above this, the decision regarding the best therapy for a high-risk patient should be made by an MDT, made up of cardiothoracic surgeons, interventional cardiologists, imaging specialists, cardiac anaesthetists, and elderly medicine specialists. One important aspect of this assessment that is not captured in the logistic Euroscore is the frailty of the patient. Certain 'scoring systems' are available for this, but often this comes down to clinical judgement. It is important to realize that although the results of surgical AVR in octogenarians are excellent, these are carefully selected patients, often with low Euroscores. In general, this is not the type of patient who would be considered for TAVI. There are also other considerations when deciding between high-risk aortic surgery and TAVI, other than 30-day mortality. One must consider the recovery period, length of stay, and utilization of high-cost hospital facilities such as the intensive care unit and the need for renal replacement therapy. These are often lower in the TAVI patient.

⊕ **Clinical tip** TAVI work-up

- Accurate measurement of the aortic annulus is critical to allow the correct sizing of the valve. This reduces the likelihood of paravalvular leaks occurring and attenuates the risk of migration of the prosthesis post-deployment.
- Multi-slice CT is currently the best method to assess the aortic root and left ventricle, in addition to identifying calcification and tortuosity of the vascular path from the aorta to femoral arteries.
- TOE is the current gold standard for measuring the aortic annulus size.

A month later, the patient's TAVI work-up data were discussed at an MDT meeting. Of the two devices that have been CE-marked, this particular centre was using the Edwards SAPIEN™ valve which is currently available in 23 and 26 mm sizes (suitable for annular sizes of 18–21 and 22–25 mm, respectively). The patient's aortic annulus at 29 mm was too large for both commercially available devices at that point in time, rendering him unsuitable for TAVI. After a lengthy discussion, it was felt he should be

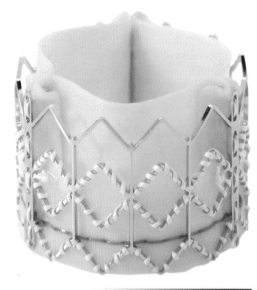

Figure 6.5 Edwards SAPIEN™ trans-catheter heart valve (courtesy of Edwards Lifesciences).

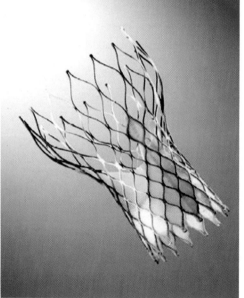

Figure 6.6 CoreValve® Trans-catheter Heart Valve (courtesy of Medtronic, Inc).

referred to a different cardiothoracic surgeon for conventional AVR. He was duly accepted for outpatient review.

Unfortunately, after discharge the patient had a number of local hospital admissions, including an intensive care admission secondary to a chest infection complicated by fast AF. This had resulted in a degree of congestive cardiac failure which was attributed to his AS as his LV systolic function remained preserved on repeat TTE. He was treated with intravenous diuretics, antibiotics, and amiodarone and made a satisfactory recovery, allowing discharge home. It was clear, however, that his aortic valve required prompt intervention and the cardiothoracic surgeons were informed of his admissions. They advised against operating immediately after an 'acute event' as this would increase the patient's peri-operative mortality, but they offered to expedite his outpatient date.

Two months after discharge from his initial TAVI work-up, he underwent successful AVR with a 29 mm Perimount tissue aortic valve prosthesis, followed by an uneventful post-operative period. He was transferred back to his local hospital for rehabilitation on day 5 and eventually discharged home. At his 6-month follow-up appointment, he was making excellent progress.

Discussion

Symptomatic severe AS is a fatal condition if left untreated. In developed countries, the prevalence of the condition mirrors the ageing population. No form of medical treatment has been shown to be beneficial in these patients as it is a mechanical obstruction to LV outflow and hence requires a mechanical solution. To this day, surgical AVR under cardiopulmonary bypass remains the gold standard and can return the patient's life expectancy to that of an unselected population [2].

Recent innovative percutaneous methods such as TAVI have shown promising short-term (2-year) results in high-risk patients turned down for conventional surgery. This is an emerging therapeutic field, and techniques and technologies for TAVI are evolving rapidly with newer, smaller devices designed to ease positioning.

As these advances strive to improve the safety and widen the applicability of the procedure, what is now needed is robust, randomized controlled trial data, comparing TAVI with conventional AVR. This is crucial to assess its safety, efficacy, durability, and its long-term clinical outcomes. The first of such trials, the PARTNER US (Placement of Aortic Trans-catheter Valves) trial [13,14] has published favourable results for TAVI (see Landmark Trial at end of case). An additional future role for TAVI may be the concept of implanting percutaneous valves into failing aortic bioprostheses ('valve-within-valve technique'). Of course, this represents a much smaller target population for the procedure, but it could end the traditional practice of implanting metallic aortic valves in younger patients. This would have the advantage of eliminating the attendant risks of anticoagulation and thrombosis with mechanical valves, but the caveat would be that one or more TAVI procedures would be required in a patient's lifetime as a consequence of degeneration of their bioprosthesis.

If the results of other future trials are favourable, percutaneous methods could revolutionize the treatment of haemodynamically significant and symptomatic AS. The treatment could potentially be applied to lower risk groups, and ultimately, may have the potential to supersede traditional open-heart surgery.

> **⚙ Landmark trial** Placement of Aortic Trans-catheter Valves (PARTNER US) [13,14]
>
> A large, multi-centre, randomized control trial predominantly conducted in the USA with a total of 1057 patients.
>
> **Inclusion criteria:** patients with severe symptomatic AS who had a high predicted rate of operative mortality (STS score 10 or more).
>
> **Methods:** this study had two arms: the first (Arm A) enrolling high-risk AS patients randomized to either AVR or TAVI, and the second (Arm B) including inoperable patients randomized to medical management (BAV allowed) or TAVI with a 1-year mortality endpoint.
>
> **Results:** TAVI is non-inferior to surgical AVR for the primary end-point of all cause mortality at 1 year (24.2% vs. 26.8%, p=0.001 for non-inferiority) in Arm A. Results for Arm B were also impressive with TAVI showing markedly higher survival and reduced risk of mortality or repeat hospitalization as compared to medical therapy (including BAV).
>
> It should be noted, however, that neurological events were more frequent with TAVI whilst major bleeding and new onset atrial fibrillation were more frequent with AVR. These differing peri-procedural risks should influence the decision making process when considering which treatment is suitable for high-risk patients with severe AS.
>
> *continued*

⚬ Expert comment

If a centre uses one particular type of TAVI device, but the patient has characteristics that would favour an alternative device used at another centre, the patient should be referred to that appropriate centre. I have done this myself on two occasions.

⚬ Expert comment

Having treated the chest infection and AF, BAV could perhaps have been considered in this situation as the surgeons did not want to operate. Indeed, aortic surgery or TAVI should be avoided in any 'acute situation'; however, BAV is a very effective method of 'buying time', especially in patients with poor LV function.

Conclusion: TAVI is already an alternative treatment option for inoperable patients with severe AS. These results now provide evidence for its safety and efficacy, and supports its role as a robust alternative strategy for a group of carefully selected patients deemed too high-risk for standard surgical AVR.

A final word from the expert

This case is a good example of the complex decision-making that is now required in high-risk patients with severe symptomatic AS. Ultimately, an MDT should make the recommendation on the best form of treatment and teamwork as a whole is crucial for the delivery of a top quality 'aortic service'. Multiple new trans-catheter aortic devices are currently in development. These will allow smaller delivery systems and the potential for retrievability and repositioning. In the future, there may be a move towards lower risk patients, but this should be done with great caution. Surgical AVR is an excellent treatment. Any change towards a lower risk group should be made with our surgical colleagues, within a multidisciplinary environment or clinical trial. Given the current cost of the trans-catheter devices, it would be very difficult to make TAVI cost-effective in lower risk patients. In addition, there are little data currently available on the durability of the trans-catheter valves. There has been no reported structural failure of the valves to date, with the longest implant being *in situ* for over five years.

Ultimately, it is highly likely that TAVI will be used in an increasing proportion of the AS population, but this must be done in a prudent, carefully judged way, and in an evidence-based manner.

References

1 Bonow RO, Carabello BA, Chatterjee K, et al. ACC/AHA 2006 guidelines for the management of patients with valvular heart disease. *J Am Coll Cardiol* 2006; 48: e1–148.
2 Carabello BA, Paulus WJ. Aortic stenosis. *Lancet* 2009; 373: 956–966.
3 Pellikka PA, Sarano ME, Nishimura RA, et al. Outcome of 622 adults with asymptomatic, haemodynamically significant aortic stenosis during prolonged follow-up. *Circulation* 2005; 111: 3290–3295.
4 Amato MC, Moffa PJ, Werner KE, et al. Treatment decision in asymptomatic aortic valve stenosis: role of exercise testing. *Heart* 2001; 86: 381–386.
5 Das P, Rimington H, Chambers J. Exercise testing to stratify risk in aortic stenosis. *Eur Heart J* 2008; 26: 1309–1313.
6 Alborino D, Hoffmann JL, Fournet PC, et al. Value of exercise testing to evaluate the indication for surgery in asymptomatic patients with valvular aortic stenosis. *J Heart Valve Dis* 2002; 11: 204–209.
7 Roques F, Nashef SA, Michel P, EuroSCORE study group. Risk factors for early mortality after valve surgery in Europe in the 1990s: lessons from the EuroSCORE pilot program. *J Heart Valve Dis* 2001; 10: 572–577.
8 STS National Database. STS US Cardiac Surgery Database: 1997 aortic valve replacement patients: preoperative risk variables (2000) Chicago: Society of Thoracic Surgeons.
9 Vahanian A, Alfieri O, Al-Attar N, et al. Trans-catheter valve implantation for patients with aortic stenosis: a position statement from the European Association of CardioThoracic Surgery (EACTS) and the European Society of Cardiology (ESC), in collaboration with the European Association of Percutaneous Cardiovascular Intervention (EAPCI). *Eur Heart J* 2008; 29: 1463–1470.
10 Cribier A, Eltchaninoff H, Bash A, et al. Percutaneous trans-catheter implantation of an aortic valve prosthesis for calcific aortic stenosis: first human description. *Circulation* 2002; 106: 3006–3008.
11 Thomas, M. Trans-catheter aortic valve implantation in the United Kingdom: NICE guidance. *Heart* 2009; 95: 674–675.
12 Sherif MA, Tolg R, Richardt G. Percutaneous aortic valve replacement: results update, future trends and new challenges. *Clin Res Cardiol* 2009; 4(Suppl 2): 102–107.
13 Leon MB, Smith CR, Mack M, et al. Transcatheter aortic-valve implantation for aortic stenosis in patients who cannot undergo surgery. *N Engl J Med* 2010; 363: 1597–1607.
14 Smith CR, Leon MB, Mack M, et al. Transcatheter versus Surgical Aortic-Valve Replacement in High-Risk Patients. *N Engl J Med* 2010; 364: 2187–2198.

7 Assessment and management of mitral regurgitation

Christopher Steadman

◔ **Expert commentary** Professor Petros Nihoyannopoulos

Case history

A 76-year-old man was under annual cardiology follow-up for mitral regurgitation (MR). This had been diagnosed five years previously, when a murmur was detected incidentally at preoperative assessment for a routine urological procedure. He had no cardiac symptoms. On initial transthoracic echocardiography (TTE), the MR was classified as moderate with prolapse of the posterior mitral valve leaflet (PMVL). Both left ventricular (LV) function and dimensions were normal.

> ⊕ **Learning point** Aetiology of MR
>
> MR is now the second most common valve lesion after aortic stenosis (AS).
> - **Organic MR** (leaflet abnormalities are the primary cause of the disease):
>   - Degenerative;
>   - Mitral valve prolapse;
>   - Rheumatic valve disease;
>   - Infective endocarditis;
>   - Collagen vascular disorders.
> - **Ischaemic MR:**
>   - Acute due to papillary muscle rupture;
>   - Chronic due to restriction of leaflet motion.
> - **Functional MR** (failure of leaflet coaptation due to LV dilatation):
>   - Cardiomyopathy;
>   - Ischaemic heart disease.

At his latest clinic visit, the patient remained asymptomatic. He had recently had a TTE, but the acoustic windows were of suboptimal quality, making the visual assessment of the MR difficult and no quantitative measurements were possible. In the parasternal long axis (PLAX) view, however, a significant jet of MR on colour Doppler was detected. LV function and dimensions had remained within normal limits with no significant change from the previous scan. Right ventricular (RV) function was impaired with a reduced tricuspid annular plane systolic excursion (TAPSE) of 10 mm.

> ⊕ **Clinical tip** Indicators of mitral valve prolapse
>
> - Superior displacement of the mitral leaflets > 2 mm above the annular plane during systole;
> - The prolapse is classic if the leaflet thickness is ≥ 5 mm and non-classic if < 5 mm;
> - Prolapse should only be diagnosed in the parasternal and apical long-axis views and not the apical 4-chamber view due to the saddle shape of the mitral valve annulus;
> - Using these criteria, the prevalence is 2.4% (1.3% classic, 1.1% non-classic) [1].

> ⊕ **Clinical tip** Serial follow-up of asymptomatic MR
>
> The aim of serial follow-up is to assess subjectively for changes in symptomatic status, and objectively for changes in cardiac function, which may be present in the absence of symptoms.
>
> **European Society of Cardiology (ESC) guidelines [2]**
> - Moderate MR and preserved LV function: yearly clinical review with 2-yearly echocardiography;
> - Severe MR and preserved LV function: 6-monthly clinical review and yearly echocardiography.
>
> **American College of Cardiology/American Heart Association (ACC/AHA) guidelines [3]**
> - Moderate MR: yearly clinical and echocardiographic evaluation;
> - Severe MR: 6- to 12-monthly clinical and echocardiographic evaluation.

🍏 **Expert comment**

MR may remain asymptomatic for a long time as the left ventricle undergoes remodelling to accommodate the extra blood volume. An early indicator of LV volume overload is a hyperdynamic left ventricle; this can be confirmed if the fractional shortening is above 40%.

Discriminating between those patients who are truly asymptomatic and those who are actually symptomatic, but have adapted their lifestyle subconsciously to remain 'asymptomatic', is difficult. It requires a careful clinical examination, noting objective clinical signs (e.g. paroxysmal atrial fibrillation, pulmonary hypertension) and ultimately, requires good clinical judgement.

🍏 **Expert comment**

Echocardiography for the evaluation and quantification of MR is very important. Full quantification is essential, but has to be performed by experts fully accredited by the British or European Society/Association of Echocardiography. If despite these basic requirements, quantification is still not possible, then a transoesophageal examination is mandatory.

In this case, the fact that RV function was impaired hints that the RV pressure was elevated, an indication that the MR is significant enough to require intervention. One may also ask why suddenly the echocardiographic examination became suboptimal during years of regular follow-up. Was the evaluation of MR in fact suboptimal from the beginning?

⭐ **Learning point** Echocardiography to assess MR

A comprehensive TTE examination, and in some cases, transoesophageal echocardiography (TOE), is extremely important at diagnosis in order to determine the anatomy, severity, and potential for repair.

Published guidelines for full quantification of MR severity have been agreed between the European Association of Echocardiography and the American Society of Echocardiography [4]. While the guidelines are unequivocal for symptomatic MR, for asymptomatic MR, they are not [5]. For example, current recommendations suggest that surgery should only be considered for asymptomatic patients with moderate MR if there is a high likelihood of valve repair (rather than replacement), together with a low operative risk (<75 years).

At diagnosis, echocardiography is the single most important investigation and aims to:
- Describe the mitral apparatus (which includes leaflets, annulus, chords, papillary muscles, and myocardial function);
- Determine the aetiology and the mechanisms of MR;
- Quantify the severity of MR, including comprehensive haemodynamics;
- Evaluate left and right ventricular function;
- Assess the suitability for mitral valve repair.

In the presence of good windows, a full assessment of MR severity can be made with TTE.

A full assessment should include:
- LV dimensions and ejection fraction (EF);
- Left atrial (LA) dimensions;
- Assessment of mitral valve anatomy;
- Colour flow Doppler for assessment of the mitral regurgitant jet:
  - Vena contracta (regurgitant jet width at narrowest point through mitral valve);
  - Colour jet area (absolute value and as percentage of LA area).
- RV dimensions and function;
- Tricuspid regurgitation continuous-wave Doppler for estimation of pulmonary artery pressure;
- Pulmonary vein pulsed-wave Doppler looking for systolic flow reversal;
- Quantitative measurements (explained in more detail later in the case):
  - Proximal isovelocity surface area (PISA) radius;
  - Effective regurgitant orifice (ERO) area;
  - Regurgitant volume;
  - Regurgitant fraction.

➕ **Clinical tip** Pitfalls in echocardiographic assessment of MR

Machine settings
Remember that Doppler gain, pulse repetition frequency, and machine settings influence the size of the regurgitant colour jet.

Coanda effect
The Coanda effect is a hydrodynamic phenomenon where a jet which flows near a surface has reduced expansion due to adherence to that surface. Therefore, eccentric jets directed along the LA wall may often appear narrow with a small area on two-dimensional (2D) imaging. This is particularly common in MR associated with single leaflet prolapse and may lead to an underestimation of the severity of the MR if multiple parameters are not measured.

Left ventricular ejection fraction (LVEF)
In severe MR, a large volume of blood is being ejected backwards into the left atrium. LVEF is, therefore, often normal and may even be supranormal. This does not necessarily mean that the underlying LV systolic function is normal. More sophisticated techniques such as strain rate imaging can show that the LV systolic function is abnormal in this situation [6]. This is not currently part of routine clinical practice; however, it should be remembered that normal LVEF is not necessarily reassuring in the context of MR.

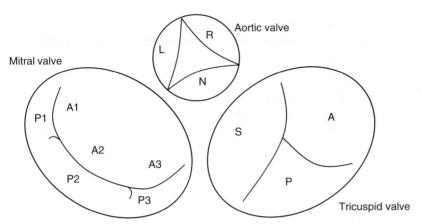

Figure 7.1 Mitral valve anatomy. The mitral valve consists of anterior and posterior mitral valve leaflets, each of which are separated into three segments. Compare this to the aortic valve cusps (R = right ; L = left ; N = non-coronary) and tricuspid valve leaflets (S = septal ; A = anterior ; P = posterior).

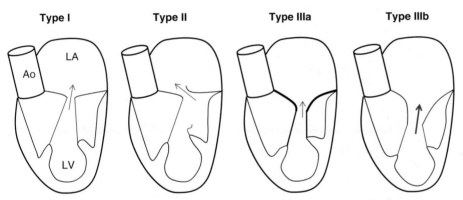

Figure 7.2 Carpentier's functional classification of mitral regurgitation. Type I: normal leaflet motion (annular dilatation); Type II: increased leaflet motion (leaflet prolapse); Type III: restricted leaflet motion, a–systolic and diastolic restrictions (rheumatic, inflammatory), b–systolic restrictions (dilatation, ischaemic).

⊕ **Clinical tip** Indications for TOE in MR

The main advantage of TOE over TTE is improved image quality. However, this is an invasive procedure usually requiring sedation and is not always tolerated by the patient. It should only be done if it will provide information not obtained by TTE that is required to manage the patient appropriately. TOE allows for an accurate assessment of mitral valve anatomy (Figure 7.1). The mechanism of MR should be described using the Carpentier classification (Figure 7.2) [7]. **ACC/AHA guidelines [3]**

Class I
- To establish the anatomic basis for severe MR in patients in whom surgery is recommended, to assess feasibility of and to guide surgical repair;
- For the evaluation of MR in patients in whom TTE provides non-diagnostic information regarding the severity of MR, mechanism of MR, and/or status of LV function.

Class IIa
- In asymptomatic patients with severe MR who are considered for surgery, to assess feasibility of repair.

In view of the suboptimal TTE images, a TOE was requested, firstly to confirm the severity of the MR and secondly to assess the valve anatomy in detail. The TOE confirmed normal LV dimensions and systolic function with prolapse of the PMVL (Carpentier type II) (Figure 7.3), and anteriorly directed MR (Figure 7.4).

The TOE images were then further analyzed using three-dimensional (3D) echocardiography techniques. This method can be performed on transthoracic studies, but is increasingly being used with TOE. The benefits are 3D visualization of anatomy and manipulation of the 3D data set, allowing 2D slices to be created in any plane. This allows a precise localization and an accurate quantification of the prolapsing portion of the leaflet [8]. Additionally, the dynamic 3D colour flow Doppler provides information superior to 2D imaging regarding regurgitant jet size and direction [9]. In this case, the prolapse was mainly of the P2 segment and was due to primary chord rupture (Figure 7.5).

❝ **Expert comment**

This comprehensive echocardiographic evaluation should have been performed at the initial diagnosis.

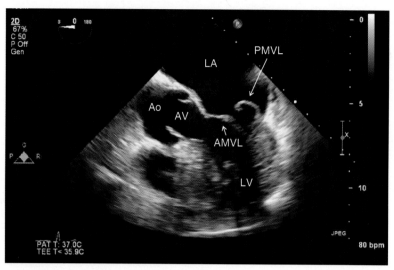

Figure 7.3 Prolapse of the posterior mitral valve leaflet (PMVL) on TOE. AMVL = anterior mitral valve leaflet; LA = left atrium; LV = left ventricle; Ao = aorta; AV = aortic valve.

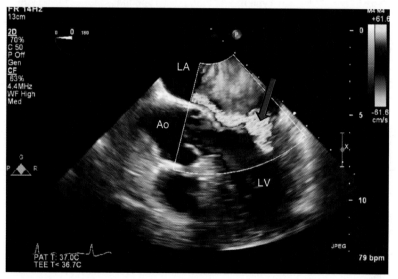

Figure 7.4 Eccentric jet of anteriorly directed MR (arrow) due to posterior mitral valve leaflet prolapse on TOE. LA = left atrium; Ao = aorta; LV = left ventricle.

Quantitative assessment of the MR (Figure 7.6) demonstrated a PISA radius of 1.8 cm with an aliasing velocity of 36.8 cm/s. Continuous-wave Doppler of the MR (not shown) showed a V_{max} of 624 cm/s, the calculated ERO, therefore, being 1.2 cm². Vena contracta was 0.7 cm. Therefore, MR was classified as severe (Table 7.1). The RV function was mildly impaired with no tricuspid regurgitation and hence, an assessment of the pulmonary artery pressure was not possible.

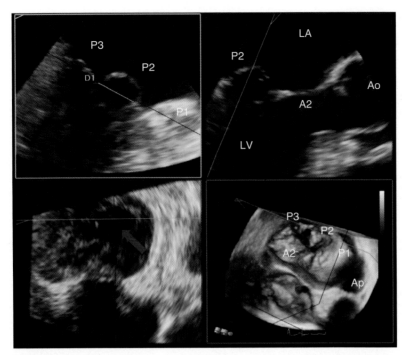

Figure 7.5 3D TOE representation of the mitral valve. From the LA (lower right), there is prolapsing of P2 with red, green, and blue planes marked. Red plane (upper right) transecting A2 and P2 showing P2 prolapse. Green plane (upper left) transecting posterior leaflet showing P2 prolapse. Blue plane transecting the valve en-face showing orifice created by prolapsing valve (arrow). Ap = left atrial appendage.

Expert comment

Transoesophageal 3D echocardiography provides excellent imaging and description of the MV, including the annulus size and commissures. This is vital information for the cardiothoracic surgeon with regards to intervention.

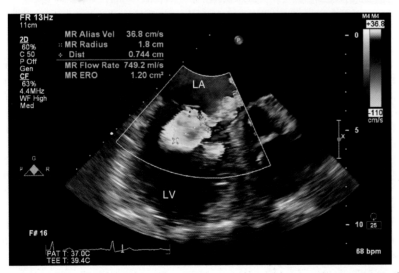

Figure 7.6 The PISA method for assessing the ERO. The X markers run between the regurgitant orifice and the PISA hemispheric shell at the blue red aliasing interface. The baseline is shifted upwards with an alias velocity of 36.8 cm/s (upper right scale). The + markers show the vena contracta.

Clinical tip Practicalities of measuring ERO using the PISA method

1. Zoom in to focus on the colour flow through the MV into the left atrium.
2. Shift the colour flow baseline to optimize the hemispheric PISA; the aliasing velocity is usually between 20 and 40 cm/s. Note that the baseline needs to be shifted downwards when using TTE (regurgitant flow away from the transducer) and upwards when using TOE (regurgitant flow towards the transducer).
3. Scroll through several cardiac cycles to find the most hemispheric PISA at mid-systole, and measure the radius (from the orifice to the red-blue aliasing interface) along the direction of the ultrasound beam.
4. Measure the MR velocity using continuous-wave Doppler.

Quantification of MR is important and should be performed routinely by accredited individuals, (often accredited sonographers are usually better placed to succeed because they are more objective, methodical, and do these assessments more often and consistently). No single measurement will reliably give an accurate assessment of the severity, so it is important to use several parameters to provide a more complete assessment. All parameters and methods are important, and must be used wisely whilst understanding each of their limitations.

Quantitative assessment is almost possible on TOE, but it is also often possible on TTE in patients with good acoustic windows as demonstrated in an example from a different case (Figure 7.7).

In the acute scenario, assessment is easy because the pathology is often dramatic. In these cases, quantification is rarely important, as what is needed is rapid surgery.

In the chronic situation, the values that are needed for patients' follow-up are the effective regurgitant area and volume/fraction. In addition, the size and function of the LV are important (volume overload), as well as the determination of LV filling pressures and RV systolic pressures.

⭐ **Learning point** Quantitative assessment of MR: PISA explained

- The PISA method is based on the principle of conservation of flow and the continuity equation, commonly used (and more frequently understood) for the assessment of valve area in aortic stenosis.
- As blood in the LV converges towards the mitral regurgitant orifice, blood velocity gradually increases, forming a series of hemispheric waves of equal velocity (isovelocity).
- Colour flow imaging can identify a PISA because the red-blue aliasing interface corresponds to the surface of the hemisphere whose flow velocity is the same as the aliasing velocity.
- Using the continuity equation:
  Flow rate at PISA = flow rate across the regurgitant orifice
- The surface area of a sphere is $4\pi r^2$ (where r is the radius), hence the surface area of the PISA hemisphere is half this:

  Surface area of PISA hemisphere = 2π (PISA radius)^2

- Regurgitant volume = ERO x MR VTI
- Regurgitant fraction = MR regurgitant volume / flow volume across MV
- Flow volume across MV = MV area (0.25 x π x annular diameter^2) x MV VTI

Table 7.1 Grading the severity of MR

	Mild	Moderate	Severe
Jet area (cm^2)	<4		>10
Jet area/LA area (%)	<20		>40
Vena contracta (cm)	<0.3		≥0.7
PISA radius (cm) (Nyquist 40 cm/s)	<0.4		>1
ERO (cm^2)	<0.2	0.2–0.39	≥0.4
Regurgitant volume (mL)	<30	30–59	≥60
Regurgitant fraction (%)	<30	30–49	≥50

ACC/AHA guidelines [3] also used by the British Society of Echocardiography (BSE).

In view of the severity of MR and the impairment to RV function, the patient was referred to the cardiac surgeons for consideration of MV surgery (the indications for MV surgery for chronic organic severe MR are detailed in Table 7.2 with notable differences between the European and American guidelines highlighted).

After discussion with the cardiac surgeons, it was felt that the patient was suitable for valve repair with low associated risks due to the absence of significant comorbidities (Class IIa indication in the American guidelines and Class IIb in the European guidelines detailed in Table 7.2). Additionally, although the impairment of RV function is not specifically mentioned in current guidelines, this information gave additional impetus for intervention at this stage.

In view of his age, the patient underwent preoperative cardiac catheterization. This demonstrated minor atheroma only, and meant that concomitant coronary artery bypass grafting was not required. The patient proceeded to MV repair without any complications.

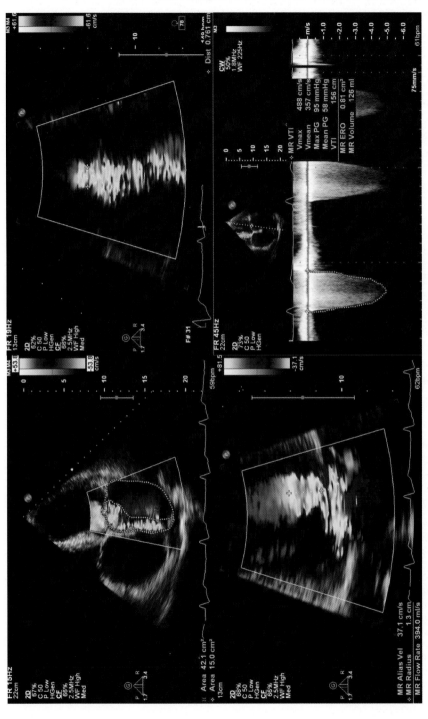

Figure 7.7 An example of assessing the severity of MR using TTE with good acoustic windows. MR colour jet area and LA area (upper left plate); vena contracta (upper right); PISA radius (lower left, baseline shifted *down*); MR velocity with ERO calculation (lower right). Note all the measurements class the MR as severe except for the colour jet area when expressed as 36% of the LA area; the actual jet area is severe (15 cm²) and the percentage is likely to be falsely low due to a dilated LA and the Coanda effect.

⊕ **Clinical tip** Preoperative cardiac catheterization

Cardiac catheterization should be performed if there are risk factors for coronary disease, but the availability of high-quality non-invasive imaging means it is rarely required for assessment of LV parameters or the severity of MR. If conducted, right heart catheterization should also be performed for the assessment of pulmonary artery pressure.

Table 7.2 Indications for MV surgery for chronic organic severe MR (the differences in parameters set by the international societies are highlighted).

	ESC guidelines [2]	ACC/AHA guidelines [3]
Class I	Symptomatic patients with LVEF >30% and LVESD <55 mm (LoE: B)	Symptomatic patients (>NYHA II) with LVEF >30% and/or LVESD <55 mm (LoE: B)
	Asymptomatic patients with LV dysfunction (LVEF ≤60% and/or **LVESD >45 mm**) (LoE: C)	Asymptomatic patients with mild to moderate LV dysfunction (LVEF 30–60% and/or **LVESD ≥40 mm**) (LoE: B)
Class IIa	Asymptomatic patients with preserved LV function and AF or pulmonary hypertension (PAP >50 mmHg at rest) (LoE: C)	Asymptomatic patients with preserved LV function and new onset AF or pulmonary hypertension (PAP >50 mmHg at rest, 60 mmHg on exercise) (LoE: C)
		Asymptomatic patients with preserved LV function (LVEF >60% and LVESD <40 mm) in experienced centres where likelihood of successful repair is >90% (LoE: B)
	Patients with severe LV dysfunction (LVEF <30% and/or LVESD >55 mm) refractory to medical therapy with high likelihood of repair and low comorbidity (LoE: C)	Patients with severe LV dysfunction (LVEF <30% and/or LVESD >55 mm) with primary abnormality of mitral apparatus, with NYHA Class III–IV symptoms in whom repair is likely (LoE: C)
Class IIb	Asymptomatic patients with preserved LV function, high likelihood of repair and low risk for surgery (LoE: B)	
	Patients with severe LV dysfunction (LVEF <30% and/or LVESD >55 mm) refractory to medical therapy with low likelihood of repair and low comorbidity (LoE: C)	MV repair may be considered for patients with severe LV dysfunction (LVEF <30%) who are NYHA Class III–IV despite optimal heart failure treatment (including biventricular pacing) (LoE: C)

LVEF = left ventricular ejection fraction; LVESD = left ventricular end systolic diameter; NYHA = New York Association; LoE = level of evidence.

⑥ **Expert comment**

There are predominantly two methods of MV repair for those with posterior leaflet prolapse. The first is the simple quadrangular resection of part of the posterior leaflet, which produces good long-term results, but causes reduced mobility of the posterior leaflet. The second is to preserve the leaflet without resecting it, and add a number of artificial chords between the papillary muscles and leaflet tips. The advantage of this procedure is that the leaflet's mobility is fully preserved, but long-term results are not yet available for comparison.

In either procedure, an intra-operative TOE study is important in order to evaluate the valve anatomy, confirm the diagnosis, plan the surgical procedure, and also to evaluate surgical results.

⭐ **Learning point** MV surgery

There are three main options for the correction of MR:
- MV repair;
- MV replacement with preservation of part or all of the MV apparatus;
- MV replacement with removal of the mitral apparatus.

MV repair
Operation of choice if:
- The valve is suitable for repair and;
- Appropriate surgical expertise is available.
Benefits:
- Lower post-operative mortality (under 2% vs approximately 6% for replacement) [10,11];
- Better post-operative LV function due to preservation of MV apparatus [12,13];
- Long-term durability up to 25 years [14,15];
- Avoids the need for anticoagulation in the majority with low rates of thromboembolism (if in sinus rhythm);
- Resistance to endocarditis.
Suitability for MV repair:
- Posterior leaflet prolapse can usually be repaired with resection and annuloplasty;
- Involvement of the anterior leaflet makes repair less likely (often requires chordal shortening, chordal transfer, or innovative anatomical repair);
- Rheumatic involvement with leaflet and/or annular calcification makes repair less likely.

continued

MV replacement

The MV apparatus should be preserved in all cases unless this is not feasible, e.g. due to a severely distorted native valve and apparatus, as this ensures post-operative competence, preserves LV function, and reduces mortality [16-18].

Mechanical vs biological prostheses

Mechanical prostheses	Advantages	Durability
	Disadvantages	Need for anticoagulation
		Increased risk of thromboembolism
Biological prostheses	Advantages	No need for anticoagulation
	Disadvantages	Decreased durability, possibly leading to re-operation

Mechanical valves have traditionally been used for patients under the age of 65. Biological prostheses are usually chosen if anticoagulation is contraindicated or in patients over 65, due to a reduced need of re-operation. Recent data suggest that second-generation biological valves may have increased durability than originally thought [19]. The choice of valve will depend on an individual's attributes and preferences, taking into account the advantages and disadvantages of different prostheses.

⭐ **Learning point** Concomitant AF surgery

The development of AF in the context of MR is independently associated with a high risk of cardiac death or heart failure [20], and is a Class IIa indication for MV surgery in asymptomatic patients.

Maze procedures

Scar lines created in the atria at the time of MV surgery can restore sinus rhythm in permanent AF. Efficacy is well established and most studies quote success in groups with a variety of valve pathology. Freedom from AF rates are typically >80%, depending on the method of assessment; using long-term ambulatory ECG monitoring to assess outcome produces lower success rates compared with single electrocardiogram (ECG) assessment [21].

* Surgical: multiple incisions are made in the atria which are then sewn back together [22];
* Cryothermy: 80% chance of cure from permanent AF at five years in a *mixed group* of MV disease [23];
* Radiofrequency ablation: 80% sinus rhythm at one year in patients with *rheumatic mitral valve disease* undergoing MV surgery [24].

⭐ **Learning point** Ischaemic and functional MR

Chronic organic MR is commonly seen in clinical practice and has well established management guidelines. In contrast, management of ischaemic and functional MR is guided by limited data. The following are some important facts regarding these conditions:

* Acute symptomatic MR due to papillary muscle rupture requires urgent surgery.
* Nitroprusside, with the addition of inotropic agents in the event of hypotension, can be used as a bridge to surgery.
* Chronic ischaemic MR is due to restriction in leaflet motion.
* Patients with ischaemic MR tend to have more comorbidities and the outcome is worse compared to organic MR [25].
* Current consensus suggests that severe MR should be corrected at the time of coronary artery bypass grafting, but the management of moderate ischaemic MR remains controversial.
* Functional MR occurs due to LV dilatation in severe LV dysfunction or cardiomyopathy.
* Data are even more limited in functional MR and there is no clear consensus on management.
* Valve repair with a downsized annuloplasty ring is the treatment of choice if undertaken for either condition [26].

Discussion

MR is the second most frequent valvular disorder after aortic stenosis. Management depends on the serial evaluation of symptom development and deterioration in cardiac function assessed with echocardiography. There is no established role for medical therapy and no evidence to support the use of vasodilators, including angiotensin-converting enzyme (ACE) inhibitors, for chronic MR with preserved LV function. If present, atrial fibrillation (AF) and LV systolic dysfunction should be treated by standard protocols. In addition, AF can be treated at the time of MV surgery (see below).

Valve repair is the treatment of choice in all cases of MR where possible. Echocardiography is the mainstay of assessment, but when this is hampered by poor acoustic windows on TTE or intolerability of TOE, newer techniques such as cardiac magnetic resonance provide additional options for a full assessment of MR [27]. Additionally, novel interventional therapies are being introduced for the treatment of MR, which may lead to a change in practice over the coming years.

ⓖ Expert comment

Percutaneous procedures to treat MR are rapidly advancing. At present, enthusiasm amongst cardiologists is far ahead of technological capability, although this is catching up fast. Ultimately, there should be no patient of any age, or indeed any comorbidity, who is denied treatment for MR. A good MV repair in expert surgical hands cannot be replaced by any percutaneous technique now or in the future. Surgical MV repair or percutaneous repair must and should be a joint decision between surgeons and cardiologists, putting the patient's interests first. It is crucial that percutaneous techniques are developed in centres where there is also enough surgical expertise for MV repair.

✪ Learning point Emerging therapies for MR

Percutaneous MV repair with edge-to-edge techniques

- Right heart catheterization and a trans-septal puncture allow the MV to be approached via the left atrium.
- The middle of the anterior and posterior MV leaflets are joined, creating a double orifice MV.
- A clip device has been used in humans with a procedural success in 79 out of 107 patients (74%). A total of 50 of 76 (66%) successfully treated patients were free from death, MV surgery, or MR >2+ at 12 months (primary efficacy endpoint) [28].
- More recently, a suture-based technique has been shown to be feasible, but with technical difficulties and limited durability currently [29].

Percutaneous transvenous mitral annuloplasty

- Right heart catheterization allows a nickel-titanium alloy implant to be placed between the coronary sinus and great cardiac vein.
- The implant has shape-memory properties which result in shortening at body temperature, reducing the mitral annular diameter.
- Implantation has been successful in four out of five patients attempted with reduction in MR, although there were subsequent technical problems with the device in three out of the four implants [30].

💬 A final word from the expert

Patients with even moderate MR have higher mortality rates than patients without. At diagnosis, the single most important investigation is a comprehensive echocardiographic examination which will almost always include a transoesophageal study.

The three 'take home' messages from this case are:

1. Assess symptoms carefully and make sure that 'asymptomatic' patients are truly asymptomatic.
2. Perform a comprehensive echocardiographic examination by an accredited individual.
3. Discuss the findings with an MDT, including cardiac surgeons, for suitability and methods of repair.

There is no doubt that in the future, the assessment of the MV, both anatomical and functional, lies in 3D echocardiography. Although spectacular pictures are currently produced, there are limitations. Real-time 3D echocardiography is currently just adequate from the transoesophageal approach and requires the images obtained to be reconstructed over several beats. The spectrum of MV pathology is just being realized and in the future, 3D valve morphology and function will be obtained from just one beat and in real time and the clarity of the images will be unparalleled.

References

1 Freed LA, Levy D, Levine RA, et al. Prevalence and clinical outcome of mitral valve prolapse. *N Engl J Med* 1999; 341: 1–7.

2 Vahanian A, Baumgartner H, Bax J, et al. Guidelines on the management of valvular heart disease: the Task Force on the management of valvular heart disease of the European Society of Cardiology. *Eur Heart J* 2007; 28: 230–268.

3 Bonow RO, Carabello BA, Chatterjee K, et al. 2008 focused update incorporated into the ACC/AHA 2006 guidelines for the management of patients with valvular heart disease: a report of the American College of Cardiology/American Heart Association Task Force on practice guidelines (Writing Committee to revise the 1998 guidelines for the management of patients with valvular heart disease). Endorsed by the Society of Cardiovascular Anaesthesiologists, Society for Cardiovascular Angiography and Interventions, and Society of Thoracic Surgeons. *J Am Coll Cardiol* 2008; 52: e1–142.

4 Zoghbi WA, Enriquez-Sarano M, Foster E, et al. Recommendations for evaluation of the severity of native valvular regurgitation with two-dimensional and Doppler echocardiography. *J Am Soc Echocardiogr* 2003; 16: 777–802.

5 Lung B, Gohlke-Barwolf C, Tornos P, et al. Recommendations on the management of the asymptomatic patient with valvular heart disease. *Eur Heart J* 2002; 23: 1253–1266.

6 Marciniak A, Claus P, Sutherland GR, et al. Changes in systolic left ventricular function in isolated mitral regurgitation. *A strain rate imaging study. Eur Heart J* 2007; 28: 2627–2636.

7 Carpentier A. Cardiac valve surgery—the 'French correction'. *J Thorac Cardiovasc Surg* 1983; 86: 323–337.

8 Delabays A, Jeanrenaud X, Chassot PG, et al. Localization and quantification of mitral valve prolapse using three-dimensional echocardiography. *Eur J Echocardiogr* 2004; 5: 422–429.

9 Sugeng L, Spencer KT, Mor-Avi V, et al. Dynamic three-dimensional color flow Doppler: an improved technique for the assessment of mitral regurgitation. *Echocardiography* 2003; 20: 265–273.

10 The Society of Cardiothoracic Surgeons of Great Britain and Ireland National Adult Cardiac Surgical Database Report 2003. The Society of Cardiothoracic Surgeons 2004. Available from: http://www.scts.org/documents/PDF/5thBlueBook2003.pdf.

11 STS adult cardiac surgery database: executive summary. Society of Thoracic Surgeons 2008. Available from: http://www.sts.org/documents/pdf/ndb/4thHarvestExecutiveSummary.pdf.

12 Enriquez-Sarano M, Schaff HV, Orszulak TA, et al. Valve repair improves the outcome of surgery for mitral regurgitation. A multivariate analysis. *Circulation* 1995; 91: 1022–1028.

13 Tischler MD, Cooper KA, Rowen M, LeWinter MM. Mitral valve replacement versus mitral valve repair. A Doppler and quantitative stress echocardiographic study. *Circulation* 1994; 89: 132–137.

14 Fedak PWM, McCarthy PM, Bonow RO. Evolving concepts and technologies in mitral valve repair. *Circulation* 2008; 117: 963–974.

15 Mohty D, Orszulak TA, Schaff HV, et al. Very long-term survival and durability of mitral valve repair for mitral valve prolapse. *Circulation* 2001; 104(12 Suppl 1): I1–I7.

16 David TE, Uden DE, Strauss HD. The importance of the mitral apparatus in left ventricular function after correction of mitral regurgitation. *Circulation* 1983; 68(3 Pt 2): II76–82.

17 Horskotte D, Schulte HD, Bircks W, Strauer BE. The effect of chordal preservation on late outcome after mitral valve replacement: a randomized study. *J Heart Valve Dis* 1993; 2: 150–158.

18 Rozich JD, Carabello BA, Usher BW, et al. Mitral valve replacement with and without chordal preservation in patients with chronic mitral regurgitation. Mechanisms for differences in post-operative ejection performance. *Circulation* 1992; 86: 1718–1726.

19 Demirag M, Kirali K, Omeroglu SN, et al. Mechanical versus biological valve prosthesis in the mitral position: a 10-year follow-up of St. Jude Medical and Biocor valves. *J Heart Valve Dis* 2001; 10: 78–83.

20 Grigioni F, Avierinos JF, Ling LH, et al. Atrial fibrillation complicating the course of degenerative mitral regurgitation: determinants and long-term outcome. *J Am Coll Cardiol* 2002; 40: 84–92.

21 Ad N, Henry L, Hunt S, Barnett S, Stone L. The Cox–Maze III procedure success rate: comparison by electrocardiogram, 24-hour holter monitoring and long-term monitoring. *Ann Thorac Surg* 2009; 88: 101–105.

22 Cox JL, Schuessler RB, D'Agostino HJ, Jr., et al. The surgical treatment of atrial fibrillation. *III. Development of a definitive surgical procedure. J Thorac Cardiovasc Surg* 1991; 101: 569–583.

23 Funatsu T, Kobayashi J, Nakajima H, et al. Long-term results and reliability of cryothermic ablation-based maze procedure for atrial fibrillation concomitant with mitral valve surgery. *Eur J Cardiothorac Surg* 2009; 36: 267–271.

24 Breu Filho CA, Lisboa LA, Dallan LA, et al. Effectiveness of the maze procedure using cooled tip radiofrequency ablation in patients with permanent atrial fibrillation and rheumatic mitral valve disease. *Circulation* 2005; 112(9 Suppl): I20–25.

25 Lung B. Management of ischaemic mitral regurgitation. *Heart* 2003; 89: 459–464.

26 Bax JJ, Braun J, Somer ST, et al. Restrictive annuloplasty and coronary revascularization in ischaemic mitral regurgitation results in reverse left ventricular remodelling. *Circulation* 2004; 110(11 Suppl 1): II103–II108.

27 Chan KJ, Wage R, Symmonds K, et al. Towards comprehensive assessment of mitral regurgitation using cardiovascular magnetic resonance. *J Cardiovasc Magn Reson* 2008; 10: 61.

28 Feldman T, Kar S, Rinaldi M, et al. Percutaneous mitral repair with the MitraClip system: safety and mid-term durability in the initial EVEREST (Endovascular Valve Edge-to-Edge REpair Study) cohort. *J Am Coll Cardiol* 2009; 54: 686–694.

29 Webb JG, Maisano F, Vahanian A, et al. Percutaneous suture edge-to-edge repair of the mitral valve. *EuroIntervention* 2009; 5: 86–89.

30 Webb JG, Harnek J, Munt BI, et al. Percutaneous transvenous mitral annuloplasty: initial human experience with device implantation in the coronary sinus. *Circulation* 2006; 113: 851–855.

Streptococcus mutans endocarditis: a cautionary tale

William Moody and Aung Myat

Ⓒ **Expert commentary** Dr Bernard Prendergast

Case history

A 43-year-old Afro-Caribbean man was admitted with a 2-month history of worsening lethargy, malaise, night sweats, and weight loss. He was a known hypertensive and had a bicuspid aortic valve (AV) with evidence of mild stenosis. An echocardiogram 12 months previously had revealed a peak gradient of 21 mmHg associated with trivial aortic incompetence and normal biventricular function. There was no history of a recent invasive procedure, foreign travel, or rheumatic fever and no risk factors for human immunodeficiency virus (HIV) infection. He was taking amlodipine, bendroflumethiazide, and doxazosin. He did not smoke and the family history was unremarkable.

On admission, he was pyrexial at 38.6°C and a wide pulse pressure was noted at 160/42 mmHg associated with a large-volume collapsing pulse. Corrigan's sign was evident in his neck. Whilst he was slow in his cerebration, there was no focal neurology of note. There were no peripheral stigmata of infective endocarditis (IE) although dentition was poor. On auscultation, he had a grade 3/6 short high-pitched early diastolic murmur and a soft first heart sound (S1) consistent with severe aortic regurgitation (AR). There was no splenomegaly. Clinically, he had a degree of pulmonary congestion, but his chest X-ray excluded any significant oedema, effusions, or consolidation. Urinary dipstick was negative for blood or protein. Blood results are noted in Table 8.1. An electrocardiogram (ECG) revealed sinus rhythm with borderline left ventricular (LV) hypertrophy, but no evidence of heart block.

Given the clinical context, three sets of peripheral blood cultures were taken within 12 hours of admission. The first became positive within 24 hours, revealing Gram-positive rods. The isolate was initially reported as 'diphtheroids' and the laboratory presumed these to be contaminants. In view of the clinical findings, however, and ongoing fever, intravenous (IV) gentamicin (1.0 mg/kg every eight hours) and benzylpenicillin (2.4 g every six hours) were initiated. An urgent transthoracic echocardiogram (TTE)

Table 8.1 Blood results on admission

Haematology		Biochemistry	
Hb	**8.6 g/dL**	C reactive protein	**105 mg/L**
MCV	**72.1 fL**	Albumin	**30 g/L**
WCC	9.24×10^9/L	Bilirubin	16 micromol/L
Neutrophils	**7.77** $\times 10^9$/L	Alanine aminotransferase	12 IU/L
Platelets	254×10^9/L		
INR	1.2		
Reticulocytes	69×10^9/L		

was arranged within 24 hours of admission, demonstrating a vegetation attached to the bicuspid AV. Severe AR with aortic root turbulence, mild impairment of LV function, and a small anterior pericardial effusion were also noted.

The remaining two sets of blood cultures became positive within 36 hours. Gram-positive rods were again seen and on review of the original Gram stains, the organisms were deemed more likely to be streptococci. After four days, the reference laboratory confirmed the isolates in all three culture sets to be a fully sensitive *Streptococcus (S.) mutans* species.

> ⭐ **Learning point** Comment on *S. mutans*
>
> This is not the first report of a case of *S. mutans* endocarditis in which the organisms were initially dismissed as a diphtheroid species. This re-emphasizes the importance of sound clinical judgement in the face of test results that do not equate with the clinical picture. As far back as 1977, Emmerson and Eykyn highlighted two cases in which they acknowledged this potential blunder as a 'trap for the unwary' [1]. More recently, Schelenz, et al. commented on a delay in diagnosing their case of *S. mutans* endocarditis in a man who had previously undergone a Ross procedure (pulmonary valve autograft to the aortic position) [2]. *S. mutans* was initially described in 1924 by Clarke in the aetiology of dental caries [3]. He noted the variation in morphology with the pH of the culture medium. It is on the basis of their rod-shaped appearance in blood culture medium that allows them to be misidentified as diphtheroids which tend to be regarded as non-pathogenic skin commensals.

The patient was known to have learning difficulties, but in view of the objective increase in cognitive impairment, an urgent brain computed tomography (CT) scan was conducted to rule out cerebral abscess formation secondary to septic emboli from the aortic vegetation. Right frontal encephalomalacia with an atrophic right temporal lobe together with asymmetry in the vault were noted (Figure 8.1). This was later attributed to hypoxic brain injury suffered by the patient *in utero*.

> ⭐ **Learning point** Making the diagnosis of IE
>
> The hallmark immunologic vascular features of subacute bacterial endocarditis as described originally in its Oslerian form are becoming increasingly infrequent in contemporary medicine. Whilst it is still worthwhile looking for them, it is rare nowadays to see signs such as Osler's nodes, Janeway lesions, petechiae, Roth spots, and splenomegaly. This is largely because IE is invariably seen in its acute form where there has not been time for the development of immunologic phenomena to evolve. It is of utmost importance, however, that IE is considered early in any patient with a new cardiac murmur together with the presence of fever coupled with other systemic symptoms of septicaemia. Central to the diagnosis of IE is the demonstration of the offending organism on blood culture. Three sets of blood cultures obtained at intervals of more than one hour within the first 24 hours is the recommended norm. In selected patients, more sets may be required, particularly before making a diagnosis of culture-negative endocarditis. It should be noted that up to 30% of blood cultures are negative when obtained after the first dose of antibiotic [4]. This clearly has implications on the ability to deliver targeted therapy. For this reason, blood cultures should be obtained in all patients with suspected endocarditis prior to receiving antibiotics.
>
> The absence of vegetations on echocardiography does not refute the diagnosis of IE and in these cases, the complete clinical syndrome should be considered. That said, echocardiography remains the benchmark investigation both in the diagnosis of vegetations as well as identifying potential valvular and other structural complications. It is well established that the sensitivity for visualization of vegetations for transthoracic echocardiography (TTE) is inferior to that of transoesophageal echocardiography (TOE) (60–77% rising to 96% in sensitivity). This is especially pertinent in the

continued

---

assessment of prosthetic valves. For this reason, if the suspicion of IE is high, the European Society of Cardiology (ESC) recommends a TOE should be performed in all of the following patients:

- Those with a negative TTE;
- Those with suspected prosthetic valve endocarditis;
- Those with suspected complications in TTE-positive patients;
- Those awaiting cardiac surgery (class IB recommendation) [4].

Size and precise location of vegetations and aortic root abscesses can only be defined with TOE. In cases where there is difficulty in making a diagnosis, it is worth employing the accepted Duke or modified Duke criteria (Table 8.2).

Table 8.2 Modified Duke criteria for the diagnosis of IE (adapted from Habib et al. [4])

Definite diagnosis of IE	Possible diagnosis of IE
Pathological criteria	**Clinical criteria**
Pathological lesions confirmed by histological examination or culture of a vegetation directly	1 major and 1 minor criterion; or 3 minor criteria
Clinical criteria	
2 major criteria; or	
1 major and 3 minor criteria; or	
5 minor criteria	
Major criteria	**Minor criteria**
Blood culture positive for IE:	**Predisposition, predisposing heart condition or IVDU**
Typical microorganisms consistent with IE from two separate blood cultures: *Viridans streptococci*, *S. bovis*, HACEK group, *S. aureus*, or community-acquired enterococci in the absence of a primary focus; Microorganisms consistent with IE from persistently positive blood cultures (i.e. at least two positive cultures drawn >12 h apart; or	**Fever >38°C**
	Immunologic phenomena:
	Glomerulonephritis, Osler's nodes, Roth's spots, and rheumatoid factor
All of three or a majority of ≥4 separate cultures of blood); Single positive blood culture for *Coxiella burnetti*; or Anti-phase 1 IgG antibody titre >1:800	**Vascular phenomena:**
Evidence of endocardial involvement:	Major arterial emboli, septic pulmonary emboli, mycotic aneurysm, intracranial bleed, Janeway lesions, conjunctival haemorrhages
Oscillating intracardiac mass on valve or supporting structures, in the path of regurgitant jets, or on implanted material; Abscess formation; New partial dehiscence of a prosthetic valve; or New valvular regurgitation (worsening or changing pre-existing murmur deemed insufficient)	**Microbiological evidence:**
	Positive blood culture, but not meeting major criterion on serological evidence of active infection with an organism consistent with IE

🔁 Expert comment

S. mutans is a non-haemolytic Gram-positive commensal of the oral cavity and a primary cause of dental caries. The organism can survive in the bloodstream and virulence factors for IE include a fibronectin-binding protein (AtlA autolysin), serotype-specific polysaccharides associated with phagocytosis resistance, and cell surface protein antigen C which is involved in platelet aggregation. Conventional laboratory identification techniques can misidentify the organism and 16S ribosomal sequencing may be required for formal identification.

➕ Clinical tip Mycotic aneurysms (MA)

- These are a complication of IE resulting from septic embolization of vegetations to the arterial vasa vasorum or the intraluminal space with subsequent seeding of infection beyond the vessel wall via the intima.
- Arterial branching points are the commonest sites for the development of MA as they favour the impaction of emboli.
- MA caused by IE occur most frequently in the intracranial arteries (ICMA), followed by the visceral arteries (splenic and hepatic abscesses) and the arteries of the upper and lower extremities.

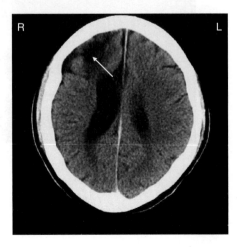

Figure 8.1 Computed tomography of the brain with contrast demonstrating the result of hypoxic brain injury in utero (arrow), but no evidence of cerebral abscess formation.

Although the so-called 'Oslerian' manifestations of IE are now rare in industrialized nations, they are frequently found in the developing world where rheumatic valve disease and streptococcal infection remain common and delays before medical assessment are frequent.

Embolic complications of IE are common and no vascular bed is spared, the cerebral circulation being most frequently affected. Silent emboli may often arise and a low threshold of suspicion is recommended, particularly in patients with subtle neurological signs or persistent fever. Routine CT scanning of the head and abdomen is common practice in many centres, particularly in the US and mainland Europe where such investigations are readily available.

✪ Learning point Intracranial MA: when to perform a brain CT?

Neurological complications develop in up to 40% of patients with IE [5,6]. ICMA represents a relatively small, but extremely dangerous, subset of these complications. Whilst cerebral angiography remains the gold standard imaging modality with a sensitivity of 90–95% for intracerebral bleeding [7], an urgent non-contrast CT brain as the initial investigation is reasonable [8]. The clinical presentation of patients with ICMA is highly variable and this was the rationale behind our brain CT request. Patients may develop severe headache, altered sensorium, or focal neurological deficits such as hemianopia or cranial neuropathies; neurological signs and symptoms are non-specific and may suggest a mass lesion or an embolic event. Some ICMA can leak slowly, producing mild meningeal irritation (a 'herald bleed') before finally rupturing. Frequently, the spinal fluid in these patients is sterile, often containing a mixture of erythrocytes, leucocytes, and elevated protein. In other patients, there are no recognized red flags before often catastrophic subarachnoid or intraventricular haemorrhage [9]. In the absence of clinical signs or symptoms of ICMA, routine screening with imaging studies is not warranted. Symptomatic cerebral emboli often, but not always, precede the finding of an ICMA [10]. In those with focal neurological signs, localized or severe headaches, and in those with 'sterile' meningitis (especially if erythrocytes or xanthochromia is present), imaging to rule out ICMA is clearly warranted. The reported occurrence of ICMA in 1.2–5% of cases is probably underestimated because some ICMA remain asymptomatic and resolve with antimicrobial therapy [11,12].

Despite prompt antimicrobial therapy, the patient's fever persisted and diuretic therapy was soon required for increasing pulmonary congestion. Four days into admission, a TOE was organized, confirming severe AR and an echo-free space around the non-coronary cusp of the AV consistent with an abscess (Figures 8.2 and 8.3). Vegetations were seen attached to both leaflets. Given the severity of AR, abscess formation, and imminent cardiac decompensation, he was transferred urgently to a surgical centre for consideration of AV replacement (AVR). The patient proceeded to exploratory aortic root and valve surgery (Figure 8.4 and Operation note).

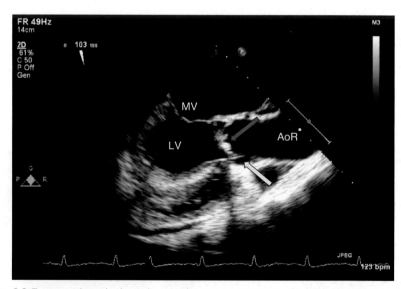

Figure 8.2 Transoesophageal echocardiogram showing vegetations attached to both aortic valve leaflets (blue arrow) and an echo-free space (yellow arrow) around the non-coronary cusp. MV = mitral valve; LV = left ventricle; AoR = aortic root.

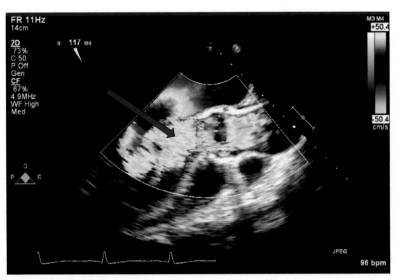

Figure 8.3 Transoesophageal echocardiogram with colour flow across aortic valve, confirming a broad jet of severe aortic regurgitation (arrow).

> ⭐ **Learning point** Comment on the haemodynamics of acute aortic insufficiency
>
> In acute AR, for instance, secondary to a perforation of the AV due to endocarditis, there is a sudden increase in the volume of blood in the left ventricle. In terms of the Frank–Starling curve, the end-diastolic volume becomes very high such that further increases in volume result in a deleterious effect on stroke volume (SV). This results in less efficient contraction. As the filling pressure of the left ventricle increases, this causes pressure in the left atrium to rise, resulting in the development of acute pulmonary oedema.
>
> Acute AR usually presents as florid congestive heart failure, but will not have any of the signs associated with chronic AR since the left ventricle has not yet developed the eccentric hypertrophy and dilatation that allows for an increased SV leading to bounding peripheral pulses. On auscultation, there may be a short diastolic murmur and a soft S1. The first heart sound is soft because the elevated filling pressures close the mitral valve (MV) in diastole (rather than the MV being closed at the beginning of systole).

⭕ **Operation note**

'The aorta was cross-clamped and the ascending aorta was opened. The AV has almost been completely destroyed by infection and vegetations. An abnormal area at the base of the anterior MV leaflet not thought to represent an abscess, but the result of the severe AR jet. Further vegetations seen on the aortic wall itself just distal and to the left of the left coronary ostium, itself abnormally displaced to the right. This area was scraped clear and cleaned with rifampicin. No cavity seen; only cracks in the endothelium. The valve was replaced with a 23 mm Sorin Slimline Bicarbon bileaflet mechanical prosthesis with interrupted Teflon sutures. Sutures were utilized to close off the roughened area at the base of the MV.'

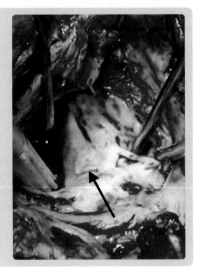

Figure 8.4 Aortic annulus abscess (arrow). With permission from Al-Attar N. Infective endocarditis. *E-Journal of the ESC Council for Cardiology Practice* 2008;7(15).

✚ **Clinical tip** Emergency indications for urgent same-day surgery

- Acute AR causing refractory pulmonary oedema and echocardiographic signs of poor haemodynamic tolerance (early closure of MV);
- Rupture of the sinus of Valsalva into right heart;
- Rupture of a pseudoaneurysm into the pericardium.

❝ Expert comment

So I was right! The AR was clearly severe at presentation and decompensation requiring surgery almost inevitable. Hindsight is a wonderful thing, but TOE and transfer to a surgical centre (or at least consultation) should have been considered earlier. It is interesting to note that the initial ECG was normal; newly developed first-degree atrioventricular block is a highly specific indicator of aortic root abscess and a daily ECG is mandatory in patients with IE affecting the AV.

✪ Learning point On whom and when should we operate in IE?

Surgery for native valve endocarditis
There is a distinct paucity of robust data available to guide clinicians on specific indications for surgery in IE. To date, there are no available randomized trials or any registries addressing this issue. The best available evidence is from a study addressing IE complicated by cardiac failure. This showed that in patients with severe congestive cardiac failure secondary to acute aortic incompetence or mitral incompetence, mortality was reduced from 56–86% in those who received medical treatment alone to 11–35% in those who received a combined medical and surgical approach. NYHA class III–IV symptoms in such patients remain the most common and best validated indication for surgery with haemodynamic status being the best determinant of peri-operative mortality [15]. Heart failure secondary to acute AR has a worse outcome compared with failure secondary to acute MR, but both entities merit surgery.

Surgery is indicated in those patients who have persistent fever with demonstration of bacteraemia for more than eight days despite adequate antibiotic therapy [16].

Demonstration of abscesses, pseudoaneurysms, fistulas, conduction disturbances, or other findings indicating an uncontrolled local spread of infection warrant surgical intervention [16].

On the basis of an increasing risk of septic embolization, early surgery should be considered in those with vegetations larger than 10 mm on the MV if they are increasing in size despite antimicrobial therapy or if they represent kissing vegetations (Table 8.3). For right-sided vegetations, the cut off is set at 20 mm [17].

Surgery should be considered in those infected with microorganisms which are frequently not cured by antibiotic therapy (e.g. fungi, *Brucella*, and *Coxiella*) or organisms with a potential for rapid destruction of cardiac structures (e.g. *S. lugdunensis*).

Surgery for active prosthetic valve endocarditis
There is an agreed early indication for surgery in patients with a prosthetic valve implanted less than 12 months previously as these patients tend to deteriorate rapidly.

Timing of surgery
The exact timing of surgical intervention is based on even more limited data, the best of which stem from a subset of patients with cerebral embolism. In a case involving ischaemic neurological injury, there is reasonable evidence to operate within the first 72 hours and if this is not possible, then surgery should be delayed for at least two weeks (or four weeks in the case of haemorrhagic stroke) [18].

Severe acute aortic insufficiency is considered a medical emergency. There is a high mortality rate if the individual does not undergo immediate surgery for AVR. If the acute AR is due to aortic valve endocarditis, there is a risk that the new valve may become seeded with bacteria. However, this risk is small [19].

The patient made a speedy post-operative recovery and was transferred back to the referring hospital in order to complete a further two weeks of IV gentamicin (3.0 mg/kg/day) and a further four weeks of IV benzylpencillin (2.4 g every six hours). Ten days following his surgery, however, he developed a significant neutropaenia (1.14 × 10^9/L) and began spiking temperatures. All repeat cultures, including three sets of blood, one sputum, and two urine, came back negative. A repeat TTE at that time showed the valve to be well seated and functioning well and no obvious vegetations. He was now 21 days post-starting high dose beta-lactam therapy. After testing positive on an antihuman globulin-containing gel test for haemagglutinating pencillin antibodies, the microbiologists advised a change in his antibiotic therapy to four weeks of oral rifampicin (450 mg every eight hours) and IV vancomycin (15 mg/kg every 12 hours). Within 72 hours, his neutrophils had recovered to normal levels and he became afebrile.

Table 8.3 Indications and timing of surgery in left-sided native valve infective endocarditis (NVE) [4]

Recommendations: indications for surgery	Timing[†]	Class[a]	Level[b]
A–HEART FAILURE			
Aortic or mitral IE with severe acute regurgitation or valve obstruction causing refractory pulmonary oedema or cardiogenic shock	Emergency	I	B
Aortic or mitral IE with fistula into cardiac chamber or pericardium causing refractory pulmonary oedema or cardiogenic shock	Emergency	I	B
Aortic or mitral IE with severe acute regurgitation or valve obstruction and persisting heart failure or echocardiographic signs of poor haemodynamic tolerance (early MV closure or pulmonary hypertension)	Urgent	I	B
Aortic or mitral IE with severe regurgitation and heart failure	Elective	IIa	B
B–UNCONTROLLED INFECTION			
Locally uncontrolled infection (abscess, false aneurysm, fistula, enlarging vegetation)	Urgent	I	B
Persisting fever and positive blood cultures >7–10 days	Urgent	I	B
Infection caused by fungi or multiresistant organisms	Urgent/elective	I	B
C–PREVENTION OF EMBOLISM			
Aortic or mitral IE with large vegetations (>10 mm) following one or more embolic events despite appropriate antibiotic therapy	Urgent	I	B
Aortic or mitral IE with large vegetations (>10 mm) and other predictors of complicated course (heart failure, persistent infection, abscess)	Urgent	I	C
Isolated, very large vegetations (>15 mm)*	Urgent	IIb	C

[a] Class of recommendation; [b] Level of evidence * Emergency surgery: surgery performed within 24 hours; Urgent surgery: within few days; Elective surgery: after at least one or two weeks of antibiotics; * Surgery may be preferred if procedure preserving the native valve is feasible.

Adapted with permission from Habib G, Hoen B, Tornos P et al. Guidelines on prevention, diagnosis and treatment of infective endocarditis (new version 2009); the task force on the prevention, diagnosis and treatment of infective endocarditis of the European Society of Cardiology (ESC). *Eur Heart J* 2009; 30: 2369–2413 with permission and copyright Oxford University Press.

⊕ **Learning point** Defining classes of recommendations and levels of evidence

Class of recommendation	Definition
I	Conditions for which there is evidence, general agreement, or both that a given procedure or treatment is useful and effective
II	Conditions for which there is conflicting evidence, a divergence of opinion, or both about the usefulness/efficacy of a procedure or treatment
IIa	Weight of evidence/opinion is in favour of usefulness/efficacy
IIb	Usefulness/efficacy is less well established by evidence/opinion
III	Conditions for which there is evidence, general agreement, or both that the procedure/treatment is not useful/effective and in some cases, may be harmful

Level of evidence

A Data derived from multiple randomized clinical trials
B Data derived from a single randomized trial or non-randomized studies
C Consensus opinion of experts

The mantra of six weeks post-operative antibiotic therapy has been challenged by recent European guidelines [4] and it is now recommended that the date of initiation of appropriate and effective antibiotic therapy is designated the first day of treatment and not the day of surgery. The only exception to this is when microscopy and culture of the excised valve (or other material) demonstrates persistent viable organisms when a 6-week course of post-operative treatment remains appropriate. Discussion with microbiological colleagues is recommended when the most appropriate regime is uncertain.

⭐ **Expert comment**

The sequence of post-operative complications was relatively unusual and it is possible that the original postulated penicillin reaction was the first indicator of persistent infection in the aortic root. In any event, repeat surgery was clearly appropriate and should always be actively considered in patients with early prosthetic valve endocarditis. A homograft was a very reasonable choice of second prosthesis, but it should be borne in mind that late complications (notably prosthetic calcification) over the next decade may require further technically challenging surgery in this young man. He will also require rigorous dental care and I would have sought a dental consult at an earlier stage. Whether he should have antibiotic prophylaxis at the time of invasive dental procedures is controversial; this would certainly be recommended by the current European guidelines [4], but not by the UK National Institute of Health and Clinical Excellence (NICE) recommendations [20]. If it were me (or one of my family), I think I would adopt the European view until a randomized controlled trial demonstrated that antibiotic prophylaxis was unnecessary.

⭐ **Learning point** Incidence of beta-lactam-induced neutropaenia

Benzylpencillin (penicillin G) given in large doses, often for as long as six weeks, has been the cornerstone of bacterial endocarditis management. Indeed, it is still recommended as part of empirical therapy before cultures are available. Severe neutropaenia with onset during the third or fourth week has been reported in up to 15% of treated episodes [13]. A clinical syndrome of neutropaenia, abundant neutrophil precursors, a lack of well differentiated myeloid elements on bone marrow aspiration, and a lack of complete recovery one to seven days after discontinuation of beta-lactam therapy has been reported in several series. The mechanism remains poorly understood although drug-specific antibodies to penicilloyated neutrophils remain an attractive proposition not dissimilar to that which occurs in penicillin-induced immune haemolytic anaemia. It is suggested that the antigenicity of penicillin preparations is caused by giving penicillin G solutions that are not freshly prepared, allowing degradation products to form which gives rise to antigenically active metabolites [13,14]. The advice is to use freshly prepared solutions that may potentially reduce all kinds of immune-mediated adverse reactions to penicillin.

He remained well for three weeks and was on the verge of discharge when he began to spike further temperatures. Within 48 hours, his inflammatory markers, including white cells and C reactive protein, rose significantly. Once again, he grew nothing from cultures, but in view of a persisting pyrexia, an urgent repeat TOE was organized (Figures 8.5 and 8.6). This indicated a small paravalvular leak together with a swollen aortic root at the level of the sinus of Valsalva and echo-free spaces seen anteriorly and posteriorly, suggesting further abscess formation. He was immediately transferred back to the cardiac surgeons and underwent emergency homograft aortic root replacement after excision of the aortic root abscess and mechanical valve. Cultures from the pericardial fluid, aorta, and the mechanical valve subsequently proved negative. The microbiologists were again involved and a joint decision was made with the cardiac surgeons to start a 6-week course of IV daptomycin. He subsequently made an uneventful post-operative recovery and the LV function was shown to be preserved on his latest echocardiogram. He was discharged home to complete the last two weeks of antibiotic therapy and an outpatient dental consult was arranged.

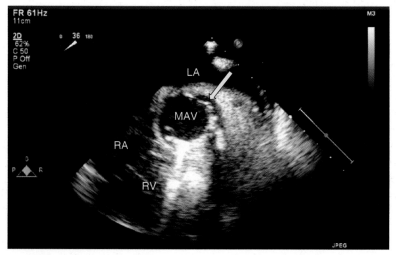

Figure 8.5 Transoesophageal echocardiogram in short axis view showing a large area of echo-free space (yellow arrow). RA = right atrium; RV = right ventricle; LA = left atrium; MAV = mechanical aortic valve.

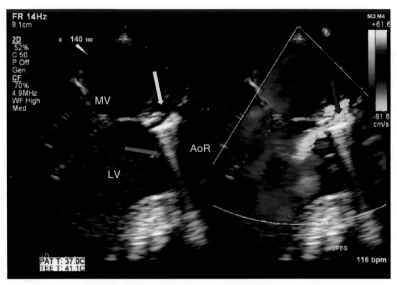

Figure 8.6 Transoesophageal echocardiogram revealing a small paravalvular leak (red arrow) around the periphery of the mechanical aortic valve (green arrow) secondary to an echo-free space (yellow arrow), suggesting abscess formation. MV = mitral valve; LV = left ventricle; AoR = aortic root.

Discussion

Endocarditis remains a serious and often fatal disease with multiple cardiac and extracardiac sequelae. The management of IE should be based primarily on sound clinical judgement and where at all possible, should involve a coordinated team approach comprising a cardiologist, microbiologist, and cardiac surgeon in order to maximize the chances of a successful outcome. Blood cultures should be obtained in all patients with suspected IE prior to therapy with antibiotics. In patients requiring lengthy courses of high-dose beta-lactam therapy, the possibility of myeloid suppression resulting in a clinical syndrome of neutropaenia should be borne in mind. This case also underlines the important rule of not dismissing the growth of Gram-positive rods in blood cultures as a skin contaminant while the clinical diagnosis remains in doubt. IE should always be considered early in patients presenting with unexplained fever, particularly in the presence of an abnormal native valve such as a bicuspid AV or an intracardiac prosthesis.

Any review of endocarditis would not be complete without mention of the recent controversy surrounding prophylaxis. It is noteworthy that after the introduction of the recent NICE guidance, the widespread use of antibiotic prophylaxis for IE is no longer supported [20]. Whilst NICE identifies patients at increased risk of developing IE, it does not advocate prophylaxis for any dental or respiratory procedures and reserves the use of antibiotics for gastrointestinal and genitourinary procedures that are being performed for an underlying infection (in which case the antimicrobials chosen should cover IE-causative organisms). This approach reflects the virulence of enterococcal organisms. The NICE guidelines were initially met with dissatisfaction by many cardiologists who, in dealing directly with the complications of IE in their patients, were naturally fearful of its consequences and so upheld the dogma of prevention by antibiotic prophylaxis before invasive procedures.

Table 8.4 Cardiac conditions at highest risk of endocarditis for which prophylaxis is recommended when a high-risk procedure is performed [4]

Recommendations: prophylaxis	Class[a]	Level[b]
Antibiotic prophylaxis should only be considered for patients at high risk of IE	IIa	C
1. Patients with a prosthetic valve or prosthetic material used for cardiac valve repair		
2. Patients with previous IE		
3. Patients with congenital heart disease		
• Cyanotic congenital heart disease, without surgical repair, or with residual defects, shunts or conduits		
• Congenital heart disease with complete repair with prosthetic material (surgery or percutaneous technique) up to six months after the procedure		
• When a residual defect persists at the site of implantation of a device or prosthetic material (surgery or percutaneous technique)		
Antibiotic prophylaxis is no longer recommended in other forms of valvular or congenital heart disease	III	C

Adapted with permission from Habib G, Hoen B, Tornos P et al. Guidelines on prevention, diagnosis and treatment of infective endocarditis (new version 2009); the task force on the prevention, diagnosis and treatment of infective endocarditis of the European Society of Cardiology (ESC). *Eur Heart J* 2009; 30: 2369–2413 with permission and copyright Oxford University Press.

Table 8.5 Recommendations for prophylaxis of IE in high risk patients according to the type of procedure at risk [4]

	Class[a]	Level[b]
A–Dental procedures:		
Antibiotic prophylaxis should only be considered for dental procedures requiring manipulation of the gingival or periapical region of the teeth or perforation of the oral mucosa	IIa	C
Antibiotic prophylaxis is not recommended for local anaesthetic injections in non-infected tissue, removal of sutures, dental X-rays, placement or adjustment of removable prosthodontic or orthodontic appliances or braces. Nor is it recommended following shedding of deciduous teeth or trauma to the lips and oral mucosa.	III	C
B–Respiratory tract procedures[†]:		
Antibiotic prophylaxis is not recommended for respiratory tract procedures, including bronchoscopy or laryngoscopy, transnasal or endotracheal intubation.	III	C
C–Gastrointestinal or urogenital procedures[†]:		
Antibiotic prophylaxis is not recommended[†] for gastroscopy, colonoscopy, cystoscopy, or TOE	III	C
D–Skin and soft tissue[†]:		
Antibiotic prophylaxis is not recommended for any procedure	III	C

[†] Except in cases where an invasive procedure is performed in the context of an established infection, e.g. drainage of an abscess; [a] Class of recommendation; [b] Level of evidence.
Reproduced with permission from Habib G, Hoen B, Tornos P et al. Guidelines on prevention, diagnosis and treatment of infective endocarditis (new version 2009); the task force on the prevention, diagnosis and treatment of infective endocarditis of the European Society of Cardiology (ESC). *Eur Heart J* 2009; 30: 2369–2413 with permission and copyright Oxford University Press.

The ESC conducted a review of the existing evidence for the efficacy of endocarditis prophylaxis and published its updated guidelines in 2009 [4]. Previous guidance had been issued on the basis of non-uniform expert opinion, data from animal work, case reports, and contradicting observational studies. Given the lack of prospective randomized controlled data, the ESC no longer supports the blanket use of antibiotic prophylaxis as was recommended previously. Prophylaxis should now be limited to the highest risk patients. In contrast to NICE, the ESC does advocate consideration of prophylaxis for complex dental procedures (Tables 8.4 and 8.5). Optimal dental hygiene and regular dental review still play an important role in preventing the development of IE.

> **A final word from the expert**
>
> This case certainly confirms the complexity and dangers of IE. Despite advances in diagnosis, antibiotic treatment, and surgery, the mortality of the condition remains high (30% at one year and higher in certain subsets) with frequent devastating complications and the need for cardiac surgery in 50% of patients. The disease remains a challenge to cardiologists, microbiologists, and cardiac surgeons and best outcomes are obtained by the interaction of an expert multidisciplinary team.

References

1 Emmerson AM, Eykyn S. *Streptococcus mutans* endocarditis–a trap for the unwary. *Br Med J* 1977; 1: 905.

2 Schelenz S, Page AJF, Emmerson AM. *Streptococcus mutans* endocarditis: beware of the 'diphtheroid'. *J R Soc Med* 2005; 98: 420–421.

3 Clarke JK. On the bacterial factor in the aetiology of dental caries. *Br J Exper Pathol* 1924; 5: 141–147.

4 Habib G, Hoen B, Tornos P, et al. Guidelines on prevention, diagnosis and treatment of infective endocarditis (new version 2009); the task force on the prevention, diagnosis and treatment of infective endocarditis of the European Society of Cardiology (ESC). *Eur Heart J* 2009; 30: 2369–2413.

5 Francioli P. Central nervous system complications of infective endocarditis. In: Scheld WM, Whiteley RJ, Durack DT, editors. Infections of the Central Nervous System. New York, NY: Raven Press. 1991; 515–559.

6 Heiro M, Nikoskelainen J, Engblom E, et al. Neurologic manifestations of infective endocarditis: a 17-year experience in a teaching hospital in Finland. *Arch Intern Med* 2000; 160: 2781–2787.

7 Camarata PJ, Latchaw RE, Rufenacht DA, et al. Intracranial aneurysms. *Invest Radiol* 1993; 28: 373–382.

8 Huston J III, Nichols DA, Luetmer PH, et al. Blinded prospective evaluation of sensitivity of MR angiography to known intracranial aneurysms: importance of aneurysm size. *Am J Neuroradiol* 1994; 15: 1607–1614.

9 Lerner P. Neurologic complications of infective endocarditis. *Med Clin North Am* 1985; 69: 385–398.

10 Moskowitz MA, Rosenbaum AE, Tyler HR. Angiographically monitored resolution of cerebral mycotic aneurysms. *Neurology* 1974; 24: 1103–1108.

11 Clare CE, Barrow DL. Infectious intracranial aneurysms. *Neurosurg Clin N Am* 1992; 3: 551–566.

12 Wilson WR, Giuliani ER, Danielson GK, et al. Management of complications of infective endocarditis. *Mayo Clin Proc* 1982; 57: 162–170.

13 Neftel KA, Hauser SP, Muller MR. Inhibition of granulopoiesis *in vivo* and *in vitro* by beta-lactam antibiotics. *J Infect Dis* 1985; 152: 90–98.

14 Neftel KA, Walti M, Schulthess HK, et al. Adverse reactions following intravenous penicillin G related to degradation of the drug *in vitro*. *Klin Wochenschr* 1984; 62: 25–29.

15 Mylonakis E, Calderwood SB. Infective endocarditis in adults. *N Engl J Med* 2001; 345: 1318–1330

16 Devlin RK, Andrews MM, von Reyn CF. Recent trends in infective endocarditis: influence of case definitions. *Curr Opin Cardiol* 2004; 19: 134–139.

17 DiSalvo G, Habib G, Pergola V, et al. Echocardiography predicts embolic events in infective endocarditis. *J Am Coll Cardiol* 2001; 37: 1069–1076.

18 Angstwurm K, Borges AC, Halle E, et al. Timing the valve replacement in infective endocarditis involving the brain. *J Neurol* 2004; 251: 1220–1226.

19 al Jubair K, al Fagih MR, Ashmeg A, et al. Cardiac operations during active endocarditis. *J Thorac Cardiovasc Surg* 1992; 104: 487–490.

20 National Institute for Health and Clinical Excellence. Prophylaxis against endocarditis. NICE guidance CG64 [issued March 2008]. Available from: www.nice.org.uk.

A word to the wise: not all chest pain is ischaemic

Amal Muthumala

⊕ **Expert commentary** Dr Iqbal Malik

Case history

A 64-year-old man presented overnight to Accident and Emergency (A&E) at his local hospital. He complained of severe chest pain at rest, radiating to his jaw. The pain lasted for 15 minutes, before subsiding spontaneously. He admitted feeling very dizzy prior to the onset of pain, but had had no other associated symptoms. There was no previous history of ischaemic heart disease or diabetes, but he was hypertensive. He had never smoked, and there was no history of excessive alcohol intake. His medical history included benign prostatic hypertrophy and mild osteoarthritis. He was taking bendroflumethiazide and tamsulosin. He was otherwise fit and healthy. There was no family history of vascular disease.

On examination, the patient was free of pain and well perfused. He had a regular pulse of 84 beats per minute (bpm). His jugular venous pressure (JVP) was not visible, and the blood pressure (BP) in the right arm was 120/60 mmHg. Heart sounds were documented as normal except for the addition of a diastolic murmur. The chest was clear, and abdominal examination was unremarkable. There was no focal neurology.

An electrocardiogram (ECG) demonstrated sinus rhythm with no dynamic changes and a chest radiograph demonstrated clear lung fields, with no other obvious abnormalities. In view of the history of cardiac-sounding chest pain, he was treated for an acute coronary syndrome (ACS) with aspirin, clopidogrel, and low molecular weight heparin (LMWH). Blood tests revealed normal full blood count, urea and electrolytes, and liver function tests. Troponin T at 12 hours was mildly elevated at 0.31 ng/mL, as was the D-dimer.

He was reviewed on the post-take ward round, when he was noted to have a collapsing pulse and the left radial pulse was found to be slightly weaker than the right. There was no difference in upper limb blood pressures. He continued to be pain-free and was haemodynamically stable. In light of the new examination findings raising the suspicion of aortic dissection, urgent imaging was requested and treatment for ACS was discontinued.

⭐ **Learning point** Presentation of aortic dissection

Aortic dissection can present in a variety of manifestations. The differential diagnosis can, therefore, be wide and may include acute myocardial infarction, pulmonary embolism, acute left ventricular failure, and pericardial tamponade. Severe acute chest pain radiating to the back is the classical presentation. Symptoms and signs may also relate to a particular complication of the dissection, e.g. leg weakness (with spinal artery compromise), abdominal pain (with mesenteric artery involvement), or an ischaemic limb (peripheral artery complication).

⊕ **Expert comment**

This patient's pain appeared 'coronary' in nature, but with a normal ECG. There would be no suspicion of dissection without the murmur of aortic regurgitation, but that single finding should lead to a more thorough examination to exclude dissection. Although dissection classically presents with a tearing pain going between the shoulder blades, more subtle presentations are commoner. It takes little effort to record a blood pressure in both arms and to document all peripheral pulses, particularly if there is the slightest hint that aortic dissection may be the underlying pathology in those cases that present atypically. Pre-syncope is not a classical feature of dissection, but should raise suspicion of non-ischaemic pain.

⊕ **Expert comment**

The clinical findings on the post-take ward round may have been more pronounced than when the patient was first admitted. This is because the dissection, and hence the aortic regurgitation, may have progressed. This highlights the need to act quickly when the diagnosis is first suspected.

⊕ **Clinical tip** Important clues in aortic dissection

- In the context of acute chest pain, the presence of syncope/pre-syncope or a diastolic murmur should immediately arouse suspicion of non-ischaemic chest pain.
- Pulse deficits and differences in upper limb blood pressures are other important signs to look for.

⬤ **Expert comment**

D-dimers are often elevated and so should be done if the diagnosis is suspected. If positive, it does not mean there is a pulmonary embolism!

⊕ **Clinical tip** Confirming the diagnosis of aortic dissection

- Several imaging modalities, including contrast CT, transoesophageal echocardiography (TOE), or magnetic resonance imaging may be used to confirm aortic dissection.
- All these modalities have a very high diagnostic accuracy, with almost 100% sensitivity and specificity [3].
- The current practice in most hospitals, especially out of hours, is to use contrast CT. This is probably the most accessible and safest option.
- TTE has a lower accuracy for type A dissections with a sensitivity that varies from approximately 80–100% [4]. However, it can identify accurately, high-risk features such as aortic regurgitation, pericardial effusion, and regional wall motion abnormalities, together with the presence of a dilated aortic root with or without a dissection flap [5]. Nevertheless, in a patient with a good history and signs suggestive of aortic dissection, a normal TTE cannot rule out this diagnosis, and more definitive imaging will be necessary.

⊗ **Learning point** The ECG and chest X-ray (CXR)

The ECG can be helpful and may show signs of ischaemia in patients with aortic dissection. For example, inferior ST-elevation may be seen in those with anterograde extension of a dissection flap into the right coronary ostium, compressing the right coronary artery. However, in general, the ECG has very poor predictive value. In one series, 20% of patients with type A dissection had ECG evidence of ischaemia and 33% of patients with coronary involvement had a normal ECG [1]. Troponins may also be elevated as a result of myocardial ischaemia or cardiac dysfunction.

The CXR classically demonstrates a widened mediastinum or left-sided pleural effusion (rupture into the pleural space), but an abnormal CXR is only seen in between 60–90% of suspected cases [2].

⊗ **Learning point** D-dimers

D-dimers are cross-linked fibrin degradation products which are released when the endogenous fibrinolytic system breaks down the fibrin matrix of fresh venous thromboemboli. D-dimers are often used to help diagnose venous thromboembolism, but due to their low specificity, they should be evaluated in the appropriate clinical context as raised levels can also be detected in the following conditions:
- Any inflammatory process
- Infection
- Trauma
- Disseminated intravascular coagulation
- Vaso-occlusive sickle-cell crisis
- Acute cerebrovascular accident
- Acute myocardial infarction
- Many cancers, including lung, prostate, cervical, and colorectal.

Whilst waiting for a computed tomography (CT) scan, a bedside transthoracic echocardiogram (TTE) demonstrated a markedly dilated aortic root (60 mm in diameter) with a jet of moderate aortic regurgitation (Figure 9.1). The non-coronary cusp was seen to be prolapsing into the left ventricular outflow tract (LVOT). A linear echo, most likely a dissection flap, was also seen to prolapse back into the LVOT. The left ventricle was mildly dilated and hyperdynamic. In the apical 4-chamber view, the descending aorta was dilated and clearly seen. A linear echo was also clearly seen in the descending aorta, consistent with a possible dissection flap.

Subsequently, a contrast enhanced CT scan of the aorta demonstrated dilatation of the ascending and descending aorta with multiple dissection flaps (Figure 9.2). On these findings, the patient was diagnosed with a type A (or De Bakey type I) aortic dissection.

⊗ **Learning point** Classification of aortic dissection (Figure 9.3)

Aortic dissection occurs when a tear in the aortic media results in an intimo-medial flap with an entrance tear. This lumen is then exposed to elevated aortic pressures, which cause delamination of the media from the aortic wall, forming a false lumen which runs alongside the true lumen. The elevated pressures can lead to propagation of the dissection proximally or distally, or in both directions.

The Stamford classification of aortic dissections is very simple, with type A dissections representing those that involve the ascending aorta and aortic arch, and type B involving those that only involve the descending aorta [6]. This classification lends itself to different management strategies, where type A dissections should be repaired surgically, and type B dissections should initially be managed conservatively. The De Bakey classification is slightly more complex, as there is a distinction between the involvement of only the ascending aorta and the aorta distal to ascending aorta [7].

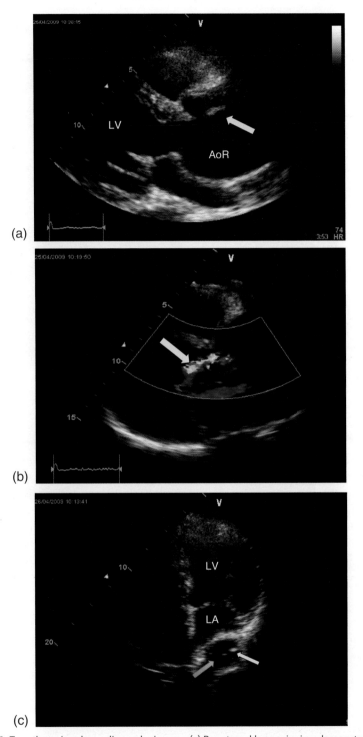

Figure 9.1 Transthoracic echocardiography images. (a) Parasternal long axis view demonstrating a severely dilated aortic root with a dissection flap (arrow). LV = left ventricle; AoR = aortic root; (b) Parasternal long axis view with colour flow Doppler demonstrating aortic regurgitation (arrow); (c) Apical 4-chamber view demonstrating a dilated descending aorta (blue arrow) with possible dissection flap (yellow arrow). LV = left ventricle; LA = left atrium.

Aortic dissection is part of a spectrum of disorders that comprise the acute aortic syndromes (AAS). AAS embraces a heterogeneous group of patients with a similar clinical profile, presenting with one of the following acute aortic pathologies: penetrating aortic ulcer, intramural haematoma, and classic aortic dissection. All can progress to aortic rupture and death. [8]

Aortic dissection is characterized by a separation of the aortic media. The outer part of the aortic media together with the adventitia forms the false channel outside the wall, whereas the rest of the aortic media with the intimal layer form the intimo-medial flap. Therefore, the 'intimal flap' is a misnomer. The proportion of media that remains at the external wall of the false channel is a determining factor in the risk of rupture. The false channel rupture is the most common mechanism of death in patients with classic aortic dissection. With the use of endovascular techniques becoming more common, recognizing which is the true lumen is increasingly important.

➕ Clinical tip Importance of recognizing aortic dissection promptly

- The diagnosis of aortic dissection can be very challenging, reflecting the variety of clinical presentations. The mortality from type A dissection is very high at 1–2% per hour for the first 48 hours, and increases rapidly with time. [9] This reflects the need for a rapid diagnosis.
- Sometimes, an incorrect diagnosis of ACS or pulmonary embolism is made, prompting the initiation of anti-thrombotic therapy. This inevitably exacerbates the problem.

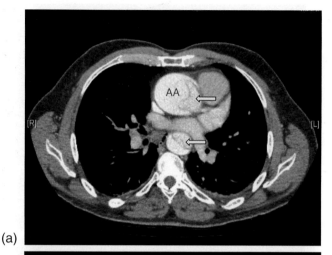

(a)

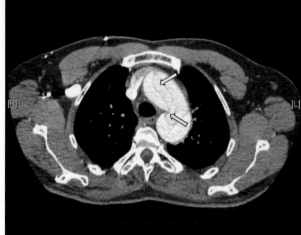

(b)

Figure 9.2 Contrast CT aortograms. (a) A dilated ascending aorta (AA) and descending aorta with dissection flaps in both (arrows); (b) Multiple dissection flaps in a dilated aortic arch (arrows).

⭐ Learning point Risk factors for the development of aortic dissection

- Trauma
- Hypertension
- Atherosclerosis
- Collagen disorder
- Inflammatory (e.g. Takayasu's arteritis, giant cell arteritis, and syphilis)
- Ankylosing spondylitis
- Bicuspid aortic valve
- Coarctation of the aorta
- Pregnancy
- Iatrogenic (e.g. post-angiography or post-cardiac surgery).

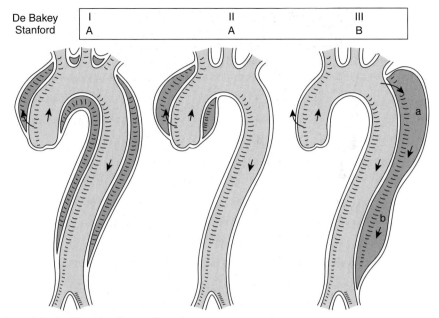

De Bakey	I	II	III
Stanford	A	A	B

Figure 9.3 Classification of aortic dissection.

> ⊗ **Learning point** Mechanisms of aortic regurgitation in aortic dissection
>
> - Prolapse of the aortic leaflet when the dissection extends into the root;
> - Prolapse of the dissection flap through the aortic valve;
> - Dilatation of the annulus, causing incomplete valve closure;
> - Pre-existing disease (e.g. bicuspid aortic valve disease, annular dilatation secondary to collagen disease).

The patient's vital signs were strictly monitored, including urinary output. His systolic blood pressure had risen to 140 mmHg and he was subsequently started on a labetolol infusion. He was urgently transferred to the local cardiothoracic centre for surgical intervention. Despite this, he suffered a cardiorespiratory arrest secondary to pulseless electrical activity while awaiting theatre. A prolonged attempt at cardiorespiratory resuscitation was unsuccessful.

> ⊗ **Learning point** General management of aortic dissection
>
> *Supportive care and close monitoring*
> These patients require close observation in a high dependency or intensive care environment. Rigorous BP control (keeping systolic BP between 100 and 120 mmHg) is essential to try to prevent further propagation of the dissection. This is achieved through intravenous beta-blockade, with either labetolol or esmolol. Beta-blockers reduce the force of left ventricular contraction, ameliorating the effect on the arterial wall. In cases of severe hypertension, the addition of vasodilators such as sodium nitropusside or glyceryl trinitrate may be used, but they can cause a reflex increase in contractility or tachycardia. Analgesia with opiates is often necessary.
>
> *continued*

Specific management of type A aortic dissection

All type A dissections should be immediately referred to the local cardiothoracic centre. Surgery is undertaken to prevent aortic rupture or development of pericardial effusion which may lead to cardiac tamponade. It is also necessary to eliminate aortic regurgitation and to avoid myocardial ischaemia. Basic surgical management involves transection of the involved area of the ascending aorta with cuffs of true and false lumen sutured. A new Dacron® aortic graft is inserted, and either the native valve is re-suspended or the aortic valve is replaced along with root replacement. Re-implantation of the coronary arteries may also be required.

Specific management of type B aortic dissection

The mainstay is medical treatment with tight BP control. Surgical treatment has a high reported mortality of up to 65% with a high risk of paraplegia in approximately 30% [10]. The indication for surgery in type B dissection is limited to signs of aortic rupture: persistent or recurrent chest pain, aortic expansion, and/or periaortic haematoma [11].

Endovascular therapy

In selected patients at a number of specialist centres in Europe and North America, endovascular techniques have been used to treat type B aortic dissections. The objective is to cover the intimo-medial flap and seal the entry site. In a meta-analysis of 39 studies, including over 600 patients with type B dissections (of which a minority were chronic dissection), there was 98% procedural success. The major complication rate was 20%, but the mortality rate was only 5%, with figures comparable to medical management [12]. Recent studies have demonstrated a possible role for endovascular therapy in type B dissection where there are specific complications, such as late expansion or distal malperfusion. As for uncomplicated type B dissections, endovascular therapy has not been shown to be superior to medical therapy, and one must remember that there is exposure to a definite complication risk [13].

✦ Learning point International Registry for acute Aortic Dissections (IRAD) [2]

In view of the high mortality and morbidity of aortic dissections, together with its low incidence, it has been difficult to collect comprehensive prospective data in this group of patients. In 1996, IRAD was established to gather data on all aspects of patients with aortic dissection, including presentation, diagnosis, treatment, and outcomes. It is the largest such international multicentre registry and by 2008, more than 2,000 patients have been recruited from over 26 sites with over 30 papers published.

The IRAD has revealed valuable information in the epidemiology of aortic dissection [2]. It has demonstrated the variety of clinical presentations, and has shown that pre-existing hypertension is present in 70% of patients with dissection [2]. It has also confirmed that in type A dissection, surgical treatment is superior to medical treatment, and that medical treatment remains the mainstay therapy for type B dissection [2,14].

Discussion

Aortic dissection, due to its varied clinical presentation, can be a very difficult diagnosis to make. The differential diagnosis can include myocardial ischaemia and other intrathoracic catastrophes that may present in a similar manner. The mortality is dependent on time from presentation, with death rates from type A dissections up to 50% at 48 hours. Rapid confirmation of the diagnosis is essential. Sinister histories and abnormal physical signs should not be ignored. TTE can demonstrate high-risk features, namely pericardial effusion and aortic regurgitation, but this should not delay definitive imaging, namely contrast-enhanced CT in most current hospital settings. It is important to note that despite the high diagnostic accuracy of CT imaging, they are still very much operator-dependent. Therefore, if there is a high degree of clinical suspicion, but the CT scan is non-diagnostic, one must consider repeating the scan or carrying out an alternative diagnostic imaging test. Once a dissection has been diagnosed, immediate discussion with the local cardiothoracic centre should take place. Patients with type A dissections should undergo immediate surgical intervention and those with type B dissections should be initially managed conservatively. There may be a role for endovascular repair, especially in type B dissection, but this needs further evaluation in future randomized trials.

> **A final word from the expert**
>
> This case highlights the fact that delay in diagnosis leads to increased mortality. This is more of a medical emergency than an inferior myocardial infarction. Unfortunately, there is no equivalent of the ECG to establish the diagnosis quickly. The diagnosis has first to be thought of and then the appropriate test ordered. In most cases, this will be a CT scan. Use of contrast significantly increases diagnostic quality. Once the diagnosis is made, transfer to the local cardiothoracic centre should be with a 'blue light' ambulance; better still would be transfer to a specialist 'aortic centre'. Even in large cities such as London, each surgeon will only see one or two cases a year. It would be better to have the expertise of the multidisciplinary cardiovascular team, including interventional radiology and vascular surgery, consolidated in fewer centres. This would give the patient the best chance of a successful outcome, with either an open surgical, endovascular, or combined approach.

References

1 Kamp TJ, Goldschmidt–Clermont PJ, Brinker JA, et al. Myocardial infarction, aortic dissection, and thrombolytic therapy. *Am Heart J* 1994; 128: 1234–1237.

2 Hagan PG, Nienaber CA, Isselbacher EM, et al. The International Registry of Acute Aortic Dissection (IRAD): new insights into an old disease. *JAMA* 2000; 283: 897–903.

3 Shiga T, Wajima Z, Apfel C, et al. Diagnostic accuracy of transoesophageal echocardiography, helical computed tomography, and magnetic resonance imaging for suspected thoracic aortic dissection: systematic review and meta-analysis. *Arch Int Med* 2006; 166: 1350–1356

4 Miller D. Surgical management of aortic dissections: indications, peri-operative management, and long-term results. In: Doroghazi RM, Slater EE, editors. Aortic Dissection. New York: McGraw-Hill, 1983; 193–243.

5 Meredith EL, Masani ND. Echocardiography in the emergency assessment of acute aortic syndromes. *Eur J Echocardiogr* 2009; 10: i31–39.

6 Crawford ES, Svensson LG, Coselli JS, et al. Surgical treatment of aneurysm and/or dissection of the ascending aorta, transverse aortic arch, and ascending aorta and transverse aortic arch. Factors influencing survival in 717 patients. *J Thorac Cardiovasc Surg* 1989; 98: 659–674.

7 De Bakey ME, McCollum CH, Crawford ES, et al. Dissection and dissecting aneurysms of the aorta: twenty-year follow-up of five hundred and twenty-seven patients treated surgically. *Surgery* 1982; 92: 1118–1134.

8 Vilacosta I, P Aragoncillo, V Cañadas, et al. Acute aortic syndrome: a new look at an old conundrum. *Heart* 2009; 95: 1130–1139.

9 Chirillo F, Marchiori M, Andriolo L, et al. Outcome of 290 patients with aortic dissection. *A 12-year multicentre experience. Eur Heart J* 1990; 11: 311–319.

10 Elefteriades JA, Lovoulos CJ, Coady MA, et al. Management of descending aortic dissection. *Ann Thorac Surg* 1999; 67: 2002–2005.

11 Erbel R, Alfonso F, Boileau C, et al. Diagnosis and management of aortic dissection. Recommendations of the Task Force on Aortic Dissection, *European Society of Cardiology Eur Heart J* 2001; 22: 1642–1681.

12 Eggebrecht H, Nienaber CA, Neuhäuser M, et al. Endovascular stent graft placement in aortic dissection: a meta-analysis. *Eur Heart J* 2006; 27: 489–498.

13 Nienaber CA, Rousseau H, Eggebrecht H, et al. Randomized comparison of strategies for type B aortic dissection: the INvestigation of STEnt Grafts in Aortic Dissection (INSTEAD) trial. *Circulation* 2009; 120: 2519–2528.

14 Tsai TT, Evangelista A, Nienaber CA et al. Long-term survival in patients presenting with type A acute aortic dissection: insights from the International Registry of Acute Aortic Dissection (IRAD). International Registry of Acute Aortic Dissection (IRAD). *Circulation* 2006; 114(1 Suppl): I350–1356.

10 Assessment and management of the breathless patient

Badrinathan Chandrasekaran

Expert commentary Professor Theresa McDonagh

Case history

A 67-year-old man presented to his general practitioner (GP), complaining of progressive shortness of breath and reduced exercise tolerance over the preceding three months. He denied any exertional chest pain. He was a smoker of 20 pack years, having stopped five years earlier, and had no history of excess alcohol. His past medical history was otherwise unremarkable and he was taking no regular medications.

On examination, he was well perfused and his pulse was 98 beats per minute (bpm) and regular. His jugular venous pressure (JVP) was not visible and blood pressure (BP) was 110/80 mmHg. Heart sounds were normal with a soft systolic murmur. There was reduced air entry at both bases with a mild expiratory wheeze. His GP attributed his symptoms primarily to obstructive airways disease, and hence, prescribed inhaled bronchodilator therapy and arranged pulmonary function tests.

There was some initial improvement in his symptoms and pulmonary function testing did reveal a mild obstructive defect. However, his breathlessness suddenly deteriorated significantly, necessitating admission to the emergency department (ED). On arrival, he was dyspnoeic at rest and his JVP was raised to the angle of the jaw. He had a third heart sound with a systolic murmur, and there was pitting oedema to his calves. A diagnosis of decompensated HF was made and he was admitted under the care of the medical team. His ECG revealed left bundle branch block with a broad QRS width (Figure 10.1) and a chest radiograph showed cardiomegaly with upper lobe venous diversion and clear lung fields. His BP was 120/80 mmHg and he was treated with intravenous furosemide to good effect. On admission, he had a mild normocytic anaemia and his renal function was impaired (MDRD eGFR of 32 mL/min/1.73 m² based on a serum creatinine of 186 micromol/L); however, the rest of his baseline biochemistry was normal (Table 10.1). A transthoracic echocardiogram (TTE) showed a dilated left ventricle with severe left ventricular systolic dysfunction (LVSD) and an akinetic anterior wall. The valves were normal; however, there was moderate to severe functional mitral regurgitation (MR) into a dilated left atrium. The estimated pulmonary artery pressure from his tricuspid regurgitation jet was 54 mmHg + right atrial pressure.

Expert comment

The GP has opted to perform respiratory investigations first. However, this man has an abnormal cardiac examination in the form of a murmur. In this scenario, I would recommend that an electrocardiogram (ECG) and a brain natriuretic peptide (BNP) test should be performed first to exclude heart failure confidently.

Clinical tip Clinically diagnosing HF

The symptoms of HF are common to a number of conditions. A high index of suspicion is needed in order not to miss the diagnosis. Physical signs which have a relatively high predictive value for HF are:
- Raised JVP;
- Gallop rhythm, particularly in patients over the age of 30 years;
- Pulsus alternans.

➕ **Clinical tip** Diuretics in decompensated HF with renal impairment

Diuretics are often withheld or underused in decompensated HF patients with renal impairment. However, when a patient is clearly fluid-overloaded, they need an adequate dose of loop diuretic to achieve a negative fluid balance and weight loss, with the renal function often improving or remaining stable. In some cases, it may be necessary to stop the angiotensin-converting enzyme inhibitor/angiotensin receptor blockers (ACEi/ARBs) and aldosterone antagonists temporarily while diuresis is achieved. This is particularly the case in those with a systolic BP of <90 mmHg. They should be restarted when the patient's BP and renal function have recovered. All patients being treated for decompensated HF should have the following:

- Daily weights;
- Fluid chart;
- Fluid restriction of 1.5–2 L;
- Regular monitoring of renal function.

A continuous infusion of furosemide is sometimes more effective than bolus doses in certain patients, but particularly those with refractory oedema. The combination of a loop diuretic and thiazide is also useful in those resistant to diuresis. Once the patient is euvolaemic, they should be stable on oral diuretics for 48 hours prior to discharge. Oral diuretics should be kept to the minimum dose necessary to avoid fluid retention and prevent further activation of the renin-angiotensin-aldosterone system (RAAS). Oral bumetanide should be considered in patients who decompensate on oral furosemide as the gastric absorption is better.

Table 10.1 Blood results on admission

Hb	12 g/dL	C reactive protein	12 mg/L
MCV	**72.1 fL**	Total protein	70 g/L
WCC	7.3 × 10⁹/L	Albumin	**34 g/L**
Neutrophils	5.4 × 10⁹/L	Bilirubin	14 micromol/L
Platelets	290 × 10⁹/L	Alanine aminotransferase	28 IU/L
INR	1.0	TSH	1.10 mu/L
Ferritin	64 mcg/L	FT4	11.9 pmol/L
Na	**133 mmol/L**	Troponin I	<0.07
K	4.2 mmol/L	Corrected calcium	2.34 mmol/L
Urea	**16 mmol/L**	Creatinine kinase	168 IU/L
Creatinine	**186 micromol/L**	MDRD eGFR	32 mL/min/1.73 m²

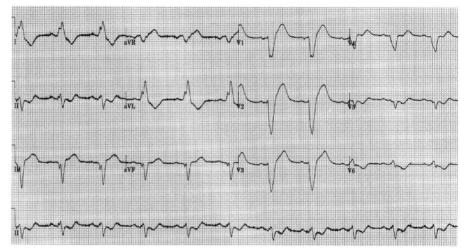

Figure 10.1 Electrocardiogram showing sinus rhythm with left bundle branch block and a broad QRS width (198 ms).

⭐ **Learning point** Diagnosis of HF

Cardiac failure is a syndrome characterized by dyspnoea, fatigue, and fluid retention. The syndrome can result from any structural or functional cardiac disorder that impairs the ability of the heart to function as a pump to support a physiological circulation. The diagnosis of HF remains a clinical diagnosis as defined in the current European Society of Cardiology (ESC) guidelines (Table 10.2) [1].

TTE is the most commonly used modality to assess cardiac function and can help exclude significant valvular and pericardial pathologies as well as quantifying chamber dimensions and estimating systolic and diastolic function. TTE can also identify regional wall motional abnormalities consistent with ischaemic heart disease (IHD) and help identify patients who are candidates for device therapy. The majority of the evidence base for the use of neurohormonal blockade or device therapy is in HF with reduced left ventricular ejection fraction (LVEF), also referred to as systolic dysfunction. A high proportion of patients with HF have preserved LVEF (also referred to as diastolic dysfunction or heart failure with normal ejection fraction [HFNEF]), where the evidence base for pharmacological or device therapy is less robust.

Where access to echocardiography is limited, a normal ECG and plasma BNP are good screening tests to exclude HF. This allows appropriate prioritisation of patients who actually require an urgent TTE. Conversely, an abnormal ECG such as a prolonged QRS duration (QRSd) is associated with a poor prognosis in patients with HF.

Table 10.2 ESC guidelines for the diagnosis of HF [1]

I	Symptoms of cardiac failure at rest or during exercise
II	Objective evidence of cardiac dysfunction at rest
III	Response to treatment directed towards cardiac failure

In order to diagnose HF, criteria I and II have to be met in all cases. Where there is doubt, criterion III is required to confirm the diagnosis [1].

He was established on an ACEi and referred to the cardiology team as an inpatient. By this time, his symptoms had improved; he was euvolaemic and stable on oral bumetanide 2 mg in addition to ramipril 5 mg once daily. His renal function had improved considerably, allowing for a diagnostic coronary angiogram to be undertaken which demonstrated unobstructed smooth coronary arteries. Spironolactone 25 mg once daily (od) was added to his regime and he was discharged with a HF specialist nurse follow-up. His ramipril was increased to 10 mg od, and he was successfully started on bisoprolol which was uptitrated to 5 mg od over a number of weeks. There was no deterioration in his breathing and repeat spirometry was unchanged.

> ⭐ **Learning point** Multidisciplinary teams (MDTs) and the role of HF specialist nurses
>
> There is good evidence to support the role of a multidisciplinary team (MDT) approach to the management of HF. After stabilizing a patient presenting with acute HF, a coordinated approach, including patient education, support, monitoring, and uptitration of evidence-based pharmacotherapy, has been shown to improve quality of life and reduce hospitalizations for HF [2]. Although individual studies were not powered to show a mortality benefit, a meta-analysis did suggest a significant reduction in mortality with interventions based on a medical input, combined with one of the following allied healthcare professionals: specialist nurse, clinical pharmacist, dietician, or social worker [3]. Although it is not clear which method of organized HF management is best, the majority involve HF specialist nurses as the main interface with the patient. HF management programmes reduce healthcare costs, mainly driven by a reduction in hospitalization. The current ESC guidelines recommend the use of an MDT approach to HF management [1].

He was reviewed as an outpatient three months after his initial admission. Although much improved, he was still breathlessness on minimal exertion, placing him in NYHA class III. He denied any chest pain and had never complained of palpitations or syncope. On examination, there were no signs of congestion, his pulse was now 50 bpm, and his BP was 90/65 mmHg with no postural drop. The ECG was unchanged, and a repeat TTE showed no improvement in left ventricular function, with a biplane Simpson's ejection fraction (EF) estimated at 25%. Cardiac dyssynchrony assessment was positive as confirmed by a prolonged aortic pre-ejection time and an interventricular delay of >40 ms. There was moderate to severe functional MR. His current medical therapy was bisoprolol 5 mg, ramipril 10 mg, spironolactone 25 mg, and bumetanide 1 mg. He was, therefore, considered a suitable candidate for device therapy. However, in order to establish the aetiology for his HF and to determine the most appropriate device, he had an outpatient stress cardiac magnetic resonance (CMR) scan. This showed a dilated left ventricle with severe LVSD, and a transmural myocardial infarction in the anterior wall (Figure 10.2). There was no evidence of a reversible perfusion abnormality with adenosine.

🗨 **Expert comment**

Although HF is a clinical diagnosis, it is imperative to prove that there is cardiac dysfunction underlying the symptoms and signs.

🗨 **Expert comment**

Management here is excellent; however, I would have started the beta-blocker in hospital. There is evidence to show that when it is commenced in hospital, patients are more likely to remain on them [2]! Spironolactone is appropriate as the patient was in New York Heart Association (NYHA) class III HF, at least on admission (see RALES trial in case 13).

➕ **Clinical tip** Neurohormonal blockade

- Beta-blockers should only be initiated when the patient is euvolaemic.
- Patients should be warned that they may experience a temporary deterioration in their symptoms when starting a beta-blocker.
- Patients established on beta-blockers admitted with fluid overload should not have the beta-blocker discontinued, if possible.
- If low BP should become symptomatic, then it is better to reduce the ACEi dose to achieve a combination with beta-blocker therapy.
- Once patients are stable on maximally tolerated medical therapy, then loop diuretics should be reduced, if possible.

Expert comment

It is not necessary to measure markers of dyssynchrony prior to consideration of device therapy. An ECG demonstrating interventricular conduction delay will suffice. A small proportion of patients entered into the CArdiac REsynchronization in Heart Failure (CARE-HF) study with a QRSd between 120 and 150 ms did have echocardiographic features of dyssynchrony. However, a more recent study suggests that measuring echocardiographic parameters is not useful when selecting patients for cardiac resynchronization therapy (CRT) as they do not correlate with a favourable response to implantation.

Whilst CMR is a very useful test for non-invasive assessment of the presence/absence of ischaemia, most centres would opt for an exercise tolerance test (ETT) or a myocardial perfusion scan.

Expert comment

This course of action is appropriate. He fulfils evidence-based criteria for CRT (see CARE-HF and COMPANION studies and the recent ESC guidelines) and for a defibrillator for the primary prevention of sudden cardiac death (as his LVEF is less than 30% and he has IHD).

Expert comment

Unfortunately, there is no reliable method to predict whether a patient will have a favourable outcome from CRT, just as with ACEi and beta-blockers. The correct strategy is to select those who meet the criteria used in the clinical trials which have proven the efficacy of CRT.

It is worth noting that the recent CORONA trial results indicate that there is no benefit in starting statin therapy in patients with established HF [22]. Therefore, this man could take one fewer drug, especially as his coronary angiogram is normal! This also suggests that the aetiology of his previous myocardial infarction must have been 'plaque rupture'.

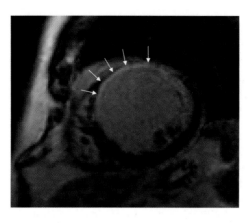

Figure 10.2 Cardiac magnetic resonance 2D short axis slice with late gadolinium enhancement confirming a dilated left ventricle with a transmural myocardial infarct (arrows).

On the basis of these investigations, the patient was presumed to have a dilated cardiomyopathy, and the systolic dysfunction was felt to be ischaemic in origin. CRT with a defibrillator (CRT-D) was advised to improve his symptoms and prognosis.

He was quoted a 70% response rate and counselled about any driving restrictions that may result from an appropriate implantable cardioverter-defibrillator (ICD) discharge. He was also started on aspirin 75 mg and simvastatin 40 mg for secondary prevention of coronary artery disease.

Learning point Indications for device therapy

The two main causes of death in patients with HF and systolic dysfunction are sudden cardiac death and pump failure. A number of studies have shown that primary prevention with ICDs in patients with systolic dysfunction is superior to medical therapy (Table 10.3) [4-7]. However, although ICDs prolong life in patients with HF, they do not improve symptoms or delay the onset of pump failure. This is the role of CRT, which is also known as biventricular pacing. CRT has been shown to improve morbidity [8,9] and mortality [10-12] in HF patients with severe systolic dysfunction, NHYA class III symptoms, and on optimal pharmacological treatment with a prolonged QRSd. CRT can improve cardiac dyssynchrony and lead to a reduction in ventricular dimensions and improvement in LVEF (reverse left ventricular remodelling) [11,12]. On its own, CRT is referred to as a CRT-pacemaker (CRT-P) or when combined with a defibrillator, it is CRT-D [13,14]. There is only one randomized trial of CRT in patients with atrial fibrillation (AF), and this did not show any benefit [15]. The COMPANION study comparing CRT with or without a defibrillator and medical therapy showed that CRT-D improved mortality [10]. However, the study was not powered to compare CRT-D with CRT-P, which itself showed a trend to improved survival. The CARE-HF study showed that CRT-P alone reduced mortality and hospitalization for HF, compared to medical therapy [12].

Selection criteria for ICD implantation (Table 10.4) [16]

The evidence base for primary prevention with an ICD is more convincing in patients with IHD [4-6]. Device insertion should be delayed after an acute myocardial infarction or revascularization [17,18]. The use of device therapy for primary prevention in patients with non-ischaemic cardiomyopathy is less clear from the randomized trials and this is reflected in the lack of clarity in the National Institute for Health and Clinical Excellence (NICE) guidelines [7,19-21]. It should be noted that patients in randomized clinical trials are younger than the average age of patients who present with *de novo* HF and usually have fewer comorbidities.

Dyssynchrony

One of the consequences of adverse left ventricular remodelling is the development of electromechanical dyssynchrony which can be between the atria and ventricles (atrioventricular), between the right and left ventricle (interventricular), or between different segments of the left ventricle (intraventricular). This reduces the efficiency of cardiac contraction and can result in functional MR,

continued

a reduction in filling time, and contraction of the ventricle after the closure of the aortic valve, leading to a reduction in cardiac output. A prolonged QRSd is a marker of cardiac dyssynchrony and remains the predominant selection criterion for CRT. Based on current guidelines (see Table 10.4), the clinical response from CRT is 70%. A number of echo parameters of dyssynchrony have been shown to predict response to CRT in small studies, but in the setting of a randomized multicentre trial, they were not reproducible or able to predict CRT responders [23]. From the CARE-HF trial, dyssynchrony on TTE (Table 10.5) identifies a group that may derive a greater benefit from CRT, but the absence of dyssynchrony did not select out non-responders [24]. Therefore, the QRSd width remains the main selection criterion for CRT.

As an outpatient, he underwent insertion of a CRT-D device on the left side, under conscious sedation with standard aseptic technique. A subcutaneous pocket was fashioned for the device. Access was by subclavian vein puncture using a Seldinger technique. A dual-coil active endocardial defibrillator lead was placed in the right ventricular apex and an active atrial lead in the right atrial appendage. The coronary sinus was intubated with a guide catheter and a balloon occlusion venogram was obtained (Figure 10.3). The posterolateral vein was deemed a suitable target vessel and a bipolar lead was positioned in the epicardial vein successfully (Figure 10.4).

Table 10.3 NICE guidelines for primary prevention with ICD in patients with systolic dysfunction (adapted from NICE technology appraisal 1995 and 2006) [16]

Greater than four weeks post-MI and LVEF <30% and:
- NYHA classes I–III
- With broad QRS (>120 ms)

Greater than four weeks post-MI and LVEF <35% and:
- NYHA classes I–III
- Non-sustained ventricular tachycardia on 24-hour tape
- A positive electrophysiological study

A familial cardiac condition with a high risk of sudden death, including long QT syndrome, hypertrophic cardiomyopathy, Brugada syndrome or arrhythmogenic right ventricular dysplasia, or have undergone surgical repair of congenital heart disease.

Note: There is no specification of what to do in patients with a non-ischaemic dilated cardiomyopathy.

Table 10.4 NICE guidelines for CRT (adapted from the NICE guidelines 2007) [25]

Indication for CRT
- **Severe LVSD (LVEF <35%)**
- **QRSd >150 ms**
- **Symptomatic NYHA class III or IV**
- **On optimal medical therapy for HF**
- For those with QRSd >120 ms but <150 ms, additional evidence of mechanical dyssynchrony is required
- For those who fulfil the criteria for CRT and an ICD, a CRT-D may be considered

---

Table 10.5 CARE-HF dyssynchrony criteria [24]

CARE-HF criteria for dyssynchrony on TTE
Patients with QRS >120 ms but <150 ms required two out of the following:
- Aortic pre-ejection time (APET) >140 ms
- Interventricular delay (IVD) >40 ms
- Evidence of delayed activation of posterolateral wall*

* Time to maximal posterolateral wall thickening (M-mode) or systolic velocity (tissue Doppler) > time to onset of E-wave (mitral inflow).

Expert comment

Selection of a suitable vein for CRT is most usually constrained by the patient's coronary venous anatomy. If possible, a posterolateral vein should be chosen. There is now some evidence to suggest that pre-screening suitable patients with CMR helps to avoid veins supplying areas of scarred territory. This may be of some help in improving the effects of CRT.

Device optimization

The device function was optimized by altering the atrioventricular delay to achieve maximal separation of the E and A waveforms without premature truncation of the A wave (Figure 10.5). It was noted that the MR had also improved and was now mild. The aortic pre-ejection time was still prolonged, but the interventricular delay was now only 35 ms.

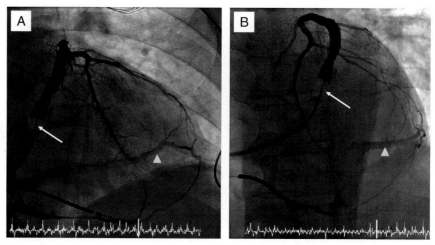

Figure 10.3 Balloon occlusion venogram of the coronary sinus (CS) in the antero-posterior (AP) (panel A) and left anterior oblique (LAO) (panel B) projection. The tip of the RV defibrillation lead is seen in the bottom left corner and the balloon occlusion catheter in the body of the CS (arrow). A posterior lateral vein (triangle) is shown to fill retrogradely.

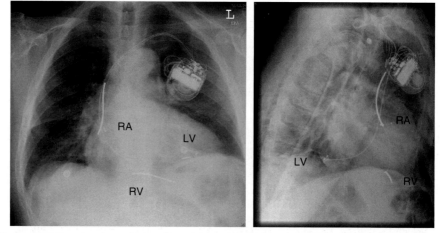

Figure 10.4 Postero–anterior (PA) and lateral chest radiographs post-CRT-D implant showing positions of right ventricular defibrillation (RV), left ventricular lead (LV), and right atrial lead (RA) leads.

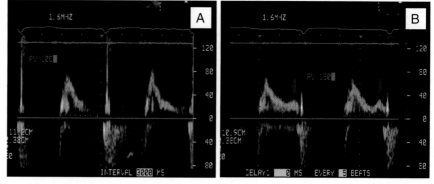

Figure 10.5 Mitral valve pulse wave Doppler. There is no A wave initially (panel A) and by changing the AV delay, the filling is improved with the emergence of an A wave (panel B, arrows).

Despite device implantation, he remained symptomatic and complained of tiredness and lassitude. Clinical examination suggested that he was dehydrated, later confirmed by his electrolyte results (urea 22 mmol/L and creatinine 150 micromol/L). His loop diuretic was discontinued, and his symptoms improved as did his renal function.

At his 6-month review, the patient was well with an unrestricted exercise tolerance. He was taking bisoprolol 10 mg, ramipril 10 mg, spironolactone 25 mg, aspirin 75 mg, and simvastatin 40 mg. He had not had any admissions with decompensated HF, and there had been no therapies from his device. The HF monitoring capabilities of his device had been activated and the trends had remained stable. A repeat echocardiogram showed a reduction in his left ventricular dimensions and improvement in his EF to 38%.

He continued to be under regular review, but noticed a sudden deterioration in his symptoms 11 months following his device insertion. His ECG showed a paced rhythm, but the morphology of the QRS was different to his post-implant ECG (Figure 10.6). The pacing check confirmed that his left ventricular lead was not capturing and a CXR confirmed a lead displacement (Figure 10.7). His HF monitoring showed a steady rise in his fluid index and a decrease in his intrathoracic impedance (Figure 10.8). He was admitted and underwent an left ventricular lead revision, after which he was re-established on his medical therapy with good effect.

❻ Expert comment

This highlights an important point that patients with HF post-CRT should be followed up carefully to optimize medication post-device insertion. Usually diuretic doses can be reduced and if the BP and renal function have improved, there is scope to uptitrate the dose of ACEi/ARB, beta-blockers, and aldosterone antagonists, thus increasing RAAS and sympathetic nervous system (SNS) blockade.

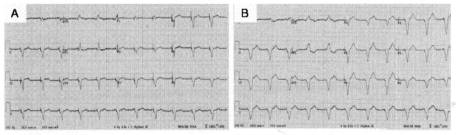

Figure 10.6 The 12-lead ECG post-implantation shows biventricular pacing (A). After LV lead displacement, there is a change in the QRS morphology with RV apical pacing (B).

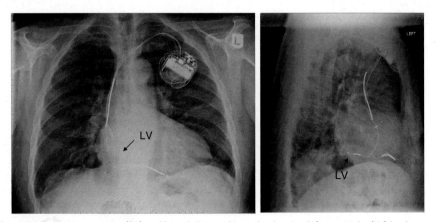

Figure 10.7 Postero–anterior (PA) and lateral chest radiographs showing left ventricular (LV) lead displacement (compare with Figure 10.4).

⊕ Clinical tip Deterioration in patients with CRT

- A sudden change in symptoms in patients previously stable with CRT warrants an urgent review.
- The left ventricular lead is epicardial and most often not actively secured, hence is prone to displacement.
- Loss of biventricular pacing can also occur if the ventricular rate is too high such as with the onset of AF or ventricular tachycardia.

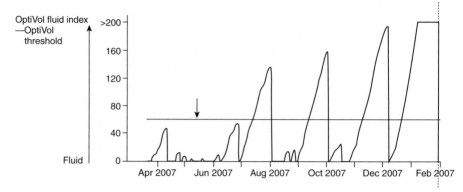

Figure 10.8 As intrathoracic impedance decreases, the Optivol fluid index rises and an audible alert can be programmed above a set threshold (arrow) to alert the patient to seek medical attention.

⊘ Landmark trial Cardiac Resynchronization in Heart Failure (CARE-HF) [12]

The CARE-HF study was a European, multicentre, randomized study of medical therapy vs CRT pacemaker implantation in 813 patients with a mean follow-up of 29.4 months. It was the first study to show a mortality benefit of CRT-P over medical therapy. The primary endpoint was a composite of unplanned hospital admissions from a cardiovascular cause with all-cause mortality, and the principle secondary endpoint was death from any cause.

Inclusion criteria: patients with sinus rhythm, NYHA class III, LVEF <35%, optimally tolerated pharmacological therapy for HF, and a QRS width of >120 ms. Those with QRS widths of 120–149 ms had to have additional echo criteria for dyssynchrony (Table 10.5). Randomization was 1:1 and the baseline medical treatment in both groups was excellent with 95% on ACEi or ARBs, 72% on beta-blockers, and 57% on aldosterone antagonists.

Results: the primary endpoint was reached in 39% of the CRT group and 55% of the medically treated group (hazard ratio 0.64, 95% confidence intervals [CI] 0.51–0.77, p < 0.001). Mortality was 20% in the CRT group compared to 30% in the medical group (hazard ratio 0.64, 95% CI 0.48–0.84, p < 0.002). Other significant secondary endpoints were a reduction in interventricular dyssynchrony, left ventricular end systolic volume index, MR area, and an increase in LVEF as measured by TTE. There was also a significant decrease in N-terminal (NT)-proBNP with CRT compared to medical therapy.

Conclusions: CRT-P alone reduces hospitalization and mortality in patients with HF, low EF, and broad QRSd compared to medical therapy. There is also evidence of favourable left ventricular remodelling with CRT-P and a reduction in natriuretic peptides.

✪ Learning point HF diagnostics and telemonitoring through devices

There are a number of surrogate markers of HF severity, which can be monitored and may help predict subclinical deterioration and prevent hospitalization for decompensated HF. Combined with the advances in telecommunications, remote monitoring through devices is a feasible alternative to hospital clinic follow-up. Devices can measure intrathoracic impedance which decreases as fluid accumulates. Preliminary studies suggest impedance measurements can predict hospitalization by 15 days [26]. Patient activity and heart rate variability are also decreased with decompensated HF, and are measured by a number of devices [27].

The use of telemonitoring requires a fundamental change in the way in which healthcare services are organized in order to follow the patients effectively. Although there are obvious practical advantages with telemonitoring through devices, the full clinical benefit and cost-effectiveness are yet to be determined by large randomized studies.

Discussion

HF secondary to LVSD is increasing in prevalence and is associated with considerable morbidity and mortality despite neurohormonal blockade. The advent of device therapy for subsets of patients with HF has added to the therapeutic arsenal available to cardiologists, allowing for a tangible improvement in symptoms and prognosis. It is likely that the indications for device therapy will expand to include less symptomatic patients and even patients who do not have a prolonged QRS. In patients who have an indication for an ICD and a prolonged QRSd, but are NYHA class II, studies have shown that CRT-D can improve exercise capacity [14], LVEF [14,28], and more recently with multicentre automatic defibrillator implantation trial with cardiac resynchronization therapy (MADIT-CRT), cause a reduction in HF events [29]. The role of non-invasive imaging will also help refine the selection of appropriate patients, and may even help predetermine the highly variable coronary venous anatomy. The emergence of HF diagnostics adds a new layer to managing HF patients, and may prove increasingly useful in the future. The debate over CRT-P or CRT-D is ongoing and requires an individual patient approach, with full discussion of the implications of each treatment option. As the major burden of HF is in the elderly, the potential to alter the mode of death with device therapy becomes an important consideration when counselling the patient, and deciding on the appropriate treatment.

☙ A final word from the expert

This case illustrates numerous important learning points in the diagnosis and management of HF. Firstly, this man's condition could have been diagnosed at an earlier stage by a simple BNP test in the primary care setting. Invariably, the BNP concentration would have been high, indicating that he was high-risk for subsequent admission. An ECG could also have been done at the time of, or immediately following, the BNP. With his prolonged QRS, this would have flagged him up for more intensive investigation and treatment. This is important as the mortality rate from incident HF is much higher than prevalent stable congestive HF.

Once diagnosed, patients with HF should have their medical therapy optimized as rapidly as possible, provided they are clinically euvolaemic and have sufficient systolic BP and renal function to tolerate uptitration of ACEi and beta-blocker therapy. Multi-professional and coordinated HF services ensure the best chance of this happening seamlessly and improve outcomes for patients. Both ACEi and beta-blockers should be started in hospital, if possible.

The use of CRT-P has a sound evidence base for improving both morbidity and mortality in patients with advanced HF (NYHA classes III/IV), systolic dysfunction, prolonged QRSd, on optimal medical therapy, and in sinus rhythm. All patients meeting these criteria should be offered CRT. Predicting those who will 'respond' is not yet possible; however, all patients who meet the criteria should be offered the therapy. The decision to implant a CRT-D should be guided by whether the patient is also a candidate for an ICD [1]. Patients in AF do not have as favourable a response rate as those in sinus rhythm, and it is important to note that most of the large outcome trials excluded those in AF. Some more recent studies have shown favourable effects in patients who are less symptomatic, i.e. those in NYHA classes I and II, with LBBB, and systolic dysfunction [29,30]. As yet, there is no evidence that those with a narrow QRS benefit from CRT.

And finally, follow-up of HF patients post-CRT is mandatory; the patient still has HF and should still have the benefit of multi-professional HF care.

References

1 Swedberg K, Cleland J, Dargie H, et al. Guidelines for the diagnosis and treatment of chronic heart failure: executive summary (update 2005): The Task Force for the Diagnosis and Treatment of Chronic Heart Failure of the European Society of Cardiology. *Eur Heart J* 2005; 26: 1115–1140.

2 Gattis WA, O'Connor CM, Gallup DS, et al. Predischarge initiation of carvedilol in patients hospitalized for decompensated heart failure: results of the Initiation Management Predischarge: *Process for Assessment of Carvedilol Therapy in Heart Failure (IMPACT-HF) trial*. J Am Cardiol 2004; 43:1534–1541.

3 Blue L, Lang E, McMurray JJ, et al. Randomized controlled trial of specialist nurse intervention in heart failure. *BMJ* 2001; 323:715–718.

4 Holland R, Battersby J, Harvey I, et al. Systematic review of multidisciplinary interventions in heart failure. *Heart* 2005; 91:899–906.

5 Moss AJ, Hall WJ, Cannom DS, et al. Improved survival with an implanted defibrillator in patients with coronary disease at high risk for ventricular arrhythmia. Multicentre Automatic Defibrillator Implantation Trial Investigators. *N Engl J Med* 1996; 335:1933–1940.

6 Buxton AE, Lee KL, Fisher JD, et al. A randomized study of the prevention of sudden death in patients with coronary artery disease. Multicentre Unsustained Tachycardia Trial Investigators. *N Engl J Med* 1999; 341:1882–1890.

7 Moss AJ, Zareba W, Hall WJ, et al. Prophylactic implantation of a defibrillator in patients with myocardial infarction and reduced ejection fraction. *N Engl J Med* 2002; 346: 877–883.

8 Bardy GH, Lee KL, Mark DB, et al. Amiodarone or an implantable cardioverter-defibrillator for congestive heart failure. *N Engl J Med* 2005; 352: 225–237.

9 Cazeau S, Leclercq C, Lavergne T, et al. Effects of multisite biventricular pacing in patients with heart failure and intraventricular conduction delay. *N Engl J Med* 2001; 344: 873–880.

10 Abraham WT, Fisher WG, Smith AL, et al. Cardiac resynchronization in chronic heart failure. *N Engl J Med* 2002; 346: 1845–1853.

11 Bristow MR, Saxon LA, Boehmer J, et al. Cardiac resynchronization therapy with or without an implantable defibrillator in advanced chronic heart failure. *N Engl J Med* 2004; 350: 2140–2150.

12 Cleland JG, Daubert JC, Erdmann E, et al. Longer-term effects of cardiac resynchronization therapy on mortality in heart failure [the CArdiac REsynchronization-Heart Failure (CARE-HF) trial extension phase]. *Eur Heart J* 2006; 27:1928–1932.

13 Cleland JG, Daubert JC, Erdmann E, et al. The effect of cardiac resynchronization on morbidity and mortality in heart failure. *N Engl J Med* 2005; 352: 1539–1549.

14 Young JB, Abraham WT, Smith AL, et al. Combined cardiac resynchronization and implantable cardioversion defibrillation in advanced chronic heart failure: the MIRACLE ICD trial. *JAMA* 2003; 289: 2685–2694.

15 Abraham WT, Young JB, Leon AR, et al. Effects of cardiac resynchronization on disease progression in patients with left ventricular systolic dysfunction, an indication for an implantable cardioverter defibrillator and mildly symptomatic chronic heart failure. *Circulation* 2004; 110: 2864–2868.

16 Leclercq C, Walker S, Linde C, et al. Comparative effects of permanent biventricular and right univentricular pacing in heart failure patients with chronic atrial fibrillation. *Eur Heart J* 2002; 23: 1780–1787.

17 National Institute for Health and Clinical Excellence. Implantable cardioverter-defibrillators for arrhythmias (review): NICE guidance TA095 [issued January 2006]. Available from: www.nice.org.uk.

18 Hohnloser SH, Kuck KH, Dorian P, et al. Prophylactic use of an implantable cardioverter-defibrillator after acute myocardial infarction. *N Engl J Med* 2004; 351: 2481–2488.

19 Bigger JT Jr. Prophylactic use of implanted cardiac defibrillators in patients at high risk for ventricular arrhythmias after coronary artery bypass graft surgery. Coronary Artery Bypass Graft (CABG) Patch Trial Investigators. *N Engl J Med* 1997; 337: 1569–75.

20 Kadish A, Dyer A, Daubert JP, et al. Prophylactic defibrillator implantation in patients with non-ischaemic dilated cardiomyopathy. *N Engl J Med* 2004; 350: 2151–2158.

21 Strickberger SA, Hummel JD, Bartlett TG, et al. Amiodarone vs implantable cardioverter-defibrillator: randomized trial in patients with non-ischaemic dilated cardiomyopathy and asymptomatic non-sustained ventricular tachycardia—AMIOVIRT. *J Am Coll Cardiol* 2003; 41: 1707–1712.

22. Kjekshus J, Apetrei E, Barrios V, et al. Rosuvastatin in older patients with systolic heart failure—CORONA Group. *N Engl J Med* 2007; 357: 2248–2261.

23 Bansch D, Antz M, Boczor S, et al. Primary prevention of sudden cardiac death in idiopathic dilated cardiomyopathy: the Cardiomyopathy Trial (CAT). *Circulation* 2002; 105: 1453–1458.

24 Chung ES, Leon AR, Tavazzi L, et al. Results of the Predictors of Response to CRT (PROSPECT) trial. *Circulation* 2008; 117: 2608–2616.

25 Richardson M, Freemantle N, Calvert MJ, et al. Predictors and treatment response with cardiac resynchronization therapy in patients with heart failure characterized by dyssynchrony: a pre-defined analysis from the CARE-HF trial. *Eur Heart J* 2007; 28: 1827–1834.

26 National Institute for Health and Clinical Excellence. Heart failure-cardiac resynchronisation: NICE guidance TA120 [issued May 2007]. Available from: http://www.nice.org.uk.

27 Yu CM, Wang L, Chau E, et al. Intrathoracic impedance monitoring in patients with heart failure: correlation with fluid status and feasibility of early warning preceding hospitalization. *Circulation* 2005; 112: 841–848.

28 Adamson PB, Smith AL, Abraham WT, et al. Continuous autonomic assessment in patients with symptomatic heart failure: prognostic value of heart rate variability measured by an implanted cardiac resynchronization device. *Circulation* 2004; 110:2389–2394.

29 Linde C, Abraham WT, Gold MR, et al. Randomized trial of cardiac resynchronization in mildly symptomatic heart failure patients and in asymptomatic patients with left ventricular dysfunction and previous heart failure symptoms. *J Am Coll Cardiol* 2008; 52: 1834–1843.

30 Moss AJ, Hall WJ, Cannom DS, et al. Cardiac resynchronization therapy for the prevention of heart failure events. *N Engl J Med* 2009; 361: 1329–1338.

11 Cardiac transplantation

Ali Vazir and Shouvik Haldar

Expert commentary Dr Jayan Parameshwar

Case history

A 55-year-old male taxi driver, with a 20-year history of dilated cardiomyopathy, presented with worsening breathlessness on minimal exertion (one to two metres on the flat), orthopnoea, and peripheral oedema to the mid-shin level. He was admitted to the Coronary Care Unit (CCU) at his local hospital, where he was treated with an intravenous furosemide infusion and optimization of his heart failure (HF) medication.

During this time, he had normal renal function and his electrocardiogram (ECG) had shown sinus rhythm with left bundle branch block, although short runs of non-sustained ventricular tachycardia (NSVT) were noted on telemetry. A transthoracic echocardiogram (TTE) demonstrated a significantly dilated left ventricle (left ventricular end-diastolic dimension 69 mm, left ventricular end-systolic dimension 60 mm), with severe left ventricular systolic dysfunction (LVSD) (biplane Simpson's ejection fraction of 37%). A coronary angiogram performed six years previously had shown normal coronary arteries. In view of the fact that he remained in New York Heart Association (NYHA) class III despite being on maximally tolerated HF therapy, coupled with the NSVT, it was felt that he would benefit from cardiac resynchronization therapy (CRT) with defibrillator (CRT-D). This was scheduled as an outpatient procedure and he was discharged home on lisinopril 20 mg once daily (od), spironolactone 25 mg od, digoxin 250 mcg od, furosemide 80 mg bd, carvedilol 25 mg bd and pravastatin 40 mg od.

Six weeks later, a CRT-D was implanted. This resulted in an initial, but short-lived, improvement in symptoms to NYHA class II. Four weeks later and despite echocardiographic optimization of his CRT-D device, he once again deteriorated back to NYHA class III with an exercise tolerance of 50–60 metres on the flat. As he remained refractory to maximum medical therapy, the local hospital referred him to the regional cardiac surgical centre to be considered for cardiac transplantation.

> **Expert comment**
>
> Guidelines for the treatment of chronic HF strongly recommend that the dose of drugs shown to be of prognostic benefit should be uptitrated to the maximally tolerated dose. The aim should be to reach the doses used in clinical trials. For example, the ATLAS study looked at lisinopril and demonstrated a significant benefit of high-dose ACE inhibition when compared with low-dose ACE inhibition. Therefore, the target dose for lisinopril should be 40 mg/day if blood pressure, renal function, and serum potassium allow [1].

> **★ Learning point** Indications for cardiac transplantation
>
> Cardiac transplantation is the treatment of choice for patients with end-stage HF who remain symptomatic despite optimal medical therapy. Unfortunately, the number of donor hearts is chronically much lower than the number of potential recipients [2]. As transplantation improves survival, the ability to estimate prognosis in patients with severe HF is a vital component of the selection process. The half-life (transplant half-life is the time at which 50% of those transplanted remain alive, or median survival) of patients' survival after cardiac transplantation was reported to be 10.3 years between 1992 and 2001 [2]. The ultimate decision to place a patient on the transplant waiting list is made by the clinicians at the transplanting centre. This is based upon the results of extensive investigations and sound clinical judgement. The indications and contraindications for cardiac transplantation are outlined in published guidelines from the American College of Cardiology/American Heart Association/International Society for Heart and Lung Transplantation (ACC/AHA/ISHLT) [3] (Table 11.1).

Apical 4 Chamber in End Diastole

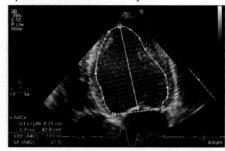

Apical 4 Chamber in End Systole

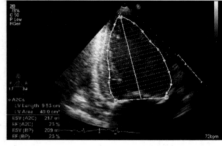

Apical 2 Chamber in End Diastole

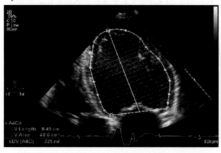

Apical 2 Chamber in End Systole

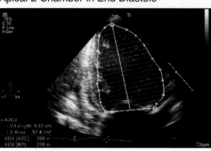

Figure 11.1 Biplane Simpson's transthoracic echocardiography images for estimation of left ventricular ejection fraction, demonstrating the tracing of endocardial borders as described.

At his initial review at the cardiac transplant centre, he underwent a repeat TTE and extensive blood tests. However, as he was tall and overweight (1.81 m, 112.5 kg, body mass index [BMI] 34 kg/m^2), a full transplant assessment was put on hold as it was felt that losing weight would improve his chances of a good outcome. The patient was advised to aim for a BMI of 30 kg/m^2 or below in order to become a more favourable candidate for cardiac transplantation. He was referred to a dietician and given an appointment for further outpatient evaluation in two months' time.

During the two months prior to his review, the patient developed atrial fibrillation (AF), resulting in a transient deterioration of his already impaired clinical status. He was electrically cardioverted to sinus rhythm and then anticoagulated with warfarin. Despite this setback, he managed to lose 13 kg of weight in this period, reducing his BMI to 30 kg/m^2. Thus, at his second review in the transplant centre, he underwent a more detailed assessment. This included a cardiopulmonary exercise test (CPET), TTE, right heart cardiac catheterization, blood tests (full blood counts, urea and electrolytes, liver and thyroid function tests), and pulmonary function tests (Table 11.2).

TTE confirmed a dilated and severely impaired LV with moderate functional mitral regurgitation (MR) and a moderate degree of pulmonary hypertension (right ventricular systolic pressure of 53 mmHg plus right atrial pressure). A CPET demonstrated a peak VO$_2$ of 13.4 mL/kg/min at anaerobic threshold.

Right heart cardiac catheterization revealed an elevated transpulmonary gradient and significant pulmonary vascular resistance (PVR). Therefore, at the same sitting, a sodium nitroprusside vasodilator study was performed in order to assess the

Table 11.1 Guidelines for cardiac transplantation adapted from the ACC/AHA/ISHLT [3]

1. Absolute indications
- Haemodynamic compromise due to HF:
  - Refractory cardiogenic shock
  - Dependence on intravenous inotropic support to maintain adequate organ perfusion and/or
  - Peak VO_2 less than 10 mL/kg/min with achievement of anaerobic metabolism
- Severe symptoms of ischaemia that consistently limit routine activity and are not amenable to coronary artery bypass surgery or percutaneous coronary intervention in patients with significantly impaired ventricular function
- Recurrent symptomatic ventricular arrhythmias refractory to all therapeutic modalities

2. Relative indications
- Peak VO_2 of 11 to 14 mL/kg/min (or 55% predicted) and major limitation of the patient's daily activities
- Recurrent unstable ischaemia not amenable to other intervention
- Recurrent instability of fluid balance/renal function not due to patient non-compliance with the pre-prescribed medical regimen

3. Absolute contraindications
- Systemic illness that will limit survival despite heart transplant (e.g. systemic lupus erythematosus and systemic sarcoid)
- Neoplasm other than skin. Low-grade prostate cancer that has not been 'cured' (by prostate-specific antigen measurement) or where the period of remission is fewer than five years is generally recognized as a contraindication
- HIV/AIDS (definition of CD4 count of <200 cells/mm³)
- Any systemic process with a high probability of recurrence in the transplanted heart
- Fixed pulmonary hypertension (both values below are arbitrary):
  - Pulmonary vascular resistance >5 Wood units
  - Transpulmonary gradient >15 mmHg

4. Relative contraindications
- Age over 65 years
- Symptomatic peripheral vascular disease
- Ankle-brachial index <0.7 or substantial risk of limb loss with diminished perfusion
- Asymptomatic carotid stenosis >75% or symptomatic carotid stenosis of less severity
- Diabetes mellitus with end-organ damage (nephropathy, neuropathy, retinopathy)
- Severe lung disease
- Systemic infection making immune suppression hazardous (HIV, hepatitis B, hepatitis C with fibrosis on liver biopsy)
- Psychosocial impairment that jeopardizes the transplanted heart (e.g. antisocial personality disorder, medication non-compliance, drug or alcohol addiction)
- Advanced liver disease (e.g. cirrhosis)
- Creatinine clearance of <40 mL/min (concern with post-transplantation immunosuppression medication such as long-term cyclosporin or tacrolimus)
- Recent pulmonary embolism (ideally need to wait at least six weeks prior to transplantation)

Clinical tip Why it is important to know the patient's vital statistics

- When referring patients for cardiac transplantation, it is imperative to know the height and weight of the patient to allow calculation of the BMI (kg/m²). The BMI is a crucial factor for two main reasons.
- Firstly, patients with a BMI >30 kg/m² have a higher morbidity and mortality after open-heart surgery [5,6]. Studies have shown that these patients are more likely to develop infections with poor wound healing, thrombosis, and pulmonary complications. However, data are still conflicting regarding these issues, as recent studies have shown no significant reduction in survival if an individual patient has a BMI >30 kg/m² [7–9]. However, the ISHLT believes that a pre-transplant BMI >30 kg/m² is associated with a poor outcome. Therefore, patients with BMI of 30–34 kg/m², if referred, are strongly encouraged to lose weight in order to improve outcomes post-transplantation.
- Secondly, size matching is important and is done differently from centre to centre. Some use height or weight alone whilst others may use both. For example, it is important not to undersize the heart for the patient by more than 5–10% of the recipient's height as the small donor heart may not be sufficient to support the circulation of a larger recipient.
- In summary, a BMI of <30 kg/m² is ideal for cardiac transplantation. Patients with a BMI of between 30–34 kg/m² are generally accepted for transplantation. However, patients with morbid obesity (BMI >34 kg/m²) will be considered too high a risk for cardiac transplantation and may be declined transplant assessment unless they demonstrate appropriate weight loss.

reversibility of the raised pulmonary arterial pressures. This showed that the PVR dropped from a baseline of 7.2 down to 2.2 Wood units with peak sodium nitroprusside infusion. The transpulmonary gradient also dropped from 24 at baseline, to 13 with peak sodium nitroprusside infusion. These results suggested that the pulmonary arterial hypertension (PAH) was reversible (see Table 11.3 for the full data set from this study).

Table 11.2 Investigations required for transplant work-up

Hb (g/dL)	13.4
WCC (x 10⁹/L)	10.4
Platelets (x 10⁹/L)	284
Na (mmol/L)	135
K (mmol/L)	4.6
Urea (mmol/L)	**11.4**
Creatinine (micromol/L)	**127**
Creatinine clearance mL/min	53
Albumin (g/L)	50
Bilirubin (micromol/L)	**26**
ALT (IU/L)	33
Alkaline phosphatase (IU/L)	65
Corrected calcium (mmol/L)	2.26
INR	**2.9**
Activated thromboplastin time (s)	**46.5**
TSH (IU/L)	4.93
T4 (pmol/L)	20
ABO blood group	A-negative
HLA	Negative
Virology	
CMV IgG	Negative
EBV IgG	Negative
Toxoplasma IgG	Negative
Hepatitis B surface antigen	Negative
Hepatitis B anti-core	Negative
Hepatitis C	Negative
Syphilis antibody	Negative
HIV-1 and -2	Negative
Spirometry	
FEV1 (L/min) (% predicted)	3.2 (88)
FVC (L/min) (% predicted)	4.4 (95)
Peak VO₂ (mL/kg/min)	12.4

⭐ **Learning point** Why is an irreversibly elevated PVR a contraindication?

Patients with an elevated PVR (>5 Wood units, see Case 23) or a transpulmonary gradient (mean pulmonary artery pressure minus mean pulmonary capillary wedge pressure) >15 mmHg, have an increased risk of right ventricular (RV) failure in the immediate post-operative period. It is in this period where the donor right ventricle is acutely subjected to a marked increase in workload [10,11].

PAH in most patients with HF is due to neurohumoral vasoconstriction, as opposed to structural changes in the pulmonary vasculature such as calcification or intimal/medial hyperplasia. Therefore, an elevated PVR may be reduced by using vasodilatory agents such as nitroprusside, dobutamine, milrinone, and inhaled nitric oxide [11–13]. Patients can be considered for transplantation if the PVR can be acutely reduced pharmacologically to below 4 Wood units. A study by Costard-Jackle, et al. showed that the 3-month mortality rate in patients whose PVR was >2.5 Wood units was higher compared to those with lower values (17.9% vs 6.9%) [11]. Their study also showed that in those with a high PVR responsive to nitroprusside, the 3-month mortality was only 3.8%. In contrast, the 3-month mortality was 41% and 28%, respectively, in those who were resistant to nitroprusside, or who only responded at a dose that caused systemic hypotension. Most importantly, their study showed that none of the patients with reversible PAH developed RV failure after transplantation.

Table 11.3 Sodium nitroprusside (SNP) vasodilator study assessing reversibility of the pulmonary arterial hypertension (Hb 12 g/dL)

	Baseline measurements	Low-dose SNP (1 mcg/kg/min)	Peak SNP dose (3 mcg/kg/min)
Non-invasive BP (mmHg)			
Systolic	100	95	90
Diastolic	70	64	57
Pulmonary arterial pressures (mmHg)			
Systolic	66	52	59
Diastolic	39	34	22
Mean	51	44	37
Mean pulmonary capillary wedge pressure (mmHg)	27	29	24
Transpulmonary gradient	24	16	13
O_2 saturation (%)	99	98	98
PA O_2 saturation (%)	58	67	71
Fick cardiac output (L/min)	3.2	5.2	5.9
PVR (Wood units)	7.4	3	2.2

Expert comment

Impaired RV function is common in the early post–transplantation period. This is thought to result from ischaemia during the period the organ is not perfused. When such a ventricle has to work against a high PVR, RV failure is more likely and patients may need inotropic support for several days post-transplantation. The degree to which 'reversibility' of a high PVR confers safety remains unclear.

Learning point Immediate complications post-cardiac transplantation

- Acute graft failure (not due to rejection, but due to an unknown cause)
- Acute rejection
- Pericardial effusion
- Arrhythmias
- Infection (cytomegalovirus, fungal, bacterial).

His case was discussed at a multidisciplinary cardiac transplantation meeting. As his elevated PVR was reversible, he was listed for cardiac transplantation. He was quoted a peri-operative mortality risk of 12%. Six months later, a suitable donor was found and he underwent successful orthotopic cardiac transplantation (OCT).

Post-operatively, he was on intensive care for five days. During this period, immunosuppression was induced by using a combination of rabbit anti-thymocyte globulin (RATG) for three days and mycophenolate mofetil (MMF) and corticosteroids (initially methylprednisolone followed by reducing doses of oral prednisolone). He was also treated with prophylactic antibacterial agents (teicoplanin, tazocin, and co-trimoxazole), antiviral agents (ganciclovir), and antifungal agents (fluconazole). Oral tacrolimus was commenced on day 4 post-operatively.

After intensive care unit (ICU), he was transferred to the high dependency unit on the transplant ward and had a complicated 2-week stay. During this period, he developed a left-sided pneumonia, with a para-pneumonic pleural effusion requiring a chest drain. He also developed renal dysfunction secondary to high tacrolimus levels. This was managed with a combination of rehydration, temporarily stopping the tacrolimus, but continuing immunosuppression with intravenous RATG, MMF, and prednisolone. At this point, he started to develop peripheral oedema with a raised jugular venous pressure, indicating possible cardiac allograft dysfunction. TTE, however, demonstrated good cardiac allograft systolic function with a small pericardial effusion. Nevertheless, he underwent an RV endomyocardial biopsy (EMB) which, after histological examination, excluded rejection. After a period of ten days, the patient's renal function and peripheral oedema improved significantly.

⊕ **Clinical tip** How to recognize and treat graft rejection

Rejection is commonest in the early period post-transplantation [14,15]. There are two types of rejection that are possible: cellular-mediated rejection and antibody-mediated rejection. The former is commoner by far, but the latter may carry a worse prognosis [16].

Rejection may manifest in several ways:

- Pyrexial illness;
- Rhythm disturbances, e.g. atrial tachycardia;
- Clinical features of HF with reduced exercise capacity or even fluid retention;
- Cardiogenic shock;
- Reduction in fractional shortening or EF on echocardiography from baseline.

If a cardiac transplant patient presents with features of HF, one must always consider the possibility of cardiac allograft rejection and consider immediate treatment with pulsed intravenous methylprednisolone (1 g for three days) whilst continuing standard oral immunosuppression. EMB is required to confirm the diagnosis and type and severity of rejection. The histological severity and presence or absence of haemodynamic compromise (e.g. reduction in cardiac output <4 L/min, a decrease in pulmonary artery saturation <50%, and raised pulmonary artery or pulmonary capillary wedge pressure), will determine the need for additional anti-rejection agents such as anti-thymocyte globulin. After an acute rejection has been treated successfully, a further EMB is required to confirm success, and the subsequent maintenance immunosuppressive regimen may need to be changed. For example, if the patient is on a combination of ciclosporin and azathioprine, the ciclosporin may be substituted with tacrolimus, which has been shown to reduce the frequency of further rejection episodes [17].

⭐ **Learning point** Arrhythmias post-cardiac transplantation

In the early post-operative period, bradyarrhythmias are common due to sinus node dysfunction secondary to surgical trauma to the sinoatrial node or its blood supply or very rarely, secondary to acute rejection. Therefore, surgeons routinely place epicardial pacing wires during the transplant to deal with this post-operative issue. A trial of theophylline may be used to try to increase the intrinsic heart rate and EMB performed to exclude acute rejection [18]. If the heart rate does not increase and acute rejection is excluded, then a permanent pacemaker should be implanted. The indications for implantation of permanent pacemakers in cardiac transplant patients are the same as for other patients. The presence of other arrhythmias such as sustained atrial flutter, atrial fibrillation, complex ventricular ectopy, or atrioventricular block may be associated with allograft rejection or graft vasculopathy [19]. Therefore, in this situation, patients should undergo EMB and receive steroids empirically, whilst awaiting the results of the biopsy. Patients with frequent and symptomatic supraventricular tachycardia should also be considered for radiofrequency catheter ablation.

Three weeks post-transplantation, he remained in a junctional bradycardia at a rate of 40–50 beats per minute despite having ten days of oral theophylline to increase his heart rate. This degree of bradycardia was felt to be inadequate for his recovery, and so a dual chamber permanent pacemaker was implanted via the left subclavian vein.

After the pacemaker was implanted, the patient was stepped down to a general cardiology ward. He was mobilized with intensive physiotherapy and made good progress. He was discharged one month after his transplant operation with the following medication; tacrolimus 1 mg twice daily (bd), MMF 1 g bd, prednisolone 10 mg od,

⭐ **Learning point**

Maintenance immunosuppression agents

Immune reactivity and tendency toward graft rejection are highest in the early period after graft implantation (within the first three to six months), and decreases with time. Thus, most drug regimens employ the highest intensity of immunosuppression immediately after surgery and decrease the intensity of therapy over the first year. The target is to prescribe the lowest maintenance levels of immunosuppression that prevent graft rejection whilst minimizing drug toxicities. The use of multiple low-dose drugs with non-overlapping toxicities is preferred over the use of higher doses of fewer drugs. Ideally, intense immunosuppression should be avoided as it may lead to a myriad of side effects, including susceptibility to infection and malignancy. An example of a typical immunosuppressive regimen consists of two or three drugs, including a calcineurin inhibitor, an anti-metabolite agent, and corticosteroids. The dose of the latter may be tapered over the first year.

Examples of maintenance immunosuppression include:

- Calcineurin inhibitors, e.g. cyclosporin and tacrolimus;
- Glucocorticoids, e.g. corticosteroids;
- Anti-metabolites, e.g. azathioprine and MMF;
- Proliferation signal inhibitors, e.g. sirolimus.

⭐ **Learning point** Long-term complications of cardiac transplantation

Most of the late occurring complications may be related to immunosuppression or related to the side effects of immunosuppressive agents:

- Hypertension
- Renal dysfunction
- Malignancy
- Osteoporosis
- Hyperlipidaemia
- Gout
- Diabetes mellitus

co-trimoxazole 480 mg od, bumetanide 2 mg bd, valganciclovir 450 mg bd, pravastatin 40 mg od, and alendronic acid 70 mg once a week.

The patient was followed up in the transplant clinic with routine TTE, ECG, CXR, and surveillance EMB which was performed on a weekly basis in the first six weeks, then fortnightly between the second and third months post-transplantation, then monthly up until the sixth month. His exercise capacity significantly improved over and above that of his pre-transplantation period to NYHA class I, alongside a moderate renal dysfunction (creatinine of 170 micromol/L) and peripheral oedema, responding to bumetanide 2 mg bd.

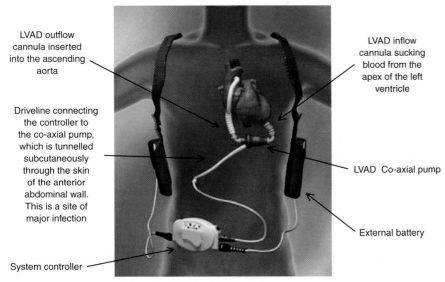

Figure 11.2 LVAD mechanism of action. With permission from Thoratec Corporation. Copyright 2010.

Discussion

Despite significant advances in the medical management of HF, some patients remain refractory to treatment. Cardiac transplantation can extend the survival and improve the quality of life for these patients. The number of transplant operations is dictated by the number of donor organs available, and despite the increasing use of older donors, organ availability has remained the rate-limiting step for the last two decades. The natural progression has been the development of cardiac support devices and currently, there are a variety of ventricular assist devices available. These devices have been successfully used as a bridge to transplantation in those deemed unlikely to survive the donor waiting list period.

Patients who are not cardiac transplant candidates due to comorbidities such as renal dysfunction may be considered for permanent LVAD implantation. This is known as destination therapy and may help maintain patients with end-stage HF for several years. Destination therapy is increasingly being used in the US and Europe; however, it is not currently funded in the UK. It is expected that the technology of LVADs will continue to improve such that a patient's cardiac function may be maintained for many years with a reducing risk of complications. This is a new area of research and is expected to play an increasing role in the survival of these patients.

Expert comment

Most patients can be weaned off steroids over the first 12 to 18 months post-transplantation. Patients with recurrent rejection or renal dysfunction (who may need low doses of calcineurin inhibitors) are often maintained on a low dose of steroid (about 5 mg/day of prednisolone).

Expert comment

Renal dysfunction is a side effect of treatment with calcineurin inhibitors, and current practice involves using lower doses than in the past. In selected patients with significant renal dysfunction (as in this case), it is possible to stop these drugs altogether, and use alternatives such as sirolimus or everolimus.

Cardiac allograft vasculopathy is a form of immune-mediated coronary artery disease, that is the biggest single cause of death in the late post-transplantation period (beyond five years). The initial lesion is intimal thickening with late lesions showing insudation of lipids and macrophages, akin to conventional atheroma. Diffuse disease is common and most patients are not suitable for treatment with angioplasty or bypass surgery. Angina does occur despite denervation, but is usually not severe. Treatment of conventional risk factors is important, and there is good evidence of improved survival with statins [20]. The only definitive therapy is re-transplantation which is an option open to very few patients.

Expert comment

The landmark ReMatch study [25] demonstrated that survival of patients with very severe HF was improved by mechanical support with the HeartMate I device, a pulsatile pump that does not require warfarin. This is still the only device approved for 'destination' therapy by the Food and Drug Administration (FDA) in the US, but has a relatively high rate of mechanical failure after the first year. A study comparing the HeartMate I device with the HeartMate II (a non-pulsatile axial flow pump) has reported significantly better survival with the latter device [26]. The HeartMate II has recently been approved by the FDA for both destination and bridge to transplantation therapy, whilst in Europe, this and other similar devices have been used for several years for these indications. With the continuing decline in the supply of donor hearts, it is expected that LVADs will play an increasing role in the long-term management of patients with advanced HF.

Learning point   Left ventricular assist devices explained

Left ventricular assist devices (LVAD) are used as a bridge to cardiac transplantation. They can be considered in patients on a cardiac transplant list who show signs of deterioration or for an individual who requires an urgent transplant where a donor heart is unavailable.

One of the commonest LVADs is an axial flow pump. This is a non-pulsatile pump that ejects blood from the left ventricle via a conduit to the aorta. These pumps are usually sewn into the apex of the left ventricle (Figure 11.2). The electrical supply to the pump is usually via a driveline that is tunnelled under the skin of the anterior abdominal wall with the external battery changed several times a day. This form of circulatory support can maintain potential transplant candidates for two to three years, or longer until an organ can be found for them.

Contraindications for LVAD implantation are similar to those of cardiac transplantation, but also include the presence of moderate to severe aortic regurgitation (AR), mechanical aortic valves, and contraindications to long-term anticoagulation [21]. If there is moderate to severe AR, blood pumped by the LVAD into the aorta will flow back into the left ventricle. This will result in volume overload for the LVAD and will impair its ability to generate forward flow. As the aortic valve does not open in the presence of an LVAD, a mechanical aortic valve is highly likely to develop thrombus on the aortic side, that can lead to thromboembolic consequences, and hence is a contraindication for LVAD implantation.

The presence of severe RV systolic dysfunction is an important determinant of post-implantation outcome, and a recent publication by Matthews, et al. has shown that an RV failure risk score (RVFRS) can be used preoperatively to determine the risk of RV failure post-LVAD implantation [22]. This scoring system includes elevated levels of aspartate transaminase >80 IU, bilirubin >2 mg/dL and creatinine >2.3 mg/dL, and the need for vasopressors. A high RVFRS identifies individuals that are at a high risk of death with LVAD implantation.

The commonest long-term complications of LVAD include localized driveline infections, infection of the LVAD, embolic strokes, and complications associated with long-term anticoagulation. It is possible that patients with severe complications from their LVAD may become unsuitable for transplant, e.g. having suffered from a severe debilitating stroke. Furthermore, the use of LVAD prior to cardiac transplantation may be associated with a small decrease in survival at one year, with the increase in mortality being most prominent in the first two weeks or six months after LVAD implantation [23,24].

A final word from the expert

Heart transplantation remains the most effective treatment modality for selected patients with advanced HF. Patients enjoy an excellent quality of life and median survival exceeds ten years in most centres. The need for lifelong immunosuppression imposes certain restrictions and long-term complications include an increased risk of malignancy (particularly skin cancer and non-Hodgkin's B cell lymphoma) and renal dysfunction. Allograft coronary artery disease is the most common cause of late graft failure, and treatment for this condition is limited. The shortage of donor organs means that this form of treatment will only be available to a minority of patients who could potentially benefit. Ventricular assist devices have been used for 25 years to support critically ill patients waiting for a heart transplant, but in the last decade, there has been increasing use of this modality as a treatment for end-stage HF. While device technology has progressed considerably, the need for an external power source and anticoagulation (often with antiplatelet agents and warfarin) remains a problem. Continuous flow devices are significantly smaller, quieter, and more patient-friendly, but survival at two years is still below 50%. Infection (particularly of the external driveline), bleeding, and thromboembolism are the main problems encountered with modern devices. Improvements in technology and increasing experience should lead to improvement in these figures over the next few years, and it is hoped that costs will fall as more devices are implanted.

References

1 Sculpher MJ, Poole L, Cleland JGF, et al. Low doses versus high doses of the angiotensin converting-enzyme inhibitor lisinopril in chronic heart failure: a cost-effectiveness analysis based on the Assessment of Treatment with Lisinopril and Survival (ATLAS) study. *European Journal of Heart Failure* 2000; 2: 447–454.

2 Taylor DO, Edwards LB, Aurora P, et al. Registry of the International Society for Heart and Lung Transplantation: twenty-fifth official adult heart transplant report—2008. *J Heart Lung Transplant* 2008; 27: 943–956.

3 Hunt SA, Abraham WT, Chin MH, et al. 2009 focused update incorporated into the ACC/AHA 2005 guidelines for the diagnosis and management of heart failure in adults: a report of the American College of Cardiology Foundation/American Heart Association Task Force on practice guidelines: developed in collaboration with the International Society for Heart and Lung Transplantation. *Circulation* 2009; 119: e391–e479.

4 Schiller NB, Shah PM, Crawford M, et al. Recommendations for quantitation of the left ventricle by 2-dimensional echocardiography. American Society of Echocardiography Committee on standards, subcommittee on quantitation of 2-dimensional echocardiograms. *J Am Soc Echocardiogr* 1989; 2: 358–367.

5 Fasol R, Schindler M, Schumacher B, et al. The influence of obesity on peri-operative morbidity: retrospective study of 502 aortocoronary bypass operations. *Thorac Cardiovasc Surg* 1992; 40: 126–129.

6 Birkmeyer NJ, Charlesworth DC, Hernandez F, et al. Obesity and risk of adverse outcomes associated with coronary artery bypass surgery. Northern New England Cardiovascular Disease study group. *Circulation* 1998; 97: 1689–1694.

7 Lietz K, John R, Burke EA, et al. Pre-transplant cachexia and morbid obesity are predictors of increased mortality after heart transplantation. *Transplantation* 2001; 72: 277–283.

8 Kocher AA, Ankersmit J, Khazen C, et al. Effect of obesity on outcome after cardiac transplantation. *Transplant Proc* 1999; 31: 3187–3189.

9 Taylor DO, Edwards LB, Boucek MM, et al. The Registry of the International Society for Heart and Lung Transplantation: twenty-first official adult heart transplant report—2004. *J Heart Lung Transplant* 2004; 23: 796–803.

10 Kirklin JK, Naftel DC, Kirklin JW, et al. Pulmonary vascular resistance and the risk of heart transplantation. *J Heart Transplant* 1988; 7: 331–336.

11 Costard–Jackle A, Fowler MB. Influence of preoperative pulmonary artery pressure on mortality after heart transplantation: testing of potential reversibility of pulmonary hypertension with nitroprusside is useful in defining a high-risk group. *J Am Coll Cardiol* 1992; 19: 48–54.

12 Givertz MM, Hare JM, Loh E, et al. Effect of bolus milrinone on haemodynamic variables and pulmonary vascular resistance in patients with severe left ventricular dysfunction: a rapid test for reversibility of pulmonary hypertension. *J Am Coll Cardiol* 1996; 28: 1775–1780.

13 Loh E, Stamler JS, Hare JM, et al. Cardiovascular effects of inhaled nitric oxide in patients with left ventricular dysfunction. *Circulation* 1994; 90: 2780–2785.

14 Nagele H, Rodiger W. Sudden death and tailored medical therapy in elective candidates for heart transplantation. *J Heart Lung Transplant* 1999; 18: 869–876.

15 Kubo SH, Naftel DC, Mills RM, et al. Risk factors for late recurrent rejection after heart transplantation: a multi-institutional, multivariable analysis. Cardiac Transplant Research Database Group. *J Heart Lung Transplant* 1995; 14: 409–418.

16 Taylor DO, Yowell RL, Kfoury AG, et al. Allograft coronary artery disease: clinical correlations with circulating anti-HLA antibodies and the immunohistopathologic pattern of vascular rejection. *J Heart Lung Transplant* 2000; 19: 518–521.

17 Yamani MH, Starling RC, Pelegrin D, et al. Efficacy of tacrolimus in patients with steroid-resistant cardiac allograft cellular rejection. *J Heart Lung Transplant* 2000; 19: 337–342.

18 Redmond JM, Zehr KJ, Gillinov MA, et al. Use of theophylline for treatment of prolonged sinus node dysfunction in human orthotopic heart transplantation. *J Heart Lung Transplant* 1993; 12: 133–138.

19 Ahmari SA, Bunch TJ, Chandra A, et al. Prevalence, pathophysiology, and clinical significance of post-heart transplant atrial fibrillation and atrial flutter. *J Heart Lung Transplant* 2006; 25: 53–60.

20 Kobashigawa JA, Katznelson S, Laks H, et al. Effect of pravastatin on outcomes after cardiac transplantation. *N Eng J Med* 1995; 333: 621–627.

21 Wilson SR, Mudge GH, Jr., Stewart GC, et al. Evaluation for a ventricular assist device: selecting the appropriate candidate. *Circulation* 2009; 119: 2225–2232.

22 Matthews JC, Koelling TM, Pagani FD, et al. The right ventricular failure risk score a preoperative tool for assessing the risk of right ventricular failure in left ventricular assist device candidates. *J Am Coll Cardiol* 2008; 51: 2163–2172.

23 Joyce DL, Southard RE, Torre-Amione G, et al. Impact of left ventricular assist device (LVAD)-mediated humoral sensitization on post-transplant outcomes. *J Heart Lung Transplant* 2005; 24: 2054–2059.

24 Drakos SG, Kfoury AG, Long JW, et al. Effect of mechanical circulatory support on outcomes after heart transplantation. *J Heart Lung Transplant* 2006; 25: 22–28.

25 Rose EA, Geljins AC, Moskowitz MD, et al. Long-term use of a left ventricular assist device for end-stage heart failure. *N Engl J Med* 2001; 345: 1435–1443.

26 Slaughter MS, Rogers JG, Milano CA, et al. Advanced heart failure treated with continuous flow left ventricular assist device. *N Engl J Med* 2009; 361: 2241–2251.

Young patients with hypertrophic cardiomyopathy: how to decide on implantable defibrillators

Ricardo Petraco

❝ Expert commentary Professor Michael Frenneaux

Case history

A 32-year-old Afro-Caribbean male patient was referred to cardiology for investigation of dyspnoea on exertion. Previously fit and well, he described 12 months of progressive deterioration in his exercise tolerance, initially noted as a lack of fitness to play football with his peers and ultimately to struggling with stairs and inclines. He denied chest pain, palpitations, and syncope, but on further questioning, he described occasional episodes of dizziness which would resolve spontaneously, mainly occurring on hot days. His previous medical history was unremarkable with no family history of cardiac disease or sudden cardiac death (SCD). His cardiovascular (CV) examination was normal at rest with a blood pressure (BP) of 130/70 mmHg and a heart rate of 75 beats per minute (bpm). His chest X-ray was normal, but the 12-lead electrocardiogram (ECG) revealed voltage criteria for left ventricular hypertrophy (LVH) with marked repolarization abnormalities (Figure 12.1).

> **➕ Clinical tip** Dyspnoea and cardiac disease
>
> - Assessing dyspnoea in a young adult with a possible inherited or congenital heart disorder can be challenging since they adapt to their level of exercise tolerance and might not report any symptoms spontaneously. A useful tip is to ask them to compare their ability to their peers. The commonly used New York Heart Association (NYHA) class may be misleading on assessing symptoms.
> - Remember that the clinical examination at rest may be entirely normal since 'heart failure' is a disease of exertion.
> - An abnormal ECG in a young patient with exertional symptoms is highly suggestive of a cardiac aetiology.

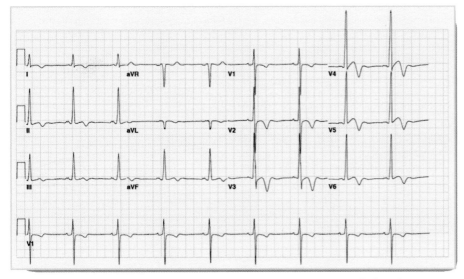

Figure 12.1 ECG showing voltage criteria for left ventricular hypertrophy and marked repolarization abnormalities in the chest leads.

A transthoracic echocardiogram (TTE) was performed and showed marked asymmetric septal hypertrophy (ASH) of 2.8 cm with normal left ventricular cavity size and preserved systolic function (Figure 12.2). Doppler study of the left ventricular outflow tract (LVOT) revealed a gradient of 20 mmHg, considered to be only mild. There was mild chordal systolic anterior motion (SAM).

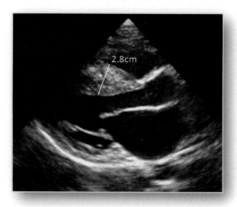

Figure 12.2 Parasternal long axis view of a transthoracic echocardiogram showing marked asymetric septal hypertrophy.

⭐ **Learning point** Differential diagnosis of left ventricular hypertrophy

Patients with LVH on echocardiography without an obvious clinical reason (aortic stenosis, aortic coarctation, longstanding uncontrolled high BP, etc) are classified as having 'unexplained hypertrophy'. The differential diagnoses are [1,2]:

1. Hypertrophy caused by sarcomeric mutations or classical hypertrophic cardiomyopathy (HCM), the commonest inherited cardiac disorder;
2. Athlete's heart, usually associated with a slightly enlarged LV cavity size, symmetrical hypertrophy, and septal thickness of <15 mm [2,3];
3. Fabry's disease (caused by alpha-galactosidase A enzyme deficiency, accounts for approximately 1% of patients with unexplained hypertrophy, and is a form of cardiomyopathy that can be treated if diagnosed early) [4];
4. Amyloidosis (in the early stages, LV systolic function can be normal);
5. Other forms of infiltrative heart disease [2].

There is no gold standard test for the diagnosis of HCM and none of the imaging findings are pathognomonic of the condition [1]. However, the finding of unexplained hypertrophy is more likely to represent HCM in the presence of the following features:

- Septal to posterior wall thickness ratio >1.5;
- Presence of SAM of the mitral valve with a dynamic LVOT gradient;
- Family history of HCM;
- Marked ECG repolarization abnormalities.

Indeed, to differentiate HCM from the physiological hypertrophy seen in athletes, the ECG is the most useful tool. The presence of an LV strain pattern and repolarization abnormalities in the left chest leads are highly suggestive of HCM and virtually exclude 'normal hypertrophy' [3,5], at least in Caucasians.

ℹ️ **Expert comment**

In Afro-Caribbeans, the ECG may show repolarization changes, even in the absence of HCM and LVH may be more marked in athletes, making the diagnosis very difficult in some cases.

> ⊗ **Learning point** Classification of cardiomyopathies: the genotypic or phenotypic approach?
>
> In the last few years, much debate has arisen on how to classify cardiomyopathies. One approach, favoured by the American Heart Association (AHA), is to define the disease by its aetiology and underlying genetic abnormality [2]. For example, HCM would be diagnosed only in those patients with proven sarcomeric protein mutations and/or after exclusion of other conditions such as storage disorders (e.g. Fabry's disease and amyloidosis). The problem with this type of classification (diagnosis by exclusion) is its lack of application in clinical practice since the majority of patients present with a symptomatic manifestation of the disease process (e.g. dyspnoea with unexplained LVH) rather than with an abnormal genetic test result. Also, it is well recognized that the same genetic abnormality can cause different phenotypic presentations (e.g. hypertrophic or restrictive cardiomyopathy, even in patients within the same family).
>
> An alternative approach, supported by the European Society of Cardiology (ESC), is to define disease as it presents to the cardiologist [6]. In our case, the term HCM would mean unexplained myocardial hypertrophy with symptoms of heart failure, independent of aetiology. This has the potential, however, to generate inaccuracy from the pathological point of view. For example, amyloidosis could be defined as HCM although no hypertrophy of myocardial fibres is seen. Also, it should be noted that HCM and amyloid heart disease have a completely different prognosis and currently available management options.
>
> Ideally, we should try to combine both strategies, aiming to initially assess the patient and the clinical presentation (e.g. unexplained LVH), but not forgetting the importance of searching for a final diagnosis (e.g. HCM or Fabry's disease) which will have important therapeutic implications.

With a working diagnosis of HCM, the patient proceeded to cardiac magnetic resonance (CMR) imaging for more accurate assessment of septal thickness and for visualization of the cardiac apex which can be commonly missed on echocardiography (Figure 12.3). It confirmed the presence of ASH with no evidence of apical hypertrophy. It also confirmed the associated mild dynamic obstruction of the LVOT at rest with a similar gradient as that found on TTE and no SAM of the mitral valve. Also, late gadolinium enhancement showed no evidence of septal fibrosis.

The patient was referred to the cardiomyopathy clinic where he was offered testing for Fabry's disease. It was felt that amyloid heart disease was clinically unlikely. In addition, first-degree relatives were also screened for any evidence of cardiomyopathy with a routine consultation, ECG, and TTE.

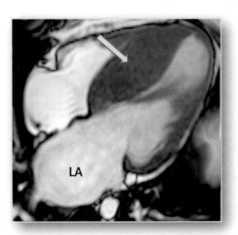

Figure 12.3 Cardiac MRI confirming the asymmetric septal hypertrophy (arrow) and no evidence of apical hypertrophy. Also, note the mildly dilated left atrium (LA).

Expert comment

The first-line treatment for symptomatic HCM patients with **LVOT obstruction** is beta-blocker therapy. This, however, is effective as monotherapy only in the minority. In the majority, the addition of disopyramide to beta-blockade is necessary to adequately relieve symptoms. In patients who remain symptomatic despite medical intervention or who cannot tolerate their side effects, alternative options include surgical septal myectomy or alcohol septal ablation.

Medical therapy for symptomatic **non-obstructive** HCM should be with non-dihydropyridine calcium channel blockers (e.g. verapamil or diltiazem) in the first instance and beta-blockers as second-line agents.

A subgroup of patients with HCM develop progressive impairment of systolic function in association with worsening symptoms. This is treated in much the same way as LV systolic dysfunction of other causes.

Learning point Derivation and management of symptoms in hypertrophic cardiomyopathy [7,8]

- In the absence of a significant resting outflow tract obstruction, symptoms of dyspnoea and chest pain in HCM are probably multifactorial, including diastolic dysfunction and microvascular disease. However, it is important to consider the possibility of a marked increase in outflow tract gradient during exercise.
- Dizziness and syncope can also be caused by LVOT obstruction, but atrial and, most importantly, malignant ventricular arrhythmias need to be excluded.
- Medical treatment is considered the first-line therapy for the relief of symptoms in HCM with associated LVOT obstruction. The general principle is to use inotropically and chronotropically negative agents, aiming to prolong diastole and increase LV diastolic volumes, which can decrease the LVOT dynamic gradient. Beta-blockers and non-dihydropyridine calcium channel blockers are usually the first choice given their safety profile.
- Avoid medications and environmental factors that could reduce pre-load or cause vasodilatation (ACE inhibitors, diuretics, dehydration, etc), except in patients with LV systolic dysfunction. They can lead to a marked drop in the pre-load-dependent cardiac output characteristic of haemodynamically significant HCM and may also exacerbate outflow tract obstruction.

For further risk stratification, the patient proceeded to a treadmill exercise test and an echocardiogram undertaken during cycle exercise. This revealed a poor exercise tolerance, the patient only managing to reach the start of stage 2 of the Bruce protocol. The BP response was appropriate (i.e. > 25 mmHg rise in systolic BP) with no exercise-induced ventricular arrhythmias. During cycle exercise, marked SAM developed and the peak instantaneous LV outflow tract gradient increased to 70 mmHg. An initial 24-hour tape recorder showed no atrial arrhythmias and only occasional ventricular premature beats (VPB). The patient was initiated on bisoprolol at 5 mg once daily (od) and was given general advice on non-pharmacological aspects of his treatment which included avoidance of competitive exercise.

Learning point Risk stratification for sudden cardiac death in hypertrophic cardiomyopathy

Identifying which patients with HCM are at greatest risk of SCD remains one of the most challenging steps in its management. Those at high risk should be offered an ICD since no medical therapy has been proven to improve prognosis in this population [1,14]. The initial problem lies in defining 'high risk'.

There is general agreement that patients with previous sustained ventricular arrhythmias or aborted SCD need an ICD (secondary prevention). No randomized controlled trial has been performed, but the reported discharge rates from implanted ICDs in this population (5–11% per year) is as high as reported in other secondary prevention trials in patients with ischaemic heart disease and heart failure [15].

One main question remains at least partially unanswered: which patients with HCM require an ICD for primary prevention of SCD? Six major risk factors for SCD have been identified [1,14]:

- Presence of NSVT on ECG monitoring (more than three beats at 120 bpm), especially in patients younger than 30 years of age, when the risk increases fourfold [16];
- Septal thickness >30 mm (this cut-off is not arbitrary since the thicker the septum, the higher the risk) [17,18];
- Family history of SCD in young first-degree relative (<45 years old);
- Abnormal BP response to exercise (failure to increase systolic BP by at least 25 mmHg) [19];
- History of unexplained syncope;
- The presence of a resting LVOT gradient >30 mmHg.

continued

Those with two or more risk factors should be offered an ICD since the reported annual rate of events is up to 5% [15]. Debate remains on which patient with one major risk factor (which represents up to 25% of patients with HCM) need an ICD. Data from more recent cohorts suggest that they are also a relatively high-risk group (1–3% per year risk of SCD), but there are no prospective data showing benefits with an ICD in this group of patients [20]. Patients with no major risk factors have a low incidence of events (0.8% per year) and there is general agreement that they should not usually be offered an ICD for primary prevention [1,14].

Other potential (minor) risk factors include: younger age at diagnosis, myocardial fibrosis seen on CMR, and certain specific sarcomeric mutations (e.g. certain troponin T and myosin heavy chain mutations). To what extent the presence of minor risk factors influences treatment decisions is yet to be determined. The general advice is to individualize treatment and to incorporate all information available to create an individual risk profile and finally decide whether an ICD is required. For example, patients with only one major risk factor might be candidates for an ICD in the presence of one or more minor risk factors [1,14,21,22].

On initial assessment, the only major risk factor for SCD was the septal thickness of 2.8 cm which was at the lower borderline limit of the established cut-off. The presence of a mild LVOT gradient at rest which increased during exercise could be included as a minor risk factor. In a multidisciplinary team (MDT) discussion, it was decided that an ICD was not indicated and the initial management should aim to control symptoms with an appropriate dose of beta-blocker.

⊕ Learning point The genetic foundation of hypertrophic cardiomyopathy

- HCM is the commonest form of inherited cardiac disease with an estimated prevalence of 0.16–0.3%. Men of Afro-Caribbean descent are affected twice as much as the general population [1,2].
- It is an autosomal dominant disease with most mutations found in one of the 12 genes that encode proteins of the cardiac sarcomere (contractile proteins). The overall prevalence of mutations in affected patients varies between study series, but ranges between 30 and 60% [23,24].
- The sarcomeric proteins involved in the aetiology of HCM include: cardiac troponin T, cardiac troponin I, myosin regulatory light chain, myosin essential light chain, cardiac myosin binding protein C, alpha and cardiac beta-myosin heavy chain, cardiac alpha-actin, alpha tropomyosin, and titin [24].
- *De novo* mutations have been described in patients with HCM without familial disease [23,24].
- The presence of Wolff–Parkinson–White (WPW) in a young patient with a phenotype of HCM could point towards the diagnosis of a glycogen storage disease (PRKAG2 and LAMP2 genes mutations), usually with a poorer prognosis. Mutation in the LAMP2 gene can cause Danon disease, a systemic syndrome, which is characterized by cardiomyopathy, skeletal myopathy, and variable mental retardation [25].
- Remember that up to 12% of patients older than 40 years of age with unexplained hypertrophy can have Fabry's disease, a treatable form of cardiomyopathy caused by a mutation in the gene encoding alpha-galactosidase A with an X-linked recessive pattern of inheritance.
- Whether or not all patients should be offered genetic testing is a matter of debate. Technical issues, relatively low prevalence of individual mutations, and related costs currently prevent its widespread use in clinical practice.

On subsequent follow-up, the patient reported that his symptoms had not improved with an optimal dose of bisoprolol. Indeed, a repeat exercise echocardiogram showed that a significant LVOT gradient was still present at peak exercise (Figure 12.4). A trial of disopyramide was unsuccessful due to poorly tolerated side effects.

Given the failure of medical therapy to control his symptoms together with the persistence of the LVOT gradient, the patient was referred to the regional tertiary centre

⊕ Clinical tip General lifestyle advice for patients with HCM

Patients with diagnosed or suspected HCM should not participate in competitive sports, given the increased risk of SCD. This recommendation is extended to all risk groups, independent of age, severity of LVH, symptomatic status, and presence of LVOT obstruction. Advising patients on the practice of recreational sports can be more challenging. In general, high-intensity activities (squash, singles' tennis, football, sprinting, weightlifting, etc) should be avoided. Cycling, doubles' tennis, swimming, and golf are generally considered safe when performed in moderation. Overall, patients with HCM should be encouraged to avoid any form of exercise which provokes limiting dyspnoea. Importantly, remember that such restrictions may also interfere with the patient's sex life [9,10].

Flying is unrestricted since there is no evidence of a specific increased risk of events in this population. However, the general recommendation to avoid dehydration must be emphasized.

Driving restrictions apply in the same manner as for other cardiac conditions and depends on the presenting history (resuscitated cardiac arrest, syncope, ventricular arrhythmias) and whether or not an implantable cardioverter-defibrillator (ICD) has been implanted. There are no individualized rules for patients with HCM [11].

⊕ Clinical tip Arrhythmias in hypertrophic cardiomyopathy

- Patients with marked ventricular hypertrophy and small cavity size may poorly tolerate atrial arrhythmias, especially AF [12].
- VPB, even if frequent (>500/ day), don't appear to be indicative of an increased risk of cardiac events in patients with HCM [13]. Non-sustained ventricular tachycardia (NSVT), however, is a risk factor for SCD.

Clinical tip What if medical therapy fails to control symptoms?

When medical therapy fails to provide relief of symptoms in the presence of a significant LVOT gradient at rest or exercise, an invasive procedure is usually indicated [1,26]. Surgical myomectomy or percutaneous septal ablation are both recognized options. No prospective, randomized trial has compared the efficacy of these interventions and most published data come from independent observational cohorts [7,8,26].

Both surgical myomectomy and septal ablation are associated with symptomatic benefit and proven LVOT gradient reduction [27,28]. However, both procedures are also associated with a risk of death and complications and there are no prospective data showing that they improve survival. Although observational data suggest that surgery might be associated with greater long-term symptomatic benefit, the choice between procedures is largely dependent on regional expertise since patients treated in high-volume centres tend to have better outcomes [29,30].

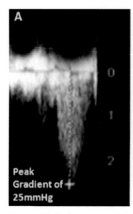 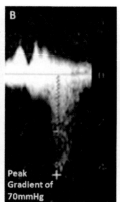 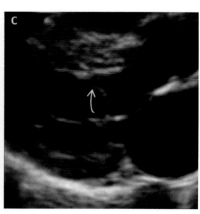

Figure 12.4 Continuous Doppler of the LVOT at rest
(A) showing only a mild gradient of 25 mmHg and at peak exercise (B) showing a significant rise to 70 mmHg. On C, 2D echo imaging during peak exercise revealing SAM of the mitral valve (arrow showing direction of the anterior mitral valve leaflet across the left ventricular outflow tract).

for percutaneous alcohol septal ablation which was performed without complications. A repeat CMR scan six months after the procedure confirmed a significant reduction in septal thickness, confirming the anatomical success of the procedure (Figure 12.5).

On subsequent follow-up, the patient reported that his exercise tolerance was significantly improved and he was finally able to perform daily activities with no restriction. A repeated exercise echocardiogram showed no evidence of SAM of the mitral valve and a significant reduction of the LVOT gradient (25 mmHg).

However, follow-up investigations prompted review of his treatment options. A 7-day event recorder revealed the presence of three isolated episodes of NSVT; all were brief (≤7 beats) and asymptomatic. Hence, together with the septal thickness of 28 mm, another major risk factor was identified. Although now diminished, the raised LVOT gradient which was originally present could also be included as a minor risk factor.

At a subsequent MDT discussion, it was decided that the patient should be offered an ICD for primary prevention of SCD on the basis of two major and one minor risk factors. After an uncomplicated ICD implantation, the patient was followed up in clinic

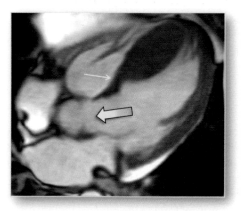

Figure 12.5 Cardiac MRI repeated post-septal ablation, showing significant thinning of the proximal septum (small arrow) and some reverse remodelling of the left ventricular hypertrophy. The net effect is a significant increase in the LVOT area which prevents SAM of the mitral valve and relieves the dynamic obstruction (large arrow).

for 12 months with no evidence of device discharge or sustained arrhythmias. His symptoms remained unchanged.

Discussion

This case describes a typical young patient with haemodynamically significant HCM and the well recognized clinical dilemmas that cardiologists face when dealing with this condition. Which patients should be offered invasive treatment for LVOT obstruction? Which patients require an ICD for primary prevention? What is the impact of individual risk factors on the decision-making process? The reason for so many unanswered questions is clearly the lack of prospective and randomized controlled trial data to guide current management decisions. Large trials are unlikely to be developed given the low prevalence of the disease and a relatively low incidence of major clinical events in affected individuals.

However, there are several key messages to be learnt from the medical literature, which have been applied in this clinical case:

- A phenotypic diagnosis is preferred and the term 'unexplained LVH' is the ideal starting point for a differential diagnosis. Remember that amyloid and more importantly, Fabry's disease can have very similar presentations.
- Assessing exertional symptoms in young patients can be challenging and the NYHA classification might be misleading. A formal exercise treadmill test ideally with an assessment of peak oxygen consumption can help to objectively assess symptoms.
- All patients should have an assessment for LVOT obstruction at rest and if necessary, during exercise.
- The two most important management decisions are how to improve symptoms and how to prevent SCD.
- For symptoms of angina and dyspnoea, medical therapy is the first option. Invasive procedures should be offered when symptoms persist AND significant LVOT obstruction is proven at rest or during exercise. The choice of the procedure should be based on local availability and more importantly, experience.
- The risk stratification for SCD should be individualized in those patients with one major risk factor. Patients with two major risk factors need an ICD.
- Follow-up with a cardiologist is very important and risk stratification for SCD should be reassessed when a new variable is added to the clinical context.
- Family screening of first-degree relatives with ECG and echocardiography is recommended.
- The precise role of genetic testing in clinical practice is yet to be determined.

💬 **A final word from the expert**

HCM is a common inherited cardiac disorder. Symptomatic management should be tailored to underlying mechanisms (obstructive/non-obstructive/systolic failure). Risk factor stratification is an important aspect of assessment and in high-risk cases, ICD implantation should be offered. Overall management requires a discussion of the treatability and implications for first-degree relatives and this is often best done in collaboration with clinical genetics services. Genetic testing is now available.

➕ **Clinical tip** Surveillance of patients with hypertrophic cardiomyopathy

The current consensus recommends yearly cardiology follow-up with the following: complete history and clinical examination, echocardiography, 24–48 hour Holter monitoring, and exercise test to assess BP response [1]. If an ICD has already been implanted, none of the risk stratification investigations are necessary. Symptoms should be assessed clinically and by resting or exercise echocardiography, looking for SAM and the presence of an LVOT gradient.

➕ **Clinical tip** Risks of implantable cardioverter–defibrillator implantation

When deciding which HCM patients should receive an ICD, it should be borne in mind that this is a treatment option associated with potential short- and long-term complications [31,32,33]:

- A 1% risk of pneumothorax if subclavian access is used;
- Up to 1% risk of device infection per year, which can be a catastrophic complication;
- The need for device change every five to ten years, which is an important consideration in young patients when many subsequent procedures are expected;
- Risk of inappropriate shocks when atrial tachyarrhythmias or even sinus tachycardia are misdiagnosed as ventricular tachycardia (VT) or ventricular fibrillation (VF).

Also, the psychological impact of such therapy should be considered. Patients can develop great anxiety related to the possibility of ICD discharge and the repercussions of an event can be life-changing. Group support can be useful along with a dedicated team to look after patients during follow-up. In the UK, the charity group, Cardiac Risk in the Young (CRY), runs specific projects to help young patients with cardiomyopathies and patients with an ICD (available from: **www.c-r-y.org.uk**).

References

1 Maron BJ, McKenna WJ, Danielson GK, et al. American College of Cardiology/European Society of Cardiology clinical expert consensus document on hypertrophic cardiomyopathy. A report of the American College of Cardiology Foundation Task Force on Clinical Expert Consensus Documents and the European Society of Cardiology Committee for practice guidelines. *J Am Coll Cardiol* 2003; 42: 1687–1713.

2 Maron BJ, Towbin JA, Thiene G, et al. Contemporary definitions and classification of the cardiomyopathies: an American Heart Association Scientific Statement from the Council on Clinical Cardiology, Heart Failure and Transplantation Committee; Quality of Care and Outcomes Research and Functional Genomics and Translational Biology Interdisciplinary Working Groups; and Council on Epidemiology and Prevention. *Circulation* 2006; 113: 1807–1816.

3 Maron BJ, Pelliccia A, Spirito P. Cardiac disease in young trained athletes. Insights into methods for distinguishing athlete's heart from structural heart disease, with particular emphasis on hypertrophic cardiomyopathy. *Circulation* 1995; 91: 1596–1601.

4 Sachdev B, Takenaka T, Teraguchi H, et al. Prevalence of Anderson–Fabry disease in male patients with late onset hypertrophic cardiomyopathy. *Circulation* 2002; 105: 1407–1411.

5 Savage DD, Seides SF, Clark CE, et al. Electrocardiographic findings in patients with obstructive and non-obstructive hypertrophic cardiomyopathy. *Circulation* 1978; 58: 402–408.

6 Elliott P, Andersson B, Arbustini E, et al. Classification of the cardiomyopathies: a position statement from the European Society of Cardiology Working Group on myocardial and pericardial diseases. *Eur Heart J* 2008; 29: 270–276.

7 Fifer MA, Vlahakes GJ. Management of symptoms in hypertrophic cardiomyopathy. *Circulation* 2008; 117: 429–439.

8 Spirito P, Seidman CE, McKenna WJ, et al. The management of hypertrophic cardiomyopathy. *N Engl J Med* 1997; 336: 775–785.

9 Pelliccia A, Fagard R, Bjornstad HH, et al. Recommendations for competitive sports participation in athletes with cardiovascular disease: a consensus document from the Study Group of Sports Cardiology of the Working Group of Cardiac Rehabilitation and Exercise Physiology and the Working Group of Myocardial and Pericardial Diseases of the European Society of Cardiology. *Eur Heart J* 2005; 26: 1422–1445.

10 Maron BJ, Chaitman BR, Ackerman MJ, et al. Recommendations for physical activity and recreational sports participation for young patients with genetic cardiovascular diseases. *Circulation* 2004; 109: 2807–2816.

11 Driver and Vehicle Licensing Agency. DVLA fitness to drive standards, 2009. Available from: www.dvla.gov.uk.

12 Olivotto I, Cecchi F, Casey SA, et al. Impact of atrial fibrillation on the clinical course of hypertrophic cardiomyopathy. *Circulation* 2001; 104: 2517–2524.

13 Adabag AS, Casey SA, Kuskowski MA, et al. Spectrum and prognostic significance of arrhythmias on ambulatory Holter electrocardiogram in hypertrophic cardiomyopathy. *J Am Coll Cardiol* 2005; 45: 697–704.

14 Elliott P, Spirito P. Prevention of hypertrophic cardiomyopathy-related deaths: theory and practice. *Heart* 2008; 94: 1269–1275.

15 Maron BJ, Shen WK, Link MS, et al. Efficacy of implantable cardioverter-defibrillators for the prevention of sudden death in patients with hypertrophic cardiomyopathy. *N Engl J Med* 2000; 342: 365–73.

16 Monserrat L, Elliott PM, Gimeno JR, et al. Non-sustained ventricular tachycardia in hypertrophic cardiomyopathy: an independent marker of sudden death risk in young patients. *J Am Coll Cardiol* 2003; 42: 873–879.

17 Spirito P, Bellone P, Harris KM, et al. Magnitude of left ventricular hypertrophy and risk of sudden death in hypertrophic cardiomyopathy. *N Engl J Med* 2000; 342: 1778–1785.

18 Elliott PM, Gimeno Blanes JR, Mahon NG, et al. Relation between severity of left ventricular hypertrophy and prognosis in patients with hypertrophic cardiomyopathy. *Lancet* 2001; 357: 420–424.

19 Sadoul N, Prasad K, Elliott PM, et al. Prospective prognostic assessment of blood pressure response during exercise in patients with hypertrophic cardiomyopathy. *Circulation* 1997; 96: 2987–2991.

20 Maron BJ, Spirito P, Shen WK, et al. Implantable cardioverter-defibrillators and prevention of sudden cardiac death in hypertrophic cardiomyopathy. *JAMA* 2007; 298: 405–412.

21 Maron MS, Olivotto I, Betocchi S, et al. Effect of left ventricular outflow tract obstruction on clinical outcome in hypertrophic cardiomyopathy. *N Engl J Med* 2003; 348: 295–303.

22 Maron BJ, Maron MS, Lesser JR, et al. Sudden cardiac arrest in hypertrophic cardiomyopathy in the absence of conventional criteria for high-risk status. *Am J Cardiol* 2008; 101: 544–547.

23 Marian AJ, Roberts R. The molecular genetic basis for hypertrophic cardiomyopathy. *J Mol Cell Cardiol* 2001; 33: 655–670.

24 Richard P, Charron P, Carrier L, et al. Hypertrophic cardiomyopathy: distribution of disease genes, spectrum of mutations, and implications for a molecular diagnosis strategy. *Circulation* 2003; 107: 2227–2232.

25 Arad M, Maron BJ, Gorham JM, et al. Glycogen storage diseases presenting as hypertrophic cardiomyopathy. *N Engl J Med* 2005; 352: 362–372.

26 Ommen SR, Shah PM, Tajik AJ. Left ventricular outflow tract obstruction in hypertrophic cardiomyopathy: past, present and future. *Heart* 2008; 94: 1276–1281.

27 Valeti US, Nishimura RA, Holmes DR, et al. Comparison of surgical septal myectomy and alcohol septal ablation with cardiac magnetic resonance imaging in patients with hypertrophic obstructive cardiomyopathy. *J Am Coll Cardiol* 2007; 49: 350–357.

28 Sorajja P, Valeti U, Nishimura RA, et al. Outcome of alcohol septal ablation for obstructive hypertrophic cardiomyopathy. *Circulation* 2008; 118: 131–139.

29 Watkins H, McKenna WJ. The prognostic impact of septal myectomy in obstructive hypertrophic cardiomyopathy. *J Am Coll Cardiol* 2005; 46: 477–479.

30 Maron BJ. Controversies in cardiovascular medicine. Surgical myectomy remains the primary treatment option for severely symptomatic patients with obstructive hypertrophic cardiomyopathy. *Circulation* 2007; 116: 196–206.

31 Kron J, Herre J, Renfroe EG, et al. Lead- and device-related complications in the anti-arrhythmics versus implantable defibrillators trial. *Am Heart J* 2001; 141: 92–98.

32 Rosenqvist M, Beyer T, Block M, et al. on behalf of the European 7219 Jewel ICD Investigators. Adverse events with transvenous implantable cardioverter-defibrillators: a prospective multicentre study. *Circulation* 1998; 98: 663–670.

33 Klug D, Balde M, Pavin D, et al. for the PEOPLE Study Group. Risk factors related to infections of implanted pacemakers and cardioverter-defibrillators: results of a large prospective study. *Circulation* 2007; 116: 1349–1355.

13 Myocarditis: an inflammatory cardiomyopathy

Owais Dar

Expert commentary Dr Rakesh Sharma

Case history

A 44-year-old white male nurse was brought in by ambulance to the Emergency Department (ED) with a 3-week history of increasing breathlessness and chest pain. He had no past medical history of note. He had never smoked, drank alcohol only occasionally, and had no family history of cardiovascular disease. He was only taking self-prescribed multivitamin tablets regularly, and had no history of illicit drug abuse.

On arrival to the hospital, he had oxygen saturations of 85% on room air, and a respiratory rate of 35 breaths per minute. His jugular venous pressure was elevated at 8 cm above the sternal angle. On auscultation, both heart sounds were present and no murmurs were detected. Bilateral widespread crackles up to the mid-zones could be heard in the chest. His blood pressure (BP) was 86/52 mmHg. An electrocardiogram (ECG) showed sinus rhythm and left bundle branch block (LBBB). A chest X-ray confirmed florid pulmonary oedema. His laboratory blood tests were unremarkable (Table 13.1), but he was significantly hypoxic on arterial blood gases taken on air (Table 13.2).

In view of the clinical context, an initial diagnosis of acute myocardial infarction complicated by pulmonary oedema and cardiogenic shock was made. The patient was given boluses of aspirin 300 mg and clopidogrel 300 mg, and taken to the cardiac

Expert comment

LBBB is common in heart failure (HF). However, remember other aetiologies, including hypertension, valvular heart disease (especially aortic stenosis), and coronary artery disease.

Expert comment

Note the elevation of C reactive protein. Remember it is an acute phase reactant. Apart from the main differential of an ischaemic cardiomyopathy, there may also be another aetiology going on here.

Table 13.1 Blood results on admission

Haematology		Biochemistry	
Hb	13.2 g/dL	C reactive protein	**66 mg/L**
MCV	90 fL	Albumin	42 g/L
WCC	8.24×10^9/L	Bilirubin	16 micromol/L
Platelets	254×10^9/L	Alanine aminotransferase	12 IU/L
INR	1.2	Na	140 mmol/L
K	3.9 mmol/L	Urea	3.2 mmol/L
Creatinine	118 micromol/L		

Table 13.2 Arterial blood gases

Arterial blood gas on air	
pH	7.38
PCO_2	5.8 kPa
PO_2	**7.2 kPa**
HCO_3^-	23 mmol/L

⊕ **Clinical tip** The intra-aortic balloon pump explained

- An IABP is a mechanical device which consists of a balloon attached to a long tube.
- The IABP is inserted via the femoral artery and positioned so that the balloon rests just distal to the origin of the left subclavian artery.
- The balloon is actively inflated in diastole and deflated during systole (counterpulsation).
- The effect is an increase in cardiac output and a decrease in myocardial oxygen demand due to a reduction in cardiac afterload and an increase in coronary blood flow, respectively.
- IABPs are typically used as a bridge to a more definitive therapy such as percutaneous coronary intervention or valve surgery in patients with cardiogenic shock.
- IABPs should be avoided in severe aortic regurgitation, aortic dissection, or peripheral vascular disease.

🎔 **Expert comment**

IABPs have a mechanical effect on diastole. They augment diastole if correctly set up, and therefore, will improve coronary artery perfusion. Due to the mechanistic effects, they are beneficial in acute decompensated HF. However, the centre needs to be able to utilize a balloon pump appropriately. In a low-volume centre or where the technology is not available, the patient should be admitted to the Intensive Care Unit (ICU) and optimized medically.

🎔 **Expert comment**

Remember other causes of a dilated cardiomyopathy include drugs (especially alcohol misuse), toxins (prior chemotherapy), and rare inherited disorders (muscular dystrophies).

🎔 **Expert comment**

In most cases an identifiable pathogen is not found.

catheter laboratory for primary coronary angioplasty. In view of the patient's clinical status, an intra-aortic balloon pump (IABP) was inserted initially. The coronary angiogram showed only very minor coronary disease, and the left ventriculogram demonstrated a globally hypokinetic left ventricle with severe systolic dysfunction.

The patient was transferred to Coronary Care Unit (CCU) where he was given intravenous furosemide (80 mg bolus, followed by an infusion of 240 mg over 24 hours) and a nitrate infusion (50 mg of isosorbide dinitrate in 50 mg 0.9% of normal saline). An urgent transthoracic echocardiogram (TTE) was arranged, and confirmed a moderately dilated left ventricle with severe systolic dysfunction.

At this point, a provisional diagnosis of acute fulminant myocarditis was made. A more detailed history from the patient's partner revealed that the patient had been complaining of a coryzal illness in the days preceding the admission. This included symptoms of fever, sore throat, cough, myalgia, fatigue, and night sweats. There was no history of recent foreign travel. Further blood tests for viral serology (including HIV, CMV, EBV, and coxsackie viruses) were ordered.

⭐ **Learning point** Definition of myocarditis

In 1995, the World Health Organization/International Society and Federation of Cardiology (WHO/ISFC) task force on the definition and classification of cardiomyopathies defined myocarditis as part of an inflammatory cardiomyopathy spectrum:

'Inflammatory cardiomyopathy is defined by myocarditis in association with cardiac dysfunction. Myocarditis is an inflammatory disease of the myocardium and is diagnosed by established histological, immunological, and immunohistochemical criteria. Idiopathic, autoimmune, and infectious forms of inflammatory cardiomyopathy are recognized [1].'

Although robust, application of this definition in clinical practice is difficult as it requires every suspected diagnosis to be confirmed with an endomyocardial biopsy (EMB).

⭐ **Learning point** Aetiology and pathogenesis of myocarditis

Many causes of myocarditis exist, of which the most common is viral. A list is given below to illustrate the variety of different aetiologies, but the list should not be considered comprehensive [2].

Viral: Coxsackie virus, HIV, CMV, parvovirus B12, hepatitis A and B, varicella zoster, influenza;
Bacterial: Staphylococcus aureus, Haemophilus pneumoniae, Mycoplasma pneumoniae, Chlamydia species;
Fungal: Candida species, Histoplasma, Cryptococcus;
Parasitic: Toxoplasma, Schistosoma, Trichina;
Toxin: Penicillins, indomethacin, spironolactone, sulfonylureas, cocaine, lithium;
Others: Radiation.

The pathogenesis of myocarditis can be divided into three different phases:

- Phase I – Direct myocardial cell damage by an insult, leading to cell death and dilatation (e.g. viral infection).
- Phase II – After the inital insult, ongoing damage to cardiac myocytes continues by autoantibodies and by the release of cytokines produced by the immune system.
- Phase III – Long-term cell damage and fibrosis leads to remodelling and progressive cardiac dilatation and loss of function, causing dilated cardiomyopathy [3].

A few hours later, there was no improvement in the patient's condition; he remained hypoxic and tachypnoeic. Non-invasive ventilation was commenced. Despite this, he failed to improve and several hours later, the patient's heart rhythm changed to VF. The patient was electrically cardioverted back into sinus rhythm with return of a spontaneous circulation and then, immediately transferred to the ICU where he was intubated and ventilated. On ICU, he was given intravenous amiodarone (300 mg bolus, followed by 900 mg over 12 hours) in an attempt to stabilize his myocardium chemically as he remained sedated on the ventilator.

> **⊕ Learning point** Diagnosis of myocarditis
>
> - The current gold standard test for diagnosing myocarditis is based on EMB, histopathology and immunohistology. Most cases of myocarditis have a mild presentation and currently, EMB is only warranted for patients with severe HF not responding to medical therapy, or those with associated haemodynamic compromise. No single test is diagnostic of milder forms of myocarditis; instead diagnosis is based on a combination of history, examination, ECG findings, cardiac enzymes, and imaging.
> - ECG: ST-elevation or T wave inversion is present in <16% of cases, abnormal Q waves in 18%, and a bundle branch block pattern in 31% of cases with myocarditis [6].
> - Cardiac enzymes: the sensitivity of a raised troponin in one study was 53%, specificity 94%, a positive predictive value of 93%, and negative predictive value of 56% [7].
> - Echocardiography: there are no specific features diagnostic of myocarditis on echocardiography. Many patients with mild myocarditis have normal echocardiograms. When abnormalities are found, they can reveal left ventricular (LV) dysfunction, LV dilatation, LV hypertrophy, thrombi, restrictive filling, or regional wall motion abnormalities [8].
> - Cardiac magnetic resonance (CMR) imaging: allows the identification of myocardial oedema using T2-weighted images, hyperaemia and capillary leakage using myocardial early gadolinium enhancement, and necrosis and fibrosis using late gadolinium enhancement. If any two of these three criteria are positive for myocarditis, then CMR has a sensitivity of 67%, specificity of 91%, and positive predictive value of 91% in diagnosing myocarditis [9].
>
> The use of CMR imaging in the diagnosis and follow-up of myocarditis is promising. Recommended indications for CMR in patients suspected with myocarditis includes the presence of all of the following:
>
> 1. Symptoms suggestive of myocarditis (dyspnoea, orthopnoea, chest pain, palpitations, malaise);
> 2. Evidence of myocardial dysfunction (raised troponin, ECG abnormalities, ventricular dysfunction);
> 3. Suspected viral aetiology (recent viral illness, absence of risk factors for coronary disease, negative ischaemic stress test, or symptoms unexplained by coronary disease on a coronary angiogram) [9].

> **⊕ Clinical tip** Continuous positive airway pressure (CPAP) in acute decompensated heart failure
>
> In patients presenting to hospital with acute pulmonary oedema, the addition of CPAP to standard medical therapy is associated with improved symptoms, reduced ICU length of stay and reduced intubation rates [4].
>
> CPAP works by preventing alveolar collapse, increasing arterial oxygenation, increasing lung compliance and reducing the effort of breathing. Whether CPAP improves short-term mortality remains controversial due to conflicting data [5].

> **⊕ Expert comment**
>
> Ventricular arrhythmias are commonly encountered in acutely decompensated HF patients. With the use of concomitant diuretics, one should pay attention to the electrolytes and correct any subsequent imbalance. This is especially true for potassium and magnesium.

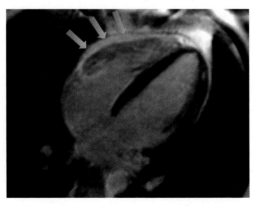

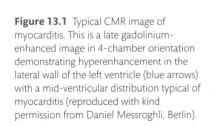

Figure 13.1 Typical CMR image of myocarditis. This is a late gadolinium-enhanced image in 4-chamber orientation demonstrating hyperenhancement in the lateral wall of the left ventricle (blue arrows) with a mid-ventricular distribution typical of myocarditis (reproduced with kind permission from Daniel Messroghli, Berlin).

During the following day on ICU, the patient's supportive needs had escalated to requiring inotropic support (noradrenaline) in addition to IABP support. By 48 hours, however, his improvement was sufficient to allow withdrawal of inotropes, IABP support, and artificial ventilation. Once extubated, the patient was transferred to the nearest tertiary cardiac centre for an EMB. This confirmed lymphocytic myocarditis as the diagnosis.

Learning point Role of endomyocardial biopsy (indications and risk)

EMB is carried out for diagnostic purposes, to guide therapy, and to define prognosis. However, the decision to carry out an EMB depends on the risks of EMB against the potential benefit gained. Factors affecting each individual patient, as well as local availability and expertise must also be considered. EMB is prone to sampling error (a diagnosis of myocarditis is still missed in over 30% of cases even when taking more than five individual EMB samples), and interpretations of biopsy specimens are prone to inter-observer variability [13].

The 2007 Scientific Statement from the American Heart Association/American College of Cardiology/European Society of Cardiology (AHA/ACC/ESC) on the role of EMB in the management of cardiovascular disease, gave a class IB recommendation for EMB in two clinical scenarios:

1. 'New onset HF of less than two weeks' duration associated with a normally sized or dilated left ventricle and haemodynamic compromise [14].'
2. 'New onset HF of two weeks' to three months' duration associated with a dilated left ventricle and new ventricular arrhythmias, second- or third-degree heart block, or failure to respond to usual care within one to two weeks [14].'

EMB in these settings allows the identification of types of myocarditis which may respond to immunosuppressant therapy (giant cell myocarditis and necrotizing eosinophilic myocarditis), and differentiate from those that do not respond to immunosuppressant therapy (fulminant lymphocytic myocarditis) [14].

Giant cell myocarditis has a poorer prognosis than lymphocytic myocarditis, with only 11% of patients alive or transplant-free at four years, compared to 44% of patients with lymphocytic myocarditis. Clinical clues to suggest giant cell myocarditis include the presence of other autoimmune disorders or thymoma, malignant arrhythmias, and failure to respond to usual care [14].

Necrotizing eosinophilic myocarditis is a rare disease with a poor prognosis. Patients present acutely and progress rapidly with haemodynamic compromise [14].

The risk of endomyocardial biopsy

The overall complication risk of right ventricular EMB via the internal jugular vein approach is 6%. Major risks include death (0.4%), perforation (1%), and arrhythmia (2.1%). Minor risks include arterial puncture, vasovagal episodes, and bleeding (3%) [15].

The patient was commenced on bisoprolol, ramipril, spironolactone, and oral furosemide. He then proceeded to ICD implantation as an inpatient, and was discharged home after three weeks of hospitalization with outpatient follow-up under the care of the HF team.

Learning point Treatment of heart failure

Patients with myocarditis and impaired LV systolic function should be treated with standard anti-HF therapies similar to those recommended for dilated cardiomyopathy, as stated in several international guidelines. These drugs have been validated in major landmark trials and the principles of treatment are based on providing symptom relief and improving prognosis by modifying the disease process:
* Medications which provide symptom relief act by offloading excessive fluid and include loop diuretics such as furosemide and bumetanide;
* Other agents, broadly known as disease-modifying drugs (such as angiotensin-converting enzyme inhibitors (ACEis), beta-blockers, and aldosterone antagonists) act by improving cardiac function, mortality rates, and quality of life [16-18].

Expert comment

Inotropes are perhaps too commonly used and should actually be used with strict caution. They may cause tachycardia and atrial or ventricular dysrrhythmias, and may paradoxically worsen pre-existing ischaemia. They exacerbate myocardial oxygen consumption and hence may potentiate cardiac ischaemia. For this reason, they should not be used without appropriate haemodynamic monitoring and prior experience. Certain inotropes may be more useful than others in acute decompensated HF. The OPTIME-CHF trial [10] demonstrated milrinone worsened the outcomes of acute HF patients; levosimendan, on the other hand, has been demonstrated to have properties beneficial to the myocardium [11,12].

Expert comment

EMBs are rarely performed nowadays in the UK, although some centres do continue to use them. However, the general consensus is that due to sophisticated imaging and the fact that in the majority of cases, it does not alter clinical management, it is not routinely used. One putative role is in rapidly progressive, treatment-refractory myocarditis to ensure both the diagnostic label is correct and to ascertain the underlying histopathology.

Expert comment

Lymphocytic myocarditis can manifest as a clinical spectrum. Some patients have a speedy uncomplicated recovery and others may progress to heart transplantation. Lymphocytic myocarditis can also be associated with other chronic inflammatory conditions.

Expert comment

After the initial diagnosis is made, further imaging should be considered at periodic intervals for reassessment of LV status.

⊘ **Landmark trial** Studies of Left Ventricular Dysfunction (SOLVD) [19]

- Effect of enalapril on survival in patients with reduced LVEF and congestive HF;
- Published in 1991: a double-blind, placebo-controlled trial randomizing 2,569 patients with symptomatic HF (NYHA classes II to IV) and LVEF ≤35% to either enalapril (2.5 to 20 mg daily) or placebo;
- After an average follow-up period of 44 months, there was a significant reduction in mortality in the enalapril group of 16% (p = 0.0036).

⊘ **Landmark trial** The Cardiac Insufficiency Bisoprolol Study II (CIBIS II) [20]

- The effect of bisoprolol on all-cause mortality in chronic HF;
- Published in 1999: a double-blind, placebo-controlled trial randomizing 2,647 patients with symptomatic HF (NYHA class III or IV) and LVEF ≤35% to either bisoprolol (1.25 to 10 mg daily) or placebo;
- This trial was stopped early as patients in the bisoprolol group had significantly lower mortality rates (11.8% vs 17.3% deaths, p<0.0001).

⊘ **Landmark trial** The Randomized Aldosterone Evaluation Study (RALES) [21]

- The effect of spironolactone on morbidity and mortality in patients with severe HF;
- Published in 1999: a double-blind, placebo-controlled trial randomizing 1,663 patients with symptomatic HF (NYHA class III or IV) and LVEF ≤35% to either 25 mg of spironolactone or placebo;
- This trial was also stopped early as patients in the spironolactone group had significantly reduced mortality rates (35% vs 46% deaths, p < 0.001).

ⓘ **Expert comment**

HF medication should be started at modest doses. Providing it is tolerated, it should be uptitrated as an outpatient in conjunction with HF specialist nurse support. In this patient's case, he had myocarditis and subsequent dilated cardiomyopathy. The coronary angiogram revealed no major underlying coronary artery disease. Therefore, from a secondary preventative stance, it is wholly appropriate that this gentleman had the insertion of an ICD whilst still an inpatient. A patient with an underlying dilated cardiomyopathy should not be treated in an analogous manner to a patient with recent acute ischaemia.

Discussion

The true incidence of myocarditis remains unknown. It can, however, be histologically detected in up to 1% of unselected autopsies in the developed Western World [22]. Subclinical myocarditis is common. In such cases, subjects are asymptomatic, but active myocardial inflammation is present. In clinically overt myocarditis, patients can present with chest pain, brady- or tachy-arrhythmias, symptoms of congestive cardiac failure with or without a dilated cardiomyopathy or SCD. Approximately 12% of dilated cardiomyopathy cases are due to myocarditis. Myocarditis may be associated with a preceding history of a viral flu-like illness with symptoms such as malaise, fever, myalgia, and upper respiratory symptoms [22,23].

Spontaneous improvement occurs in an estimated 50% of patients with biopsy-proven acute myocarditis. Progression to dilated cardiomyopathy occurs in up to 21% of patients over a 3-year period. Interestingly, the long-term prognosis (i.e. the 4-year transplant-free survival) is better for those presenting with arrhythmia or chest pain (87%) than those presenting with symptoms of HF (54%) [24]. Myocarditis can be divided into two separate groups based on the mode of presentation and histopathological diagnosis; acute myocarditis or fulminant myocarditis [25].

Acute myocarditis is characterized by a vague and protracted onset of symptoms with milder symptoms of HF, less severe systolic dysfunction and the presence of active or borderline myocarditis on EMB [25].

In contrast, fulminant myocarditis is characterized by a clear onset of symptoms, rapidly leading to cardiogenic shock or severe systolic dysfunction requiring vasopressor or mechanical circulatory support, and multiple foci of myocarditis on EMB [25]. Fulminant myocarditis is less frequent than acute myocarditis and is also associated with a better prognosis. In one study by McCarthy et al., from a cohort of 147 patients with myocarditis, 15 (10%) had fulminant myocarditis compared to 132 (90%) who presented with acute myocarditis. Transplant-free survival after 11 years of follow-up was significantly higher in those with fulminant myocarditis (fulminant myocarditis 95% vs acute myocarditis 45%, p=0.05) [25].

Myocarditis is a relatively understudied condition. Most cases are subclinical and are undetected or present with very mild symptoms. Uncommonly, it can present with symptoms of HF and cardiogenic shock. When this occurs, prognosis is poor. Diagnosis, in most cases, is based on history, ECG, cardiac enzymes, and imaging. The gold standard diagnosis is histological, requiring an EMB and for this reason, it is rarely implemented, except in research settings. For those presenting with chest pain only, treatment is based on analgesia alone. However, for those presenting with HF and impaired cardiac function, treatment is based on the use of anti-HF medication (diuretics, ACEis, beta-blockers, and aldosterone antagonists). In severe cases, cardiac assist devices and heart transplantation may be required.

> **⚙ Expert comment**
>
> It has been recognized that although LVADs are utilized and licensed as a bridge to transplantation, there has been some spontaneous recovery in patients with LVADs. This has enabled them to come off the transplant list. Further study is ongoing in this area.

> **💬 A final word from the expert**
>
> Myocarditis, although rare, is a great cardiac mimic. It can present with the entire gamut of myocardial disease, ranging from indolent LV disease to acute or even hyperacute HF. The important points are:
>
> 1. To recognize myocarditis as part of the differentials for acute decompensated HF;
> 2. To perform baseline investigations and echocardiography at the time of the index episode;
> 3. Patients require careful and appropriate follow-up in a specialist multidisciplinary format.
>
> The above case perfectly demonstrates modern day HF management. It calls for in-depth medical knowledge, the acute application of physiology, and knowledge of guidelines and long-term management. It also covers numerous cardiovascular subspecialties. Myocarditis can be rapidly progressive and if not recognized, will lead to the patient's demise. In common with other causes of acute decompensated HF, it is associated with significant morbidity and mortality. Apart from the recognition of its pathophysiology and plethora of clinical manifestations, prompt appropriate treatment should be initiated. If decline still perpetuates, then the patient should be considered for more invasive therapies, including transplantation. In those listed for transplantation, a small but particular group may benefit from mechanical assist devices. These may even induce regression of disease. Ultimately, myocarditis is a rare condition, which although infrequently encountered, should always be remembered.

References

1 Richardson P, McKenna W, Bristow M. Report of the 1995 World Health Organization/ International Society and Federation of Cardiology Task Force on the definition and classification of cardiomyopathies. *Circulation* 1996; 93: 841–842.

2 Mancini DM, Beniaminovitz A. Myocarditis and specific cardiomyopathies–endocrine disease and alcohol. In: Fuster V, Alexander W, O'Rourke R, editors. Hurst's The Heart. 10th edition. New York: McGraw-Hill; 2001. p. 2004.

3 Dennert R, Crijns H, Heymans S. Acute viral myocarditis. *Eur Heart J* 2008; 29: 2073–2082.

4 Vital FM, Saconato H, Ladeira MT, et al. Non-invasive positive pressure ventilation (CPAP or bilevel NPPV) for cardiogenic pulmonary oedema. *Cochrane Database Syst Rev* 2008; 16: CD005351.

5 Gray A, Goodacre S, Newby D, et al. Non-invasive ventilation in acute cardiogenic pulmonary oedema. *N Engl J Med* 2008; 359: 142–151.

6 Morgera T, Di Lenarda A, Dreas L. Electrocardiography of myocarditis revisited: clinical and prognostic significance of electrocardiographic changes. *Am Heart J* 1992; 124: 455–467.

7 Lauer B, Niederau C, Kühl U. Cardiac troponin T in patients with clinically suspected myocarditis. *J Am Coll Cardiol* 1997; 30: 1354–1359.

8 Pinamonti B, Alberti E, Cigalotto A. Echocardiographic findings in myocarditis. *Am J Cardiol* 1988; 62: 285–291.

9 Friedrich M, Sechtem U, Schulz-Menger J. Cardiovascular magnetic resonance in myocarditis: A JACC White Paper. *J Am Coll Cardiol* 2009; 53: 1475–1487.

10 Cuffe MS, Califf RM, Adams KF, et al. Short-term intravenous milrinone for acute exacerbation of chronic heart failure: a randomized controlled trial. *JAMA* 2002; 287: 1541–1547.

11 Follath F, Cleland JG, Just H, et al. Efficacy and safety of intravenous levosimendan compared with dobutamine in severe low output heart failure (the LIDO study): a randomized double-blind trial. *Lancet* 2002; 360: 196–202.

12 Moiseyev VS, Poder P, Andrejevs N, et al. Safety and efficacy of a novel calcium sensitizer, levosimendan, in patients with left ventricular failure due to an acute myocardial infarction. A randomized, placebo-controlled, double-blind study (RUSSLAN). *Eur Heart J* 2002; 23: 1422–1432.

13 Baughman K. Diagnosis of myocarditis: death of Dallas criteria. *Circulation* 2006; 113: 593–595.

14 Cooper L, Baughman K, Feldman A. The role of endomyocardial biopsy in the management of cardiovascular disease. A scientific statement from the American Heart Association, the American College of Cardiology, and the European Society of Cardiology. *Eur Heart J* 2007; 28: 3076–3093.

15 Deckers J, Hare J, Baughman K. Complications of transvenous right ventricular endomyocardial biopsy in adult patients with cardiomyopathy: a 7-year survey of 546 consecutive diagnostic procedures in a tertiary referral centre. *J Am Coll Cardiol* 1992; 19: 43–47.

16 National Institute for Health and Clinical Excellence. Management of chronic heart failure in adults in primary and secondary care. NICE Guideline No 5 [issued July 2003]. Available from: http://www.nice.org.uk.

17 Hunt SA; American College of Cardiology; American Heart Association Task Force on Practice Guidelines (Writing Committee to Update the 2001 Guidelines for the Evaluation and Management of Heart Failure). ACC/AHA 2005 guideline update for the diagnosis and management of chronic heart failure in the adult: a report of the American College of Cardiology/American Heart Association Task Force on Practice Guidelines (Writing Committee to Update the 2001 Guidelines for the Evaluation and Management of Heart Failure). *J Am Coll Cardiol* 2005; 46: e1–82.

18 European Society of Cardiology. ESC pocket guidelines for the diagnosis and treatment of chronic heart failure [issued 2005]. Available from: http://www.escardio.org.

19 The SOLVD Investigators. Effect of enalapril on survival in patients with reduced left ventricular ejection fractions and congestive heart failure. *N Engl J Med* 1991; 325: 293–302.

20 CIBIS-II Investigators and Committees. The Cardiac Insufficiency Bisoprolol Study II (CIBIS-II): a randomized trial. *Lancet* 1999; 353: 9–13.

21 Pitt B, Zannad F, Remme WJ, et al. The effect of spironolactone on morbidity and mortality in patients with severe heart failure. *N Engl J Med* 1999; 341: 709–717.

22 Friman G. The incidence and epidemiology of myocarditis. *Eur Heart J* 1999; 20: 1063–1066.

23 Kasper EK, Agema WR, Hutchins GM. The causes of dilated cardiomyopathy: a clinicopathologic review of 673 consecutive patients. *Am Coll Cardiol* 1994; 23: 586–590.

24 D'Ambrosio A, Patti G, Manzoli A. The fate of acute myocarditis between spontaneous improvement and evolution to dilated cardiomyopathy: a review. *Heart* 2001; 85: 499–504.

25 McCarthy RE, Boehmer JP, Hruban RH. Long-term outcome of fulminant myocarditis as compared with acute (non-fulminant) myocarditis. *N Engl J Med* 2000; 342: 690–695.

14 Arrhythmogenic right ventricular cardiomyopathy

Martina Muggenthaler

Expert commentary Dr Elijah Behr

Case history

A 35-year-old woman was admitted to her local hospital, complaining of fast and regular palpitations, light-headedness, and vomiting. These were of sudden onset whilst walking her dog. She had managed to get back home where she collapsed and was found confused, clammy, and pale. She denied loss of consciousness and chest pain. She had experienced five episodes of exercise-induced palpitations in the preceding six months since the birth of her second child. These episodes had settled spontaneously within an hour of resting. There was no history of syncope. She had a history of mild asthma and did not take any regular medication. She was an ex-smoker, did not drink any alcohol, and denied recreational drug use. Her father had a history of ventricular tachycardia (VT) and had had an implantable cardioverter-defibrillator (ICD) fitted 12 years previously. No further information was available at this stage about his condition. There was no family history of sudden cardiac death (SCD).

On arrival to the Accident and Emergency (A&E) department, she was pale, peripherally cold, with a heart rate of 230 beats per minute (bpm) and a blood pressure (BP) of 80/60 mmHg. A 12-lead electrocardiogram (ECG) revealed a broad complex tachycardia (BCT) with left bundle branch block (LBBB) morphology and an inferior axis consistent with right ventricular outflow tract (RVOT) VT (Figure 14.1). Spontaneous conversion

Expert comment

This presentation is already strongly suggestive of arrhythmogenic right ventricular cardiomyopathy (ARVC) with three minor diagnostic criteria being present: right ventricular (RV) arrhythmia, T wave inversion in the right precordial leads and beyond, and a family history of VT requiring an ICD (Table 14.1). The elevated troponin level is consistent with prolonged tachycardia rather than immediately supportive of underlying ischaemic heart disease.

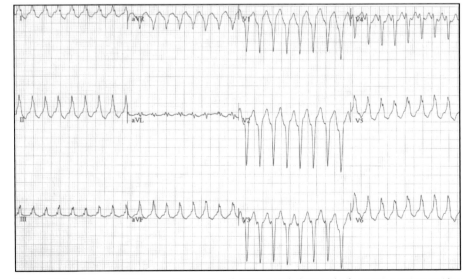

Figure 14.1 Admission ECG demonstrating VT with LBBB morphology and inferior axis consistent with a VT of RVOT type.

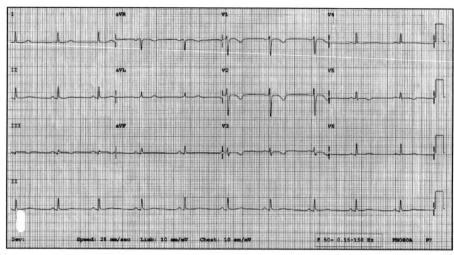

Figure 14.2 ECG post-spontaneous conversion to sinus rhythm revealing T wave inversion in leads V1–V5.

to sinus rhythm at a rate of 76 bpm occurred after a few minutes with a corresponding improvement in BP. Repeat ECG showed sinus rhythm with T wave inversion in V1 to V5 (Figure 14.2). Her chest X-ray was normal and blood tests revealed normal electrolytes and an elevated troponin I of 7.6 ng/mL.

> ⊗ **Learning point** Epidemiology and pathogenesis of arrhythmogenic right ventricular cardiomyopathy
>
> ARVC is a genetically determined cardiomyopathy with a familial background in at least 50% of cases. It is mostly transmitted as an autosomal dominant trait with incomplete penetrance and variable expression [1]. The estimated prevalence of ARVC in the general population ranges from 1 in 1,000 to 1 in 5,000. Men are more commonly affected than women with a ratio of 3:1, and the disease usually becomes overt in the second to fourth decade of life. Mutations in several genes have been discovered with most affecting desmosomal proteins, resulting in failure of cellular adhesion. Examples of affected proteins are desmoplakin, plakophillin-2, desmoglein-2, desmocollin-2 and plakoglobin. Extra-desmosomal genes linked to ARVC include the cardiac ryanodine-2 receptor, transforming growth factor-β3, and TMEM 43.
>
> Defective desmosomes are thought to result in the detachment of myocytes with consequent cell death, especially at times of increased mechanical stress, e.g. during exercise. Desmosomes are also involved in cellular signalling networks, and it has been suggested that their reduction leads to changes in gene expression, influencing the fate of cells with a shift from myocytes to adipocytes and fibrocytes [2]. This disease process may also have cutaneous manifestations including palmoplantar keratoderma and woolly hair, e.g. in Naxos disease and Carvajal syndrome. Progressive myocyte degeneration leads to fibrofatty tissue replacement, which results in the typical morphological abnormalities of ARVC and provides the substrate for ventricular arrhythmias. Fibrofatty replacement of the myocardium progresses from the epicardium to the endocardium and may then become transmural, leading to wall thinning and aneurysms [3]. The thin-walled right ventricle and the inferolateral wall of the left ventricle are thought to be more susceptible to mechanical stress, which could explain why these areas are the predominant sites of fibrofatty tissue transformation.
>
> Early myocyte death, the acute 'hot' phase, has been implicated in the occurrence of ventricular fibrillation (VF). In addition, gap junctions may become dysfunctional secondary to the effect of desmosomal mutations without obvious histological abnormalities. This is thought to result in areas of slow conduction and a substrate for re-entry tachycardias [4]. The eventual development of fibrofatty
>
> *continued*

tissue also causes conduction delay with potential for re-entry VT. Conduction abnormalities also underlie ECG characteristics such as epsilon waves (terminal notch in the QRS complex), right bundle branch block (RBBB), and late potentials on signal-averaged ECG (SAECG). The typical morphology for VT is LBBB; this indicates an origin in the right ventricle, with either an inferior axis if arising from the RVOT, or a superior axis if arising from the RV inferior wall or apex. Patients with extensive disease can exhibit several different morphologies of VT, including RBBB morphologies if there is LV involvement. The ECG typically shows T wave inversion, not only in V2–V3, but also in V4, V5, and V6 if the left ventricle is affected. In severe cases, progressive loss of contractile myocardium and replacement by fibrofatty tissue leads to dilatation and impairment of the right ventricle, as well as the left ventricle with heart failure as a consequence. Indeed, this may manifest as a dilated cardiomyopathy rather than a typical ARVC phenotype.

The patient was admitted to the Coronary Care Unit (CCU) and commenced on bisoprolol 2.5 mg once daily. A transthoracic echocardiogram (TTE) was performed and reported as normal. An exercise tolerance test (ETT) using the Bruce protocol was performed and after five minutes on the treadmill, the patient developed a BCT with LBBB pattern and an inferior axis at a rate of 200 bpm. The patient felt dizzy and systolic BP was recorded as 105 mmHg. After 25 minutes, the patient converted spontaneously to sinus rhythm again. Her bisoprolol was increased to 5 mg daily and she was transferred to a tertiary referral centre for further electrophysiological assessment.

> ⭐ **Learning point** Diagnosis of arrhythmogenic right ventricular cardiomyopathy
>
> The diagnosis of ARVC is established using standardized Task Force criteria, including morphology, histopathology, ECG, ventricular arrhythmias, and family history (Table 14.1) [5]. The original Task Force criteria [6] were proposed in 1994 at which stage clinical experience with ARVC was mostly based on symptomatic index cases and SCD victims. These criteria have recently been modified, incorporating new knowledge and genetics to improve the diagnostic sensitivity for early or minor disease. Quantitative criteria for imaging and histological examination have been added, which were lacking in the original criteria. A definite diagnosis is reached with two major, or one major and two minor criteria or four minor criteria from different categories. A case is classified as borderline with one major and one minor or three minor criteria from different categories and is possible with one major or two minor criteria from different categories.

> **Table 14.1 Revised Task Force criteria for the diagnosis of ARVC . Adapted from Marcus et al [5]**
> ....
> **1. Global or regional dysfunction and structural alterations**
> **Major**
> By 2-dimensional echo
> - Regional RV akinesia, dyskinesia, or aneurysm
> - *And* one of the following (end diastole):
>   - PLAX (parasternal long-axis view) RVOT ≥32 mm (corrected for body surface area [PLAX/BSA] ≥19 mm/m^2)
>   - PSAX (parasternal short-axis view) RVOT ≥36 mm ([PSAX/BSA] ≥21 mm/m^2)
>   - *Or* fractional area change ≤33%
> By MRI
> - Regional RV akinesia or dyskinesia or dyssynchronous RV contraction
> - *And* one of the following:
>   - Ratio of RV end-diastolic volume to BSA ≥110 mL/m^2 (male) or ≥100 mL/m^2 (female)
>   - *Or* RV ejection fraction ≤40%
> By RV angiography
> - Regional RV akinesia, dyskinesia, or aneurysm
>
> *continued*

continued

> ➕ **Clinical tip** Assessment of patients with suspected arrhythmogenic right ventricular cardiomyopathy
>
> Patients with suspected ARVC are assessed with clinical and family history, physical examination, 12-lead ECG, 24-hour Holter, SAECG, ETT, and TTE. Cardiac magnetic resonance (CMR) imaging, contrast angiography, and endomyocardial biopsy (EMB) may provide further information.

> 🕑 **Expert comment**
>
> Beta-blockers are only partially successful in the treatment of ventricular arrhythmias in ARVC with a high frequency of recurrence. Amiodarone, often in combination with a beta-blocker, is more efficacious, but less tolerable in younger patients. Sotalol is often the best alternative, but be aware of excessive QT prolongation, especially at higher doses, as this indicates a risk of torsades de pointes. No drug offers any protection from SCD, although recent evidence suggests some protection from arrhythmias in ICD patients on amiodarone.

Minor

By 2-dimensional echo

- Regional RV akinesia or dyskinesia
- *And* one of the following (end diastole):
  - PLAX RVOT ≥29 to <32 mm (corrected for body surface area [PLAX/BSA] ≥16 to <19 mm/m^2)
  - PSAX RVOT ≥32 to <36 mm (corrected for body surface area [PSAX/BSA] ≥18 to <21 mm/m^2)
  - *Or* fractional area change >33% to ≤40%

By MRI

- Regional RV akinesia or dyskinesia or dyssynchronous RV contraction
- *And* one of the following:
  - Ratio of RV end-diastolic volume to BSA ≥100 to <110 mL/m^2 (male) or ≥90 to <100 mL/m^2 (female)
  - *Or* RV ejection fraction >40% to ≤45%

2. Tissue characterization of wall

Major

Residual myocytes <60% by morphometric analysis (or <50% if estimated), with fibrous replacement of the RV free wall myocardium in ≥1 sample, with or without fatty replacement of tissue on EMB

Minor

Residual myocytes 60% to 75% by morphometric analysis (or 50% to 65% if estimated), with fibrous replacement of the RV free wall myocardium in ≥1 sample, with or without fatty replacement of tissue on EMB

3. Repolarization abnormalities

Major

- Inverted T waves in leads V1–V3 or beyond in individuals >14 years of age (in the absence of RBBB)

Minor

- Inverted T waves in leads V1 and V2 in individuals >14 years of age (in the absence of RBBB) or in V4–V6
- Inverted T waves in leads V1–V4 in individuals >14 years of age in the presence of RBBB

4. Depolarization/conduction abnormalities

Major

- Epsilon wave in leads V1–V3

Minor

- Late potentials by SAECG in ≥1 of 3 parameters in the absence of a QRS duration of ≥110 ms on the standard ECG
- Filtered QRS duration (fQRS) ≥114 ms
- Duration of terminal QRS <40 microV (low amplitude signal duration) ≥38 ms
- Root mean squared voltage of terminal 40 ms ≤20 microV
- Terminal activation duration of QRS ≥55 ms measured from the nadir of the S wave to the end of the QRS, including R', in V1, V2, or V3, in the absence of RBBB

5. Arrhythmias

Major

- Non-sustained or sustained ventricular tachycardia of LBBB morphology with superior axis

Minor

- Non-sustained or sustained ventricular tachycardia with LBBB morphology with inferior axis (RVOT configuration) or of unknown axis
- >500 ventricular extrasystoles per 24 hours (Holter)

6. Family history

Major

- ARVC confirmed in a first-degree relative who meets current Task Force criteria
- ARVC confirmed pathologically in a first-degree relative
- Identification of a pathogenic mutation categorized as associated or probably associated with ARVC in the patient under evaluation

Minor

- History of ARVC in a first-degree relative in whom it is not possible or practical to determine whether the family member meets current Task Force criteria
- Premature sudden death (<35 years of age) due to suspected ARVC in a first-degree relative
- ARVC confirmed pathologically or by current Task Force criteria in second-degree relative

At the tertiary centre, the patient underwent a CMR scan which revealed a moderately dilated right ventricle with moderate systolic impairment. The RV apex and the mid-inferolateral wall of the left ventricle showed areas of sub-epicardial fat on T1-weighted sequences and late enhancement with gadolinium, consistent with fibrotic changes (Figures 14.3 and 14.4).

ⓕ **Expert comment**

It is common that echocardiographic and CMR findings are inconsistent, particularly when undertaken in different units with varying levels of imaging experience. This reflects the differing natures of both modalities, the difficulties in achieving consistent protocols and reporting, as well as the limited understanding of normal RV physiology and, therefore, the pathological criteria.

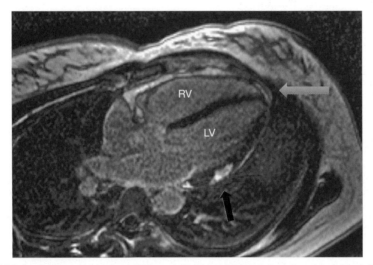

Figure 14.3 Long axis cut on cardiac MR through the RV and LV, showing sub-epicardial fat infiltration in the right ventricular apex (blue arrow) and basal left ventricular lateral wall (red arrrow)

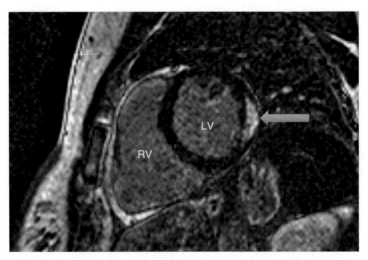

Figure 14.4 Short axis cut on cardiac MR through mid-RV and LV, showing delayed enhancement in the inferolateral LV wall (arrow). Note the significant amount of epicardial fat around the thin walled right ventricle. RV = right ventricle; LV = left ventricle.

⭐ **Learning point** Imaging in arrhythmogenic right ventricular cardiomyopathy

The standard imaging techniques used in the assessment of ARVC are echocardiography and CMR. Contrast ventriculography has been used successfully, but is less commonly required as it is invasive and usually only identifies gross abnormalities that should be picked up by the aforementioned technologies. Characteristic features include regional wall motion abnormalities (RWMA), wall thinning, focal aneurysms, global or regional dilatation, systolic impairment of the right and left ventricles, intra-myocardial fibrosis and/or fatty infiltration. Some of these features are classified as major or minor Task Force criteria, however, LV changes are not included, even though left-dominant ARVC and biventricular ARVC are now well recognized phenotypes [2]. Consensus guidelines for non-classic subtypes have yet to be established.

Echocardiography is the preferred first-line modality for assessing both index cases and family members as it is widely available and non-invasive. It is also used to monitor disease progression during follow-up [7]. Echocardiography is able to demonstrate abnormalities in patients with overt disease, but is often insensitive to subtle changes in the early 'concealed' phase of ARVC, during which individuals can already be at risk of arrhythmias or even SCD.

CMR is an important tool in the assessment of ARVC. It is non-invasive, permits simultaneous assessment of both ventricles, is superior to echocardiography in imaging the right ventricle, and permits tissue characterization [8]. It initially promised higher sensitivity, but has subsequently demonstrated some limitations. T1-weighted fast spin echo sequences in magnetic resonance imaging (MRI) allow the differentiation of myocardium and fat. However, intra-myocardial fat has been shown to be an unreliable parameter, as it is not an uncommon finding in healthy individuals of Western origin. There is also high inter-observer variability in the reporting of its presence and extent.

Cine-MRI may be used to assess ventricular volumes and RWMA, but has been criticized as the grading of RWMA is subjective. It has also been questioned whether MRI has enough spatial resolution to enable a reliable assessment of RV free wall thinning. Further challenges are the lack of standardized protocols and limited experience with scanning ARVC patients in some centres. Another limitation arises from the fact that the spectrum of normal morphology and function within the thin-walled, trabeculated, pyramidal right ventricle remains to be defined, which can give rise to over-interpretation of normal appearances [9]. The new Task Force criteria have addressed the previous lack of quantitative data with the addition of cut-off values for RVOT dimensions, RV volumes, and ejection fraction [5].

The most significant advance in CMR for ARVC has been the use of gadolinium and delayed enhancement to visualize fibrosis, which has been correlated with inducible sustained monomorphic VT and fibrofatty changes on EMB [10]. The finding of fibrotic changes can predate functional abnormalities such as RV dilatation and allows disease detection at an earlier stage [6]. The thin wall of the right ventricle can, in some cases, make it difficult to differentiate late enhancement within the RV wall from epicardial fat (Figure 14.4).

CMR has, in some cases, led to the over-diagnosis of ARVC and should always be used in conjunction with other diagnostic tools. It cannot be seen as the 'gold standard' investigation that it was initially hoped to be [8].

🔆 **Expert comment**

As ARVC is predominantly hereditary, it is vital and appropriate that blood relatives are offered appropriate evaluation. An open-minded approach is important, and more distant family members should be offered evaluation if they have symptoms such as syncope that may support the presence of disease.

An SAECG showed normal values without evidence of late potentials (see Learning Point, The signal-averaged ECG). The patient's medication was changed to sotalol 40 mg twice daily, then uptitrated to 80 mg twice daily after two days. Further information about her father now became available. He had been diagnosed with ARVC 12 years ago and had an ICD implanted for recurrent, poorly tolerated VT. Family screening, however, had never been undertaken.

The method of signal-averaging improves the signal-to-noise ratio, by processing up to several hundred QRS complexes recorded from the body surface with orthogonal XYZ leads. Additional filtering techniques contribute to a clean, average QRS complex, in which very low amplitude electrical potentials of a few microvolts (microV) can be detected.

Scarring in the myocardium creates areas of slow conduction which can be the substrate for re-entrant ventricular arrhythmias. These areas show delayed, fragmented, and low amplitude activation, which may occur after the QRS complex and is not visible on a standard ECG. SAECG can detect these late ventricular potentials of high frequency and low amplitude (1–25 microV). In ischaemic cardiomyopathies, late potentials have been shown to be a sensitive, but not specific, marker of arrhythmic risk [11]. In ARVC, a closer relationship has been found between the SAECG and the extent of disease than with the presence of ventricular arrhythmias [12]. It is common practice to consider an SAECG as abnormal if two out of the following three criteria are fulfilled:

- Filtered QRS complex duration is >114 ms;
- Root mean squared voltage of the terminal 40 ms of the QRS complex is <20 microvolts;
- The terminal filtered QRS complex remains <40 microvolts for more than 38 ms.

A recent study examined the diagnostic value of SAECG in ARVC [13]. It found that the sensitivity of SAECG for the diagnosis of ARVC was increased from 47% to 69%, if the SAECG was considered abnormal with one of the three criteria being met for a positive SAECG (rather than two of the three criteria having to be fulfilled), whilst at the same time maintaining a high specificity of 95%. This finding is incorporated in the revised Task Force criteria.

The patient underwent a further ETT on sotalol 80 mg twice daily. After six minutes of the Bruce protocol, she developed VT of similar morphology as on presentation, but at a slower rate of 200 bpm. This changed after a few minutes to another RVOT VT with a distinctively different morphology, again at a rate of 200 bpm. The patient became symptomatic with dizziness and nausea and her BP dropped to an unrecordable level. A radial pulse was palpable throughout and emergency synchronized direct current cardioversion (DCCV) re-established sinus rhythm.

Since the patient had developed haemodynamically unstable VT whilst on beta-blocker therapy, this placed her at high risk for further life-threatening arrhythmias and she was advised to have ICD implantation. As her VT had occurred at a relatively low workload on the treadmill, it was presumed that she would receive frequent therapies from her defibrillator. For this reason, a VT ablation was scheduled prior to ICD implantation in the hope that this would reduce the number of interventions from her ICD once *in situ*.

The VT ablation was performed under conscious sedation. An RV angiogram (Figure 14.5) exhibited a hypokinetic apex and areas of bulging in the RVOT. The clinical VT was induced at stage six of the Wellens protocol. Anti-tachycardia pacing changed the VT to a different morphology VT before terminating it. The VT initially induced was ablated in the RVOT using the pace-mapping technique (see Case 17). After ablation of the first VT, further programmed stimulation induced three more distinctive morphologies of VT. All three were mapped and also successfully ablated in the anterior right ventricle, anterior RVOT, and at the junction of the mid-septum and RV free wall, respectively. VT stimulation to stage 12 of the Wellens protocol did not induce any VT and the procedure was successfully completed.

⚙ Expert comment

Whilst VT ablation offers potential amelioration of symptoms due to sustained monomorphic ventricular tachyarrhythmias or ectopics, there can be a high rate of recurrence of arrhythmia. There is insufficient evidence to support its use in place of ICD implantation in patients at high risk of sudden death. Two approaches to ablation may be taken: to ablate the previously 'clinically' identified VT morphology only or ablate any other morphologies that may be induced at the time of study. There is some single-centre evidence to suggest that the latter approach may be more effective in reducing recurrence rates, but this requires further validation. The more aggressive approach in this case appears justifiable in the context of a difficult and potentially troublesome arrhythmia. The aim being to potentially reduce the amount of ICD therapy delivered, once implanted.

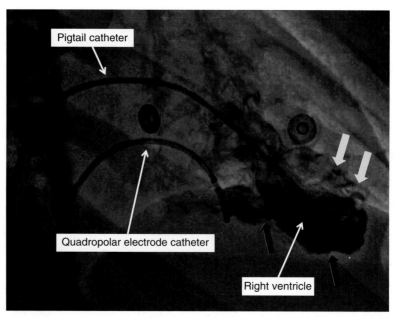

Figure 14.5 Right ventricular (RV) angiogram via pigtail catheter in the RV apex demonstrating areas of fissuring (yellow arrows) and aneurysmal appearances in the RV wall (red arrows). A diagnostic quadropolar electrode catheter is *in situ* for the electrophysiology procedure.

⊕ Clinical tip The Wellens protocol

Wellens et al. described a 12-stage induction protocol for VT [19]. This protocol (or abbreviated variations of it) is widely used during electrophysiological studies to assess the inducibility of VT. Up to three ventricular extrastimuli are introduced from a catheter that is positioned in the RV apex in sinus rhythm, following drive trains at three different cycle lengths. Typically, an 8-beat pacing drive train is used and premature extrastimuli are introduced at successively shorter coupling intervals. In general, only the induction of sustained monomorphic VT is thought to be a specific result. Some electrophysiologists use a second pacing site (RVOT or left ventricle) or isoproterenol infusion, which can improve sensitivity at the cost of specificity.

✪ Learning point Treatment of arrhythmogenic right ventricular cardiomyopathy

The main aim of the management of patients with ARVC is to prevent SCD. ICD implantation is recommended for patients with prior cardiac arrest, syncope, and haemodynamically compromising VT. Extensive RV/LV involvement and a family history of sudden death are class IIa indications in both US and European guidelines. In this patient group, the ICD intervention rate is approximately 10% per year, which improves the projected survival based on a reduction in mortality of 30% at three years' follow-up [14]. Available data suggest that asymptomatic patients or healthy gene carriers do not require any prophylactic treatment, but should be followed up regularly with clinical history, ECG, 24-hour Holter, ETT, and TTE. Well-tolerated ventricular arrhythmias are best treated with either sotalol or amiodarone and/or beta-blocker [15]. All patients should be discouraged from participation in competitive sports and endurance training as physical exercise has been shown to increase the risk of sudden death in people with ARVC and may also enhance disease progression [16]. Pregnancy is well tolerated, but an increased risk of ventricular arrhythmias has been reported in the last trimester and puerperium [17].

Catheter ablation of VT has been shown to have a high initial success rate in eliminating the clinical VT in about 80% of patients, but recurrence rates are high at up to 85% at three years' follow-up [18]. This is probably due to disease progression and the development of the arrhythmogenic substrate. VT ablation is hence usually reserved for patients with incessant VT despite anti-arrhythmic therapy or frequent shocks from their ICDs.

The patient was monitored in hospital and the sotalol was increased to 120 mg twice daily. A 12-lead ECG in sinus rhythm showed no significant QT prolongation. During a repeat ETT, the patient managed to exercise for ten minutes. ECG showed frequent ectopics of RVOT morphology early on during exercise and in recovery, but no VT.

ICD implantation was then performed under sedation. A single coil active fixation lead was introduced via the left cephalic vein, positioned in the mid-RV septum and connected to a single-chamber ICD which was implanted in a pre-pectoral pocket. A successful VF induction was carried out.

The patient was regularly reviewed in the outpatient clinic. About a year following her initial admission, she received an appropriate shock from her defibrillator for VT, but has remained well since. Both her and her father underwent genetic testing and were found to have a mutation in PKP2 which is the gene encoding plakophilin-2. The patient's three siblings were negative for the PKP2 mutation and had been discharged from clinic.

Discussion

Despite significant advances in the last decade, the clinical diagnosis of early forms of ARVC remains challenging. The revised Task Force criteria have improved diagnostic sensitivity whilst maintaining high specificity. Gadolinium late enhancement during CMR imaging enables the detection of subtle structural abnormalities consistent with minor disease, but CMR has also been implicated in over-diagnosis of ARVC. A recent study showed that electroanatomical mapping might be useful in the differential diagnosis between idiopathic RVOT tachycardia and concealed cases of ARVC, by identifying RV low-voltage regions that represent electroanatomical scars [21]. The isolation of causative mutations has enabled us to identify asymptomatic carriers and to establish a diagnosis in patients with inconclusive clinical findings.

The second challenge is risk stratification of patients who might benefit from preventative therapy, including ICD implantation. Larger studies are needed to establish whether electrophysiological studies with programmed ventricular stimulation, the extent of structural abnormalities on MRI, or certain genotypes predict the risk of ventricular arrhythmias and SCD.

A final word from the expert

ARVC is a complex genetic disease with a spectrum of clinical presentations, ranging from having a positive genetic test without any sign of the disease to sudden death and/or severe heart failure. This can be age-related, with adolescents and adults more likely to show signs of the disease than children, and may show incomplete penetrance amongst relatives from the same family. Therefore, the traditional investigative armamentarium is wide and best undertaken by units experienced in the field. Given the limitations of previous diagnostic criteria [6], the ARVC Task Force has redefined criteria to facilitate greater accuracy and reproducibility, taking into account genetic testing and incomplete penetrance [5].

Common pitfalls that lead to over-diagnosis mainly relate to imaging. For example, a mild wall motion abnormality seen at the insertion site of the moderator band into the RV free wall may have been diagnosed as a sign of ARVC, but is now recognized as a variation of normal [9]. In addition, the diagnosis of ARVC based on pathological amounts of epicardial fat on CMR imaging has been problematic, as epicardial fat without fibrosis is a normal histopathological and CMR finding, and its extent varies with age, sex, and body mass index. Involvement of the left ventricle has only recently become recognized such that some have suggested renaming the condition *arrhythmogenic ventricular cardiomyopathy* [2]. Novel diagnostic techniques are also under evaluation, including immunohistochemical analysis for depressed plakoglobin reactivity in myocardial biopsy samples [22].

Genetic testing, however, does not offer a diagnostic panacea. A 'positive' result may confirm the diagnosis, which may be helpful in borderline cases, and offer a diagnostic (or predictive) test in relatives. Unfortunately, a 'negative' result cannot exclude the condition as the test's sensitivity is 50%, even if most currently known genes are tested for. In addition, the true meaning of a positive result

continued

Expert comment

ICD implantation in this case was justified due to the involvement of both ventricles and the presentation with haemodynamically compromising VT. Well-tolerated sustained VT in itself is not an indication for ICD implantation.

Expert comment

Genetic testing should be offered to individuals with a diagnosis of ARVC who have blood relatives at risk of being carriers. Ideally, suspected but borderline cases should also undergo diagnostic testing, but in practice, resources are often insufficient to allow this to occur in every instance.

Clinical tip Role of genetic testing in arrhythmogenic right ventricular cardiomyopathy

Screening for known ARVC genes can identify mutations in around 50% of patients with a clinical diagnosis of ARVC, and both autosomal dominant and recessive forms have been identified [20]. Gene testing is useful both for suspected cases of ARVC with borderline diagnostic findings, and also for family members of gene-positive patients. Once the mutation in a specific family is known, members of this family can be tested for this mutation (predictive testing) and either identified as gene carriers or reassured that they are not affected and do not require further investigation or follow-up. Genetic testing allows identification of carriers before the appearance of any clinical signs. Regular follow-up can be instigated and lifestyle and family planning advice given.

may be unclear due to the high prevalence of previously unknown ethnically determined common genetic variants or rare variants with unknown or no pathogenic significance. In these circumstances, a more extensive evaluation of both the family and the assessment of the possible consequences of the variant will be required, but may still not provide the answer. It is also relatively common for individuals to harbour more than one variant in ARVC-associated genes, which may further complicate matters. As new genes are discovered to explain more cases of ARVC and novel high throughput sequencing technologies become available, it is possible that the role of genetic modifiers and environmental factors will be better understood, and a genetic risk stratification developed [23].

Currently, there is little prognostic benefit from genetic testing and clinical risk stratification remains straightforward and applicable to patients with a well-developed phenotype. Aggregation of databases of serially evaluated patients may provide the best chances for the discovery of novel clinical and genetic risk stratifiers. Unfortunately, in the early stages of disease, there may be few, if any, manifestations, such that even autopsies of unexplained sudden death victims (Sudden Arrhythmic Death Syndrome) may fail to identify ARVC, despite its presence in family members at subsequent evaluation [24]. These victims presumably suffered SCD during an early 'hot' phase, and identifying them is a significant diagnostic and prognostic challenge.

References

1 Nava A, Thiene G, Canciani B, et al. Familial occurrence of right ventricular dysplasia: a study involving nine families. *J Am Coll Cardiol* 1988; 12: 1222–1228.

2 Sen–Chowdhry S, Morgan RD, Chambers JC, et al. Arrhythmogenic cardiomyopathy: aetiology, diagnosis, and treatment. *Ann Rev Med* 2010; 61: 233–253.

3 Basso C, Thiene G, Corrado D, et al. Arrhythmogenic right ventricular cardiomyopathy: dysplasia, dystrophy or myocarditis? *Circulation* 1996; 94: 983–991.

4 Kaplan SR, Gard JJ, Protonotarios N, et al. Remodelling of myocyte gap junctions in arrhythmogenic right ventricular cardiomyopathy due to a deletion in plakoglobin (Naxos disease). *Heart Rhythm* 2004; 1: 3–11.

5 Marcus FI, McKenna WJ, Sherrill D, et al. Diagnosis of arrhythmogenic right ventricular cardiomyopathy/dysplasia. Proposed modification of the Task Force criteria. *Circulation* 2010; 121: 1533–1541.

6 McKenna WJ, Thiene G, Nava A, et al. Diagnosis of arrhythmogenic right ventricular dysplasia/cardiomyopathy. Task Force of the Working Group Myocardial and Pericardial Disease of the European Society of Cardiology and of the Scientific Council on Cardiomyopathies of the International Society and Federation of Cardiology. *Heart* 1994; 71: 215–218.

7 Basso C, Corrado D, Marcus FI, et al. Arrhythmogenic right ventricular cardiomyopathy. *Lancet* 2009; 373: 1289–1300.

8 Sen-Chowdhry S, McKenna WJ. The utility of magnetic resonance imaging in the evaluation of arrhythmogenic right ventricular cardiomyopathy. *Curr Opin Cardiol* 2008; 23: 38–45.

9 Sen-Chowdhry S, Prasad SK, Syrris P, et al. Cardiovascular magnetic resonance in arrhythmogenic right ventricular cardiomyopathy revisited. *J Am Coll Cardiol* 2006; 48: 2132–2140.

10 Taandri H, Saranathan M, Rodriguez ER, et al. Non-invasive detection of myocardial fibrosis in arrhythmogenic right ventricular cardiomyopathy using delayed enhancement magnetic resonance imaging. *J Am Coll Cardiol* 2005; 45: 98–103.

11 Kudaiberdieva G, Gorenek B, Goktekin O, et al. Combination of QT variability and signal-averaged electrocardiography in association with ventricular tachycardia in post-infarction patients. *J Electrocardiol* 2003; 36: 17–24.

12 Nava A, Folino F, Bauce B. Signal-averaged electrocardiogram in patients with arrhythmogenic right ventricular cardiomyopathy and ventricular arrhythmias. *Eur Heart J* 2000; 21: 58–65.

13 Kamath GS, Zareba W, Delaney J, et al. Value of the signal-averaged electrocardiogram in arrhythmogenic right ventricular cardiomyopathy/dysplasia. *Heart Rhythm* 2011; 8: 256–262.

14 Corrado D, Leoni L, Link MS. Implantable cardioverter-defibrillator therapy for prevention of sudden death in patients with arrhythmogenic right ventricular cardiomyopathy/dysplasia. *Circulation* 2003; 108: 3084–3091.

15 Wichter T, Borggrefe M, Haverkamp W, et al. Efficacy of anti-arrhythmic drugs in patients with arrhythmogenic right ventricular disease. Results in patients with inducible and non-inducible ventricular tachycardia. *Circulation* 1992; 86: 29–37.

16 Corrado D, Basso C, Rizzoli G. Does sports activity enhance the risk of sudden death in adolescents and young adults? *J Am Coll Cardiol* 2003; 42: 1959–1963.

17 Bauce B, Daliento L, Frigo G, et al. Pregnancy in women with arrhythmogenic right ventricular cardiomyopathy. *Eur J Obstet Gynecol* 2006; 127: 186–189.

18 Dalal D, Jain R, Tandri H. Long-term efficacy of catheter ablation of ventricular tachycardia in patients with arrhythmogenic right ventricular dysplasia/cardiomyopathy. *J Am Coll Cardiol* 2007; 50: 432–440.

19 Wellens HJ, Brugada P, Stevenson WG. Programmed electrical stimulation of the heart in patients with life-threatening ventricular arrhythmias: what is the significance of induced arrhythmias and what is the correct stimulation protocol? *Circulation* 1985; 72: 1–7.

20 Sen-Chowdhry S, Syrris P, McKenna WJ. Role of genetic analysis in the management of patients with arrhythmogenic right ventricular dysplasia/cardiomyopathy. *J Am Coll Cardiol* 2007; 50: 1813–1821.

21 Corrado D, Basso C, Leoni L, et al. Three-dimensional electroanatomical voltage mapping and histological evaluation of myocardial substrate in right ventricular outflow tract tachycardia. *J Am Coll Cardiol* 2008; 51: 731–739.

22 Asimaki A, Tandri H, Huang H, et al. A new diagnostic test for arrhythmogenic right ventricular cardiomyopathy. *N Engl J Med* 2009; 360: 1075–1084.

23 Sen-Chowdhry S, Syrris P, Pantazis A, et al. Mutational heterogeneity, modifier genes, and environmental influences contribute to phenotypic diversity of arrhythmogenic cardiomyopathy. *Circ Cardiovasc Genet* 2010; 3: 323–330.

24 Behr ER, Dalageorgou C, Christiansen M, et al. Sudden arrhythmic death syndrome: familial evaluation identifies inheritable heart disease in the majority of families. *Eur Heart J* 2008; 29: 1670–1680.

The sparkly heart

Jamal Nasir Khan

Expert commentary Dr Simon Dubrey

Case history

A 67-year-old Caucasian lady was admitted to hospital with a 6-month history of worsening lethargy, peripheral oedema, and dyspnoea. There was no other previous medical history. She had been commenced on furosemide 40 mg daily by her family physician three weeks previously and took no other medications.

On admission, she was borderline hypotensive at 103/65 mmHg. Clinical examination revealed a regular pulse at 64 beats per minute (bpm), raised jugular venous pressure (JVP) at 4 cm above the sternal angle, and grade 2/6 pansystolic murmur at the apex radiating to the axilla. Minimal pulmonary congestion was present clinically and radiographically. There was significant bilateral leg oedema to the level of the upper thigh. This was associated with a degree of ascites, hepatomegaly, and yellow sclerae. Blood results are noted in Table 15.1.

Urinary dipstick revealed heavy proteinuria. An electrocardiogram (ECG) demonstrated low-voltage complexes associated with poor R wave progression and Q waves across the anteroseptal leads V1–V3 (Figure 15.1). The patient denied any previous angina or myocardial infarction.

Further hepatic blood tests, including an autoimmune screen and hepatitis serology, were normal. She was commenced on intravenous (IV) furosemide 80 mg twice daily (bd) and responded well. A review of previous results revealed worsening stage 2 renal impairment over the past 18 months. In light of her deranged liver and renal function, an abdominal ultrasound was undertaken. This showed a mildly enlarged liver with a normal texture and the kidneys appeared normal. No other abnormalities were seen. A 24-hour urinalysis revealed a mildly nephrotic picture with 3.1 g of protein loss. A myeloma screen revealed raised levels of urinary Bence–Jones proteins and

> **⊕ Clinical tip** Investigating unexplained renal impairment
> - Approach this logically, considering pre-renal (commonest), intra-renal, and post-renal causes;
> - *Pre-renal*: fluid status (is the patient dehydrated?), is the patient hypotensive (this includes sepsis, cardiac pump failure);
> - *Intra-renal*: screen for nephrotoxic drugs, autoimmune/vasculitic screen, myeloma screen, dipstick/midstream urine, renal ultrasound ± biopsy;
> - *Post-renal*: investigate for evidence of obstruction (if suspected, catheterize), *per rectum* examination (prostate), renal ultrasound.

Table 15.1 Blood results on admission

Haematology		Biochemistry	
Hb	12.6 g/dL	Na	135 mmol/L
MCV	82.1 fL	K	4.8 mmol/L
WCC	6.24 × 10⁹/L	Urea	**13.1 mmol/L**
Neutrophils	4.37 × 10⁹/L	Creatinine	**185 micromol/L**
Platelets	354 × 10⁹/L	GFR	45 mL/min
INR	1.1	Bilirubin	**32 micromol/L**
		Aspartame transaminase (AST)	43 IU/L
		Alkaline phosphatase	**239 IU/L**
		Total protein	81 g/dL
		Albumin	35 g/dL

Challenging concepts in cardiovascular medicine

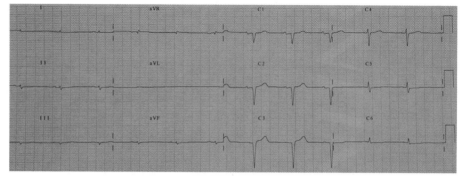

Figure 15.1 ECG on admission demonstrating low-voltage complexes and a 'pseudoinfarct' pattern.

serum electrophoresis demonstrated a monoclonal proliferation of IgG antibodies. Myeloma with renal involvement was suspected.

Serum albumin levels were only borderline low and therefore, unlikely to account for the degree of oedema. Given the context of her low-voltage ECG suggesting previous anterior myocardial infarction, it was suspected that congestive cardiac failure was a possibility.

Transthoracic echocardiography (TTE) illustrated marked concentric biventricular wall thickening associated with increased myocardial echogenicity, giving a 'speckled' or 'sparkly' appearance (Figure 15.2). Grade 2 diastolic dysfunction was seen with pseudonormalization of the mitral inflow pattern (E/A ratio 1.24) associated with reduced mitral annulus velocities on tissue Doppler imaging (TDI) (E/E' ratio 20). Left ventricular (LV) systolic function was, however, preserved with an ejection fraction (EF) of 60%. Thickening of the posterior mitral valve leaflet (PMVL) resulted in mild mitral regurgitation (MR) into a mildly enlarged left atrium (area 24 cm²). The right atrium was mildly enlarged. The overall picture suggested moderate diastolic dysfunction, resulting from restrictive cardiomyopathy.

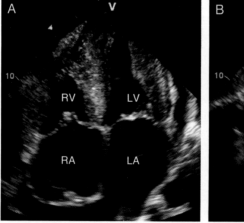
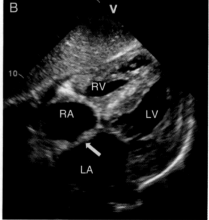

Figure 15.2 Transthoracic echocardiography (plate A: apical 4-chamber view; plate B: subcostal view) revealing marked biventricular concentric hypertrophy, biatrial dilatation, and thickening of the interatrial septum (subcostal view: arrow). LV = left ventricle; RV = right ventricle; LA = left atrium; RA = right atrium.

> ⊙ **Learning point** The E/A ratio is normal despite ventricular thickening. Is that normal diastolic function or 'pseudonormalization'? (Figure 15.3)
>
> - Diastolic dysfunction is important to identify.
> - Grade 1 (slow relaxation) manifests as a reduced E/A ratio (<1) associated with a prolonged mitral deceleration time (>200 ms) [1,2].
> - However, grade 2 dysfunction (moderate) is associated with pseudonormalization of the E/A ratio and must be excluded in all cases of ventricular wall thickening associated with a normal E/A ratio. This is confirmed by a raised E/E' ratio of >15 as follows:
>   1. *Diastolic dysfunction results in reduced velocities of mitral annular movement.*
>   2. *Select TDI on your echo machine and place the cursor across the medial annulus of the mitral valve on an apical 4-chamber view (A4C).*
>   3. *Placing the sample volume over this in pulsed wave (PW) Doppler mode reveals that two negative waves are seen in diastole.*
>   4. *The first is annular movement towards the left atrium during the initial passive filling of the left ventricle. This is analogous to a mitral E wave and is the E' wave. The second negative wave is the A' wave, analogous to the mitral inflow A wave.*
> - An E/E' ratio of >15 confirms diastolic dysfunction and E/A pseudonormalization [1,2].
> - The E/E' ratio is also useful in distinguishing restrictive cardiomyopathy from constrictive pericarditis since the former is associated with a raised E/E' ratio of >15 whereas a 'normal' ratio of <8 is seen in constriction.
> - **Abnormal pulmonary vein (PV) flow**: this provides further evidence for pseudonormalization. PW Doppler over the orifice of the left atrial PV illustrates that a normal, biphasic PV flow consists of a dominant pS wave (systolic forward flow) and smaller pD wave (diastolic forward flow). A retrograde abnormal relaxation (AR) wave is seen during atrial contraction. Diastolic dysfunction results in raised left atrial pressures. This results in changes in the D wave that parallel those of the mitral inflow E wave, initially decreasing, then increasing by grade 2 diastolic dysfunction. The AR wave increases in duration with left atrial pressure. Therefore, a reduced pS:pD ratio of <0.35 and prolonged AR wave duration of >20 ms confirm at least grade 2 diastolic dysfunction [1,2].
> - Grade 3 dysfunction (severe) reflects further reduced LV relaxation and compliance and raised left atrial pressure. This results in a rapid increase in LV pressures, shortening the early passive filling (E wave). Mitral inflow shows a raised E/A ratio (>2) in conjunction with a shortened deceleration time (<150 ms). Grade 3 dysfunction is confirmed by reversal to grade 1 or 2 on performing Valsalva manoeuvre. If no reversal is possible, this is deemed grade 4 dysfunction (very severe) [2].

Marked ventricular thickening usually results from hypertrophy, producing increased ECG voltages [3]. The presence of low-voltage ECG complexes suggested that the ventricular thickening was not due to hypertrophy. Given the 'speckled' appearance of the myocardium and biatrial enlargement, restrictive cardiomyopathy secondary to cardiac infiltration was suspected. When considered in light of the coexisting renal impairment with nephrotic syndrome and paraproteinaemia, systemic amyloidosis was a potential unifying diagnosis. Investigations for alternative causes of restrictive cardiomyopathy were negative, including normal serum ferritin (haemochromatosis), angiotensin-converting enzyme (sarcoidosis), and eosinophil levels (Loeffler's syndrome). There was no history of radiotherapy (post-radiation cardiac fibrosis) [4].

To clarify the cardiomyopathy, cardiac magnetic resonance (CMR) imaging was undertaken. This illustrated global, subendocardial late myocardial enhancement with gadolinium. Systolic function was preserved. These findings intensified the suspicion of an infiltrative restrictive cardiomyopathy, suggestive of cardiac involvement in systemic amyloidosis.

Despite an initial response to intravenous furosemide, residual oedema proved resistant to diuresis. By the fifth day of admission, she had lost 3 kg in weight, but

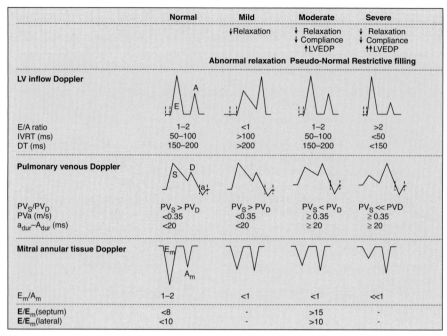

Figure 15.3 Assessment of left ventricular diastolic function (copyright British Society of Echocardiography).

merely 1 kg in the last three days. She was commenced on an intravenous furosemide infusion (240 mg over 24 hours) and later, required the addition of alternate day metolazone (2.5 mg) to achieve effective resolution of oedema. Renal function remained stable with a glomerular filtration rate (GFR) of 45 mL/min.

It was felt that AL amyloidosis (primary systemic amyloidosis) was likeliest since this was most commonly associated with cardiac and renal involvement. Since it is caused by the deposition of excess circulating immunoglobulin light chains, this could also account for the positive myeloma screen. However the diagnosis could not be made without the demonstration of amyloid protein [3,4]. Serum amyloid protein (SAP) scintigraphy was undertaken revealing amyloid protein only in the kidneys (Figure 15.4).

Management of the underlying amyloidosis would depend upon the fibril subtype. A renal biopsy sample stained red with Congo red and demonstrated apple-green birefringence under polarized light microscopy. This confirmed the presence of amyloid protein. Immunohistochemical analysis of this sample confirmed the deposition of fibrils, consisting of an excess of immunoglobulin light chains secondary to clonal proliferation. This suggested AL amyloidosis. In order to distinguish this from multiple myeloma where kappa (κ) light chains predominate, demonstration of an excess of the lambda (λ) variety was required [4]. Serum free light chains analysis revealed λ chains at 42.4 mg/L and κ chains at 13.4 mg/L (λ:κ ratio 3.16). The diagnosis of AL amyloidosis with renal and cardiac involvement was confirmed. Although SAP scintigraphy only demonstrated renal amyloid tissue, cardiac involvement was confirmed due to the characteristic ECG, TTE, and CMR findings. SAP scintigraphy cannot demonstrate amyloid in the moving heart [3].

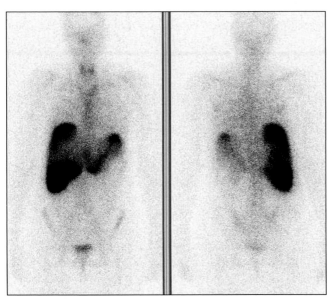

Figure 15.4 Serum amyloid protein (SAP) scintigraphy confirming amyloid protein deposition in the kidneys.

⚙ **Learning point** Diagnosing cardiac involvement in amyloidosis

ECG findings
- Cardiac involvement is often initially suspected on ECG. The characteristic pattern features low-voltage complexes associated with poor R wave progression across the precordial leads. Q waves are commonly seen producing a 'pseudoinfarct' pattern. Murtagh et al. demonstrated these in anterior (36%), lateral (14%), and inferior leads (12%) [5]. Low-voltage complexes are in direct contrast to the increased voltage that one expects in the presence of ventricular wall thickening [3-5,7].
- Atrial fibrillation is the commonest arrhythmia [5].
- Chronotropic incompetence has been demonstrated in a small case series and was shown to predict short-term mortality. This is thought to be a result of autonomic dysfunction often seen in systemic amyloidosis [6].

Echocardiography findings
- Restrictive cardiomyopathy with diastolic dysfunction is seen to some extent in all patients. Systolic failure is absent until advanced disease [3,8].
- Biventricular wall thickening with reduced chamber cavity diameters is seen in the vast majority. This results from infiltration, not hypertrophy [8,9]. In the context of diagnosing cardiac amyloidosis, sensitivities of approximately 75% and specificities of over 90% have been seen for the combination of this and low-voltage ECG complexes [7,10-12].
- Biatrial enlargement is often seen and has been described in up to 50% of cases [9,11].
- A granular or 'sparkling' or 'speckled' appearance of the myocardium is often seen as a result of increased echogenicity due to deposited amyloid fibrils. However, this is also seen in other causes of wall thickening, including LV hypertrophy [9,13].
- Thickened valve leaflets and small pericardial effusions have been described in advanced disease [9].

CMR findings
- Late gadolinium enhancement in a global, subendocardial distribution has been demonstrated by Maciera et al.. This is thought to result from the expansion of the interstitium by amyloid fibrils. Myocardial enhancement was associated with increased LV mass and impaired systolic function [14].
- The study also demonstrated reduced subendocardial relaxation time, reflecting diastolic dysfunction and restriction [14].

continued

Expert comment

Warfarin is particularly important in amyloid heart infiltration. Atrial involvement means the atria, already enlarged due to restrictive ventricular physiology, are also immobile. This results in atrial electromechanical dissociation and a high risk of thrombus formation.

Clinical tip Managing heart failure in amyloidosis

- Cardiac impairment is predominantly diastolic until advanced disease [3,8].
- The mainstay is diuretic therapy and high doses are often required, especially when nephrotic syndrome coexists [3].
- Close attention to fluid balance is vital.
- Patients should be educated to monitor weights daily and adjust diuretic doses, if required (e.g. occasional metolazone, if necessary).
- Involvement of the community heart failure nursing service is advisable.
- Beta-blockers and angiotensin-converting enzyme inhibitors must be used with extreme caution due to the risk of significant hypotension in light of autonomic dysfunction and severe restrictive cardiomyopathy that accompany cardiac amyloidosis [3,17].
- Where renal amyloidosis coexists, renal function must be monitored regularly.

Expert comment

If low BP becomes symptomatic, then careful titration of the alpha-blocker, midodrine, is frequently necessary. This drug is currently unlicensed and is used on a named patient basis. The dose starts at 2.5 mg two to three times daily and is titrated against the pressor response achieved. As this is a systemic disease, it is easy to assume that a low BP is cardiac in origin and to overlook that amyloid infiltration of the adrenals, the thyroid, or indeed the autonomic nervous system might have similar consequences in terms of hypotension.

- Recently, a more variable distribution of late gadolinium enhancement has been demonstrated by Perugini et al., extending transmurally. It was suggested that the amount of tissue demonstrating enhancement correlates with the degree of diastolic dysfunction [15].

Cardiac biomarkers
- Diastolic dysfunction in amyloidosis results in an upgraded expression of naturetic peptide genes, resulting in raised levels of brain natriuretic peptide (BNP). NT-proBNP levels are used as a marker of response to treatment. A successful response to chemotherapy has been shown to result in ≥30% reduction in NT-proBNP levels [16].

She eventually reached her dry weight after losing 11 kg and was discharged home on furosemide 80 mg bd. Liver function tests normalized and renal function remained stable. Diuretic therapy would provide symptomatic relief. However, management of the underlying amyloidosis would require chemotherapy targeting the plasma cells responsible for the proliferation of λ light chains. She would return to the amyloidosis clinic to discuss this with the haematologists in two months' time.

She failed to attend this appointment and was admitted four months later with evidence of pulmonary oedema. An intravenous furosemide infusion of 240 mg over 24 hours was commenced. ECG revealed atrial fibrillation (AF) with a fast ventricular rate (145 bpm). Since the time of onset of AF was unknown, a rate control strategy was employed. Due to her renal impairment, a loading dose of 500 mcg of digoxin over 24 hours was administered followed by 62.5 mcg daily. Despite this reduced dose, she developed symptomatic bradycardia and digoxin toxicity (vomiting, nausea, blurred vision) although serum digoxin levels were normal. Digoxin was discontinued and the patient was commenced on warfarin and amiodarone for rate control.

Beta-blockers and rate-limiting calcium channel blockers were not used due to acute heart failure with haemodynamic compromise. She responded well and had improved significantly by day 3 with a clear chest, rate-controlled AF, and of 3 kg of reduction in oedema.

Echocardiography illustrated the progression of cardiac amyloidosis. Diastolic dysfunction had increased to grade 3 (E/A ratio 3.1) and systolic function was now moderately impaired with an EF of 39%. Following successful diuresis, she was converted to oral bumetanide 3 mg bd and spironolactone 25 mg was added for right-sided failure. She remained stable on this combination and towards discharge, her BP was 97/68 mmHg. A small dose of ramipril (1.25 mg) was commenced in light of LV systolic impairment, but was not tolerated by the patient. She was eventually discharged home on bumetanide, spironolactone, warfarin, and amiodarone.

Learning point Atrial arrhythmias in cardiac amyloidosis

- AF, followed by atrial flutter, is the commonest arrhythmia [5].
- Rhythm control is desirable, where possible since atrioventricular synchrony can optimize the ventricular filling that is compromised in the often significant diastolic dysfunction in amyloidosis.
- Where this is impossible or unsuccessful, rate control can be undertaken safely with amiodarone.
- Digoxin should be avoided since it binds strongly to amyloid fibrils and can result in digoxin toxicity and significant bradycardia [18].
- Beta-blockers and calcium channel inhibitors can lead to severe bradycardia and hypotension in light of the autonomic dysfunction, restrictive cardiomyopathy, and resulting diastolic dysfunction seen in amyloidosis [3,19].
- Warfarin should be used for anticoagulation unless there are contraindications.

She was reviewed in the amyloidosis clinic two weeks after discharge and commenced on thalidomide chemotherapy with minimal response. The combination of melphalan and dexamethasone was successfully trialled three months later. She remains in complete remission two years later as evidenced by an unchanged small amount of renal amyloid tissue on SAP scintigraphy, the absence of serum or urine paraproteinaemia, and stable NT-proBNP levels under 300 pmol/L (in comparison to the 912 pmol/L prior to chemotherapy).

> ⭐ **Learning point** Management of primary systemic cardiac amyloidosis (AL amyloid)
>
> **Supportive management**
> - Management of restrictive cardiomyopathy and resulting diastolic dysfunction and later, systolic impairment;
> - Careful fluid balance;
> - Warfarinization where anticoagulation is required;
> - Management of arrhythmias, especially AF and atrial flutter;
> - A low threshold for permanent pacing since maintaining atrioventricular synchrony in severe restrictive cardiomyopathy can improve cardiac output [3]. In addition, associated autonomic neuropathy leads to a higher incidence of syncope, which may be improved with pacing in appropriate patients. Thus, ambulatory ECG monitoring should be undertaken in all patients;
> - There is no evidence of survival benefit seen from implantable cardioverter-defibrillators [20];
> - Cardiac transplantation is rarely performed due to concerns about the development of AL amyloidosis in donor hearts and poor prognosis associated with progression of systemic amyloidosis [21].
>
> **Management of the underlying amyloidosis**
> - AL amyloidosis and multiple myeloma result from the monoclonal proliferation of immunoglobulin light chains and hence share common chemotherapeutic agents.
> - Oral regimes, including melphalan, thalidomide, and steroids (prednisolone, dexamethasone) are generally well tolerated, but with variable and often delayed response [22].
> - Cardiac involvement significantly increases the risk of stem cell transplantation. Aggressive regimes involving intravenous chemotherapy and stem cell transplantation are less well tolerated, with up to 25% mortality reported following treatment [23].
>
> **Follow-up**
> - Management of AL amyloidosis requires close collaboration between haematologists, cardiologists, and nephrologists.
> - Investigations undertaken at specialist amyloid clinics typically include: renal function, liver function, clotting screen, 24-hour urinary protein, serum free light chain analysis (assesses levels and ratio of paraprotein), ECG, echocardiogram, and SAP scan.
> - In particular, NT-proBNP levels allow the assessment of response to chemotherapy [16].

Discussion

Amyloidosis is a family of conditions characterized by the extracellular deposition of abnormal, virtually insoluble proteins in tissues. Amyloid proteins derive from a range of precursors, but share a common secondary structure composed of resilient beta-pleated sheets. They stain red with Congo red under normal light, but appear apple-green under polarized light microscopy [3,4]. Amyloidoses are classified according to the protein type and can be inherited or acquired [4].

Infiltration of the heart is most commonly seen in AL (primary systemic) amyloidosis. It is less common in ATTR amyloidosis (familial amyloidosis caused by the deposition of abnormal transthyretin [TTR] protein) and 'senile cardiac amyloid' (deposition of *normal* TTR with advanced age) [3,4]. Cardiac involvement is seen in up to half

---

Expert comment

When peripheral oedema, which may be multifactorial, is problematic and BP is already low, then full length compression stockings may be necessary.

Expert comment

The gold standard for patients with AL amyloidosis who do not have severe cardiac involvement is autologous stem cell transplantation following bone marrow ablation, usually with intravenous melphalan. Eradication of the plasma cells is the aim, but it is now also recognized that the light chains are themselves toxic to organ systems. This may explain why responses to treatment (by reduction in light chains) sometimes precede any observed changes on imaging modalities.

Expert comment

In the diagnosis of AL amyloid, it is important not to miss some of the 'classic stigmata' of this disease. These include macroglossia, thickening of tissues of the muzzle region of the face, brittle nails, spontaneous peri-orbital bruising (panda or racoon eyes), the shoulder pad sign, stiff skin (the 'stiff man syndrome'), and a past history of carpal tunnel syndrome (sometime several years earlier).

Expert comment

Regression of the amyloid load on SAP scanning has shown that the amyloid matrix is not a totally insoluble entity.

of AL amyloid cases and presents as a restrictive cardiomyopathy [24,25]. It must be excluded in cases of restrictive cardiomyopathy associated with low-voltage ECG complexes. Failure to diagnose cardiac amyloidosis can have serious consequences since the majority of treatments used in diastolic and systolic impairment can result in haemodynamic compromise in the stiff, preload-dependent amyloid heart [3,17-19]. In addition, cardiac involvement in AL amyloidosis results in a particularly poor prognosis with a median survival of only 1.08 years [7].

Renal involvement has been shown to exist in over two-thirds of cases of cardiac amyloidosis with a nephrotic picture in the majority of such patients [7]. Management of cardiac amyloidosis should involve a multidisciplinary approach with close collaboration between cardiologists, haematologists, and nephrologists.

☺ A final word from the expert

AL amyloidosis is a disease that can masquerade as many others. Patients may present with one or more of the recognized 'stigmata', but many more will remain unrecognized or misdiagnosed. The important three points are:

1. To recognize that the condition is due to amyloidosis;
2. To define the exact type of amyloid disease;
3. To institute treatment rapidly.

This disease can be rapidly fatal which has meant that many patients have not lived long enough to be able to receive a curative dose of chemotherapy. Those with severe cardiac involvement at presentation tend to be those with the least treatment options available and consequently, a very poor prognosis.

In the same way that thalidomide has proved its worth in myeloma and now in AL amyloid, preliminary studies with the proteosome inhibitor, bortezomib, look encouraging following its similar success in myeloma. These drugs unfortunately have significant side effect profiles and studies are awaited that will use combinations of these therapies.

All patients with suspected or confirmed amyloid disease should be discussed with the National Amyloid Centre (NAC), located at the Royal Free Hospital in London. This ensures that patients get the latest diagnostic techniques and are availed to the latest treatment developments and are made aware of current trials and studies.

References

1 Masani N, Wharton G, Allen J, et al. (British Society of Echocardiography Education Committee). Echocardiography: guidelines for chamber quantification. 2007 (poster). Available from: http://www.bsecho.org/Guidelines%20for%20Chamber%20Quantification.pdf.
2 Galderisi M. Diastolic dysfunction and diastolic heart failure: diagnostic, prognostic and therapeutic aspects. *Cardiovasc Ultrasound* 2005; 3: 1–14.
3 Selvanayagam JB, Hawkins PN, Paul B, et al. Evaluation and management of the cardiac amyloidosis. *J Am Coll Cardiol* 2007; 50: 2101–2110.
4 Khan MF, Falk RH. Amyloidosis. *Postgrad Med J* 2002; 77: 686–693.
5 Murtagh B, Hammill SC, Gertz MA, et al. Electrocardiographic findings in primary systemic amyloidosis and biopsy-proven cardiac involvement. *Am J Cardiol* 2005; 95: 535–537.
6 Reyners AK, Hazenberg BP, Reistma WD, et al. Heart rate variability as a predictor of mortality in patients with AA and AL amyloidosis. *Eur Heart J* 2002; 23: 157–161.
7 Dubrey SW, Cha K, Anderson J, et al. The clinical features of immunoglobulin light chain (AL) amyloidosis with heart involvement. *QJM* 1998; 91: 141–157.
8 Wood MJ, Picard MH. Utility of echocardiography in the evaluation of individuals with cardiomyopathy. *Heart* 2004; 90: 707–712.

9 Siqueira–Filho AG, Cunha CL, Tajik AJ, et al. M-mode and two-dimensional echocardiographic features in cardiac amyloidosis. *Circulation* 1981; 63: 188–196.

10 Hamer JP, Janssen S, van Rijswijk MH, et al. Amyloid cardiomyopathy in systemic non-hereditary amyloidosis. Clinical, echocardiographic and electrocardiographic findings in 30 patients with AA and 24 patients with AL amyloidosis. *Eur Heart J* 1992; 13: 623–627.

11 Rahman JE, Helou EF, Gelzer–Bell R, et al. Non-invasive diagnosis of biopsy-proven cardiac amyloidosis. *J Am Coll Cardiol* 2004; 43: 410–415.

12 Carroll JD, Gaasch WH, McAdam KP. Amyloid cardiomyopathy: characterization by a distinctive voltage/mass relation. *Am J Cardiol* 1982; 49: 9–13.

13 Bhandari AK, Nanda NC. Myocardial texture characterization by two-dimensional echocardiography. *Am J Cardiol* 1983; 51: 817–825.

14 Maciera AM, Joshi J, Prasad SK, et al. Cardiovascular magnetic resonance assessment of non-ischaemia cardiomyopathies. *Eur Heart J* 2005; 92: 343–349.

15 Perugini E, Rapezzi C, Piva T, et al. Non-invasive evaluation of the myocardial substrate of cardiac amyloidosis by gadolinium cardiac magnetic resonance. *Heart* 2006; 92: 343–349.

16 Palladini G, Lavatelli F, Russo P, et al. Circulating amyloidogenic free light chains and serum N-terminal natriuretic peptide type B decrease simultaneously in association with improvement of survival on AL. *Blood* 2006; 107: 3854–3858.

17 Parikh S, de Lemos JA. Current therapeutic strategies in cardiac amyloidosis. *Curr Treat Options Cardiovasc Med* 2005; 7: 443–448.

18 Rubinow A, Skinner M, Cohen AS. Digoxin sensitivity in amyloid cardiomyopathy. *Circulation* 1981; 63: 1285–1288.

19 Gertz MA, Falk RH, Skinner M, et al. Worsening of congestive heart failure in amyloid heart disease treated by calcium channel blocking agents. *Am J Cardiol* 1985; 55: 1645.

20 Wright BL, Grace AA, Goodman HJ. Implantation of a cardioverter-defibrillator in a patient with cardiac amyloidosis. *Nat Clin Pract Cardiovasc Med* 2006; 3: 110–114.

21 Dubrey SW, Burke MM, Hawkins PN, et al. Cardiac transplantation for amyloid heart disease: the United Kingdom experience. *J Heart Lung Transplant* 2004; 23: 1142–1153.

22 Kyle RA, Gertz MA, Greipp PR, et al. A trial of three regimens for primary amyloidosis: colchicine alone, melphalan and prednisone, and melphalan, prednisone, and colchicine. *N Engl J Med* 1997; 336: 1202–1207.

23 Goodman HJ, Gillmore JD, Lachman HJ, et al. Outcome of autologous stem cell transplantation for AL amyloidosis in the UK. *Br J Haematol* 2006; 134: 417–425.

24 Kyle RA, Greipp PR. Amyloidosis (AL): clinical and laboratory features in 229 cases. *Mayo Clin Proc* 1983; 58: 665–683.

25 Appleton CP, Hatle LK, Popp RL. Demonstration of restrictive ventricular physiology by Doppler echocardiography. *J Am Coll Cardiol* 1988; 11: 757–768.

Paroxysmal atrial fibrillation

Shouvik Haldar

Expert commentary Professor John Camm

Case history

A 55-year-old man was referred to cardiology outpatients by his general practitioner (GP) with a 2-month history of intermittent palpitations. He was taking ramipril for hypertension and had no other relevant medical history. He drank 30 units of alcohol per week and was a lifelong non-smoker. There was no significant family history.

He described four recent episodes of self-terminating palpitations. They were of sudden onset, occurring both at rest and during mild exertion, and had each lasted between 15 and 60 minutes. The first episode had occurred after he had returned from a party, having consumed a significant amount of alcohol. The others had occurred whilst at work. On each occasion, he had felt his heart pounding fast and chaotically and during the more prolonged attacks, he had felt dizzy and breathless. Clinical examination revealed a regular pulse of 75 beats per minute (bpm) with a blood pressure (BP) of 145/80 mmHg. He had normal heart sounds with no signs of cardiac failure.

His 12-lead electrocardiogram (ECG) confirmed a normal sinus rhythm with a normal electrical axis. Transthoracic echocardiography (TTE) confirmed a normal cardiac structure and function with a mildly dilated left atrial size of 40 mm (normal 27–38 mm). Exercise stress testing did not induce any arrhythmias and was negative for ischaemia. Routine blood tests, including thyroid function, were normal.

At this stage, there was a high clinical suspicion of paroxysmal atrial fibrillation (PAF). However, in the absence of ECG evidence to confirm this diagnosis, treatment was not commenced. He was advised to reduce his alcohol and caffeine intake and an outpatient 7-day event recorder was requested with subsequent follow-up arranged.

By the time of his 6-week follow-up, he had had a further two symptomatic episodes. Neither of these had occurred during his 7-day event recorder which had not documented any arrhythmias. Fortunately, the patient had attended Accident & Emergency (A&E) with a symptomatic episode. Despite spontaneously reverting to sinus rhythm, an initial ECG had captured fast AF. In view of his history, the A&E specialist had given him a copy of the ECG, which he had been instructed to bring along to his follow-up appointment (Figure 16.1).

Now with firm evidence of PAF, treatment options were discussed at his outpatient review. Although his paroxysms were fairly infrequent, the patient was highly symptomatic from them. With no evidence of structural heart abnormalities or ischaemic heart disease, a class I AAD in the form of flecainide 300 mg was initiated as a pill-in-the-pocket strategy. The $CHADS_2$ criteria (Table 16.1) were used to stratify the patient's thromboembolic risk which duly scored the patient at '1'. This gave the patient a 'moderate risk' of thromboembolism and the patient was commenced on aspirin 75 mg once daily.

Expert comment

Treatment with an anti-arrhythmic drug (AAD) should not be readily considered without a definitive ECG diagnosis. However, if you have tried and failed to get a recording, it may be reasonable to try a beta-blocker.

Expert comment

It is a good idea to give the patient a letter requesting A&E to do an ECG as soon as the patient turns up complaining of an arrhythmia. A&E can then be asked to give a copy to the patient and fax a copy to the physician. If involving the GP, you should first check that they have an ECG machine and again give the patient a letter for the GP practice.

Expert comment

With a $CHADS_2$ score of 1, current guidelines allow the doctor/patient to choose aspirin or warfarin. However, the evidence base for aspirin is relatively poor.

Expert comment

A 'pill-in-the-pocket' strategy should really be tested in A&E or Coronary Care Unit (CCU) before patients can be discharged to take the medication themselves in the community.

⊕ Clinical tip Diagnosis of arrhythmias with regard to temporal relation

A thorough history and clinical evaluation is essential in diagnosing arrhythmias, but tools such as ambulatory ECG monitors can be invaluable. In those with frequent (daily) symptoms, a Holter monitor can continuously record and save data for up to 48 hours. Patients are encouraged to keep an event diary, allowing the correlation of symptoms with ECG recordings. Patients with infrequent symptoms require loop event recorders that can continuously record data, with information stored only upon activation by the patient. Once activated, they are programmed to capture the preceding and subsequent two minutes of data. Compared to Holter monitors, event recorders can be used for longer periods, have a higher yield in diagnosing arrhythmias, and have been proven to be more cost-effective and efficacious for the evaluation of palpitations [1].

If prolonged external ambulatory event monitors fail to document an arrhythmia, an implantable loop recorder (e.g. Reveal™ device) can be used. This device is implanted subcutaneously and has a battery life of up to two years. It continuously scans for arrhythmias and automatically stores tachycardia or bradycardia events for future analysis, in addition to information when activated by the patient.

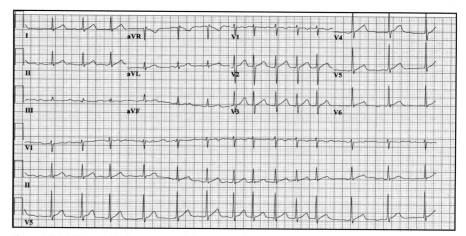

Figure 16.1 ECG on arrival to Accident & Emergency (courtesy of Jonas de Jong).

✪ Learning point Aetiology of atrial fibrillation

AF is a complex re-entrant arrhythmia based on the coexistence of multiple wavelets of electrical activity within the atria. The exact aetiology remains unclear, but multiple mechanisms have been implicated in the genesis of AF. These include ectopic activity in the form of pulmonary and non-pulmonary vein triggers, susceptible atrial substrates (e.g. atrial tissue that perpetuates AF secondary to structural or electrical remodelling, fibrosis or gap junction mutations), and areas with excessive autonomic activity. Of these, the pulmonary vein foci, which represent muscular 'sleeves' of atrial myocardium that extend into the pulmonary veins, have been shown to exhibit the majority of ectopic activity, leading to the triggering of AF [2].

Table 16.1 Adapted $CHADS_2$ scheme for the assessment of stroke risk in patients with (non-valvular) AF [3]

$CHADS_2$ risk factor	Points
Congestive heart failure	1
Hypertension (systolic >160 mmHg)	1
Age > 75 years	1
Diabetes	1
Prior stroke or TIA	2

Total $CHADS_2$ score	Risk of stroke	Annual stroke rate (%)	Antithrombotic therapy indicated
0	Low	1.9	Aspirin
1	Moderate	2.8	Warfarin or aspirin
2–6	High	4.0–18.2	Warfarin

✪ Learning point How to reduce the risk of stroke in atrial fibrillation

The most feared complication of AF is stroke secondary to thromboembolism. As the prevalence of AF increases with an ageing population, prophylaxis against thromboembolism remains the fundamental issue in the therapeutic management of AF. In practice, the risk of stroke is increased four- to five-fold in non-valvular AF. This is regardless of whether patients have paroxysmal or more prolonged bouts of AF, i.e. persistent or permanent.

Prophylaxis with antiplatelet agents or oral anticoagulants is determined by a patient's risk of thromboembolism. Well-validated and simple risk stratification models, such as the $CHADS_2$ (Table 16.1) and the NICE thromboprophylaxis guideline schemes, are commonly used to aid decision-making [4]. Both of these schemes classify patients into low-risk, moderate-risk, and high-risk categories.

continued

Low-risk patients are managed with aspirin (75–300 mg daily). Those at moderate risk can be treated with either aspirin or warfarin. The majority of patients fall into this intermediate category with the decision to anticoagulate based on risk-benefit assessments and a patient's preference rather than robust data. Patients at high risk should be anticoagulated with warfarin, aiming for a target INR of 2–3. Combination therapy with aspirin and clopidogrel should only be used in patients whose risk warrants warfarin for thromboprophylaxis, but who are unable to tolerate it.

The $CHADS_2$ score does have its limitations as it does not take into account all risk factors for stroke. Many patients fall into the moderate-risk category where data exist to show that these patients may well benefit more from warfarin than aspirin. A more risk factor-orientated approach in stroke risk stratification is the CHA_2DS_2-VASc score which refines the score by considering additional factors (refer to Case 3, Table 3.1), thus providing a more accurate assessment of thromboembolism risk.

The left atrial appendage (LAA) is the origin for a large proportion of thromboemboli. Early surgical efforts to obliterate this structure proved favourable in reducing the risk of thromboembolism and current guidelines recommend routine surgical excision of the LAA, in addition to mitral valve surgery to reduce the risk of stroke [5-8]. In those who warrant oral anticoagulation, but have contraindications, a new approach, based on this principle, has evolved. Closing the LAA with a percutaneous device (Figure 16.2) appears to be a promising alternative, with encouraging results in a recent study using the Watchman® device [9].

> ⭐ **Learning point** Pharmacological cardioversion of acute onset atrial fibrillation
>
> Pharmacological cardioversion should be considered in haemodynamically stable patients with acute onset (new or paroxysmal) AF. Class I and III AADs are the most effective in cardioversion and maintenance of sinus rhythm. Ideally, they should be used as soon as possible after arrhythmia onset for optimal efficacy. Randomized trial data comparing flecainide, propafenone, and amiodarone in cardioversion of recent onset AF found conversion to sinus rhythm occurred in 90%, 72%, and 64% of patients, respectively [10].
>
> Class I AADs are negatively inotropic, may block conduction, and can be pro-arrhythmic. Therefore, they are contraindicated in those with left ventricular impairment, significant conduction tissue disease, or a history of myocardial infarction. In this population, the drug of choice is amiodarone although cardioversion may take longer (days to weeks) [11].

> ➕ **Clinical tip** National Institute of Health and Clinical Excellence (NICE) guidelines for the 'pill-in-the-pocket' strategy [4]
>
> In patients with PAF, relatively infrequent (<1/month) symptomatic episodes of AF which do not cause significant haemodynamic compromise (e.g. hypotension) may be treated with a single loading dose of an AAD. This is known as the 'pill-in-the-pocket' strategy and should be considered in those who fulfill all of the following:
>
> - No history of left ventricular dysfunction or valvular or ischaemic heart disease;
> - History of infrequent symptomatic episodes of PAF;
> - Systolic BP >100 mmHg and a resting heart rate above 70 bpm;
> - Able to understand how and when to take the medication.
>
> Occasionally, class IC drugs may cause ventricular proarrhythmia, atrial flutter with 1:1 conduction, or profound bradycardia immediately after pharmacological cardioversion. Hence the 'pill-in-the-pocket' approach should ideally be first tested in hospital under close monitoring.

> ➕ **Clinical tip** Rate or rhythm control in paroxysmal atrial fibrillation
>
> - In those with PAF, either rhythm control or rate control may be used as the initial strategy. However, there are minimal clinical data on which is the better approach. This is due to the fact that only 25% of patients involved in the major clinical trials comparing rhythm control vs rate control had PAF. Interestingly, those who were highly symptomatic were also excluded from the trials.
> - Generally speaking, in PAF, rhythm control to reduce the number and length of paroxysms should be the initial approach. If this fails having tried the different AADs available, then a rate control strategy to control the ventricular response is acceptable. Of course, the option of a more interventional approach remains and is dealt with later in the text.

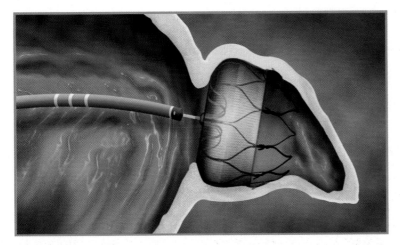

Figure 16.2 The WATCHMAN® LAA Closure Technology. The device is inserted via a catheter into the left atrial appendage. Once in the correct position, the device is expanded and remains lodged here (courtesy of Atritech, Inc. Plymouth, MN, USA).

Learning point How to maintain sinus rhythm post-cardioversion

The majority of drugs used for pharmacological cardioversion are also used to maintain sinus rhythm. Amiodarone has consistently been shown to be the most effective, but chronic use is limited due to its extensive side effect profile [12-14]. Standard beta-blockers offer an attractive combination of modest efficacy and limited adverse effects. Therefore, they are recommended as first-line in the prevention of PAF, followed by class I agents [4,15].

Sotalol is equally as effective as amiodarone in converting AF into sinus rhythm [12]. It is also effective in the maintenance of sinus rhythm [16]. Its class III action requires doses above 80 mg twice daily and the ECG should be checked after dose adjustments to look for possible QT interval prolongation. Although this is part of its therapeutic effect, when the QT_c is >500 ms, the dose should be cut back. Sotalol should be avoided in those with significant conduction disease (second- or third-degree atrioventricular block [AVB]), significant left ventricular dysfunction, and renal impairment due to the risk of QT prolongation and pro-arrhythmia.

Two months later, the patient re-presented to the A&E department. Having taken a dose of flecainide for an episode of his palpitations, he experienced a sudden acceleration in his heart rate, rendering him very symptomatic. He was found to be haemodynamically stable with a narrow complex tachycardia (NCT) and a ventricular rate of 240 bpm. He was given 6 mg of intravenous adenosine which transiently revealed atrial flutter waves at a rate of 240 bpm before reverting back to the tachycardia. At this point, a cardiology consult was requested. The specialist diagnosed atrial flutter with 1:1 AV conduction. He administered 5 mg of intravenous verapamil to the patient which achieved 2:1 AV block and slowed the flutter rate down to 150 bpm. One hour later, the arrhythmia terminated and the patient was back in sinus rhythm. Prior to discharge, the cardiology team reviewed his medical therapy. As his symptoms were becoming increasingly distressing, it was felt that the 'pill-in-the-pocket' approach was no longer appropriate. He was switched to regular flecainide, with the addition of beta-blockers to prevent accelerated AV conduction in the event of further atrial flutter.

Three months later, the patient was reviewed in outpatients. As a result of increasing lethargy and daytime somnolence, he had stopped taking beta-blockers and his GP had prescribed diltiazem as an alternative with continued flecainide. Unfortunately,

Clinical tip Class IC anti-arrhythmic drugs and co-prescribing an atrioventricular nodal blocking agent

- Class IC AADs (flecainide, propafenone, and quinidine) are sodium channel blockers and when used in atrial flutter, can slow the rate of the arrhythmia. Therefore, having administered these agents, a narrow complex atrial flutter at 300 bpm with 2:1 AV conduction at 150 bpm may paradoxically convert to a faster NCT at 200–250 bpm. This is because the atrial flutter rate may slow enough to allow the AV node to conduct in a 1:1 fashion [17].
- It is also important to note that the faster ventricular response may occasionally result in a wider QRS morphology because of enhanced sodium channel blockade at these rates. The resulting broad complex tachycardia created may be mistaken for ventricular tachycardia [18]. In a haemodynamically stable patient where this is suspected, intravenous adenosine is a safe way to establish the diagnosis; if flutter is confirmed, acute rate control with an intravenous calcium channel blocker or beta-blocker should be commenced immediately.
- In either circumstance, the resultant accelerated ventricular response may lead to haemodynamic instability and needs to be treated accordingly. Importantly, this effect can also occur in AF as these drugs can 'organize' AF into atrial flutter, as in this case. Therefore, experts advocate co-prescribing an AV nodal blocking agent with class I AADs in atrial arrhythmias to prevent accelerated ventricular responses.

despite combination therapy, his symptoms remained refractory. Although not keen on invasive procedures, the patient was keen for symptomatic relief and agreed to discuss the option of catheter ablation with an electrophysiologist.

✪ Learning point Catheter ablation for atrial fibrillation explained

Early catheter-based attempts to cure AF focussed on replicating the surgical Cox–Maze procedure. Linear lesions via radiofrequency catheter ablation were made to isolate parts of the atria, thus preventing the propagation of AF. This technique gave credence to the concept of susceptible atrial substrates [19]. It was during these procedures in 1998 when Haissaguerre et al. discovered that ectopic pulmonary vein foci played a significant role in the initiation of AF [2]. Subsequent ablation procedures were aimed at pulmonary vein isolation (PVI) to eliminate the triggering of AF. These procedures produced encouraging results, so much so that PVI has gone on to become the cornerstone of all current AF ablation techniques (Figure 16.3).

The procedure is generally done under general anaesthetic preceded by on-table transoesophageal echocardiography to exclude LAA thrombus. After transvenous femoral access, the left atrium is entered by means of trans-septal puncture. Mapping and ablation is performed in the region of the pulmonary vein antrum to isolate the veins electrically from the atrium. In more refractory cases, additional procedures may be required to check and ensure successful PVI and/or map and ablate additional susceptible atrial substrates [20].

PAF is predominantly a trigger-dependent phenomenon (particularly in recent onset cases), unlike persistent or permanent AF where electrical and structural remodelling has had time to alter the atrial substrate. Ablation techniques reflect these differences with PVI enough to 'cure' most patients with PAF whereas persistent or permanent AF requires PVI plus additional substrate modification (as mentioned above). This may entail additional linear lesions in the left atrium and/or targeting areas of abnormal electrical activity in either atrium (complex fractionated electrograms) to eliminate arrhythmogenic areas that maintain AF propagation [21].

Success rates in PAF patients are as high as 80 to 90% (1-year follow-up data) whereas in persistent/permanent AF, it is in the region of 50 to 70% (mean follow-up data of <15 months) with many patients requiring multiple procedures to achieve this. In terms of complication rates, a worldwide survey has shown a 6% risk of major complications with a 0.05% chance of peri-procedural death [22]. A more recent meta-analysis shows the following breakdown of morbidity and mortality rates:

- Cardiac tamponade (0.7%);
- Stroke or transient ischaemic attack (0.3%);
- Pulmonary vein stenosis (1.6%).

Rarer complications include phrenic nerve injury and atrio-oesophageal fistula formation [23]. Patient selection, therefore, is of paramount importance and it should be noted that ablation is generally contraindicated in those with severe heart failure, untreated coronary artery disease, valvular abnormalities, and left atrial thrombi.

Upon consultation with the electrophysiologist, he was informed that catheter ablation was an effective treatment for PAF in those whose symptoms remained refractory to drug therapy. He was quoted success rates in the order of 70% with a significant chance of requiring a second procedure. The major complication rate was quoted as <1% for stroke, death, and cardiac tamponade with a 1.6% risk of asymptomatic or symptomatic pulmonary vein stenosis [23]. On the basis of these figures, the patient chose to proceed.

Six weeks later, he had undergone a successful PVI procedure. He was able to discontinue his AADs after three months and at his 6-month review, he remained completely free of symptoms with a Holter monitor confirming sinus rhythm throughout. He was advised to remain on aspirin indefinitely and was given a further follow-up appointment at twelve months.

❝ Expert comment

Young patients often find beta-blocker therapy very debilitating, especially when trying to prevent an occasional AF recurrence. The alternative agents to protect the ventricles from a rapid rate in PAF are non-dihydropyridine calcium antagonists (verapamil or diltiazem), but digoxin should not be used in this setting since it may encourage recurrence of the arrhythmia.

❝ Expert comment

Although AF ablation is generally contraindicated in severe heart failure, in situations where the heart failure is thought to be caused by or aggravated by AF, ablation may be a very useful technique to improve left ventricular dysfunction and heart failure, even in patients with already well controlled ventricular rates.

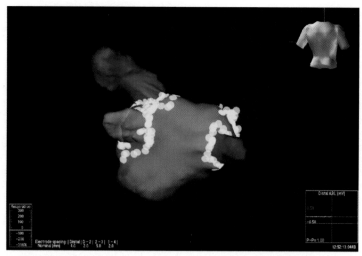

Figure 16.3 Three-dimensional electro-anatomical map of the left atrium viewed from the posterior aspect, showing ablated areas (in yellow) encircling the pulmonary veins (this figure was published in British Medical Bulletin, 88(1), Bajpai A, Savelieva I, Camm AJ, Treatment of atrial fibrillation, p. 89, Copyright Oxford University Press 2008).

⚙ **Learning point** Future directions in the management of atrial fibrillation

The need for better AADs has led to significant research into agents with novel modes of action. Dronedarone, a non-iodinated amiodarone derivative with multiple electrophysiological properties, marks an important step forward in AF management. It has lower extracardiac toxicity and has a significant impact on both maintaining sinus rhythm and controlling rate in AF when compared to placebo. In a head-to-head comparison study with amiodarone (DIONYSOS trial), dronedarone was less efficacious, but also less toxic than amiodarone in persistent AF patients [24]. The ATHENA trial put dronedarone on the map by showing a significant reduction in the risk of all-cause mortality or cardiovascular hospitalization when dronedarone was compared with placebo (54.5% vs 71.7%, respectively, hazard ratio 0.76, p value <0.001) in over 4,600 patients with AF (mean follow-up of 21 months) [25]. However, the ANDROMEDA trial demonstrated an increase in mortality when dronedarone was used in patients with recent severe heart failure, limiting its use [26]. Dronedarone appears to have advantages in those patients with stable or no significant structural heart disease and this has been reflected in the recently published European AF guidelines [27]. Longer-term safety and efficacy data are needed, but it already seems to have carved out its niche in the management of AF. In the UK, the drug has yet to be recommended in the NICE AF guidelines and so prescribing experience remains limited.

Several other agents are in the later stages of development. Vernakalant is relatively specific for atrial ion channels and delays atrial repolarization, thus prolonging the effective refractory period. It has minimal effects on ventricular tissue, a favourable side effect profile, and is currently in phase 3 trials. Other innovative modes of action under investigation are those that attempt to modulate the electrophysiological consequences of structural remodelling. This includes agents that target the regulation of intracellular homeostasis such as sodium-calcium exchanger blockade and late sodium channel blockade as well as gap junction modulators and stretch receptor antagonists [19,28].

Another interesting development has been the use of upstream therapy which aims to modify the substrate for AF pharmacologically. Inhibitors of the renin-angiotensin system (ACE inhibitors and angiotensin II receptor antagonists) as well as anti-inflammatory agents (statins and omega-3 fatty acids) may confer protection against the structural and electrical remodelling process that occurs in AF. Several studies have now shown that these agents may have a role in preventing recurrent AF and maintaining sinus rhythm post-cardioversion. Hence in the future, these drugs may be used 'upstream' in a preventative role in those deemed at high risk of developing AF [19,28].

In terms of anticoagulation, the search continues for an alternative to warfarin. Agents with similar or better efficacy without the need for monitoring and fewer bleeding complications are highly sought

continued

after. Dabigatran, a direct thrombin inhibitor, has emerged as a worthy contender in a recent trial, the Randomized Evaluation of Long-Term Anticoagulant Therapy (RE-LY) (see Landmark Trial) [29]. Advantages of the drug include its rapid onset of action, minimal drug-drug interactions, and the fact that monitoring is not required. It is already in use for primary prevention of venous thromboembolic events in adult orthopaedic surgery and has recently been approved by the US Food and Drug Administration for the prevention of stroke and systemic embolism in patients with AF. Other ongoing trials are assessing the suitability of factor Xa inhibitors in AF in both parenteral (fondaparinux, idraparinux) and oral (rivaroxaban, apixaban, edoxaban) forms.

Finally, advances to refine catheter ablation for AF continue unabated. Recurrence of AF after radiofrequency ablation often represents conduction recovery in the ablated myocardium [30]. This has led to the use of alternative, and hopefully more efficacious, energy sources such as cryoenergy, laser, and ultrasound. Alongside these energy forms are enhanced, balloon-based, radiofrequency energy delivery techniques that are designed to give greater coverage and thus reduce procedure times. Magnetic navigation systems are another exciting prospect, offering combined 3-dimensional steering and imaging capabilities in a single system. They allow remote-controlled mapping and ablation and have the potential to improve safety, reduce learning curves, and procedure times as well as limit radiation exposure. All of these technological advancements have yet to prove their effectiveness as compared to the 'traditional' RF ablation [31].

Landmark trial Randomized Evaluation of Long-term Anticoagulant Therapy (RE-LY) [29]

- A landmark study comparing the efficacy and safety of a novel oral anticoagulant called dabigatran etixilate with warfarin in the prevention of stroke in those with non-valvular AF.
- The trial was one of the largest AF outcomes trials ever conducted enrolling over 18,000 patients in 44 countries worldwide.
- Dabigatran given at 150 mg twice daily reduced the relative risk of stroke by 34% (p < 0.001) and reduced the relative risk of haemorrhagic stroke by 74% (p < 0.001) compared to warfarin.

Landmark trial The Atrial Fibrillation Follow-up Investigation of Rhythm Management (AFFIRM) [32]

- This was one of the largest randomized, multicentre studies comparing rhythm control vs rate control strategies for AF.
- The results found no statistical difference in the primary endpoint of total mortality between the two groups at five years (23.8% in the rhythm control group vs 21.3% in the rate control group, p=0.08).
- It is important to note that there was significant patient crossover from the rhythm control group to the rate control group. This was due to either failure to maintain sinus rhythm or drug intolerance.
- During the study, more patients were on warfarin in the rate control group as compared to the rhythm control group (85% vs 70%) with no difference between the two groups in the stroke rate.
- Hospitalizations occurred more frequently in the rhythm control group than in the rate control group (80.1% vs 73.0%, respectively, p<0.001). This was probably due to the need to control rhythm and perhaps reflects the poor efficacy/safety profile of current AADs.

Discussion

AF is the commonest arrhythmia worldwide and is a rising epidemic. Its sequelae can lead to significant morbidity and mortality as a result of stroke and heart failure. Physicians treating patients with this arrhythmia face a daunting array of management options. Choosing the correct one requires a careful and logical approach whilst taking into account individual circumstances and preferences. In PAF, the aim is to reduce the frequency and duration of paroxysms, and in the longer term to maintain sinus rhythm, initially by pharmacological means. This case highlights the limited efficacy and potential pro-arrhythmogenic nature of the AADs currently available, whilst re-emphasizing, that treatment of AF should be guided by symptoms.

Expert comment

In this case, only flecainide was tried as an AAD. Most physicians would try several agents and in most cases, both physicians and patients would try amiodarone. Amiodarone is the most effective drug for the prevention of AF recurrence, but it is associated with many potentially serious side effects.

> **A final word from the expert**
>
> The management of PAF is always challenging. Some cases are asymptomatic and for those, the major clinical question is whether anticoagulation is needed. There is no firm evidence base from which to make this decision, but most would agree that an asymptomatic paroxysm of six hours or more warrants a risk assessment for anticoagulation. For symptomatic cases, in addition to anticoagulation treatment according to current guidelines, it is usually recommended that patients should try at least one AAD before considering an interventional approach. In my practice, I usually try several anti-arrhythmic agents before electing for PVI because there is no solid basis on which to select any particular anti-arrhythmic agent and patients may respond to one drug whilst being completely refractory to others. However, I would not hesitate to refer active and fit people with refractory PAF for PVI, particularly if they had minimal or no heart disease. The value of left atrial ablation procedures for those with significant underlying heart disease is less certain and in these patients, rate control would be appropriate unless the patient remained highly symptomatic.

References

1 Zimetbaum P, Josephson ME. Evaluation of patients with palpitations. *N Engl J Med* 1998; 338: 1369–1373.

2 Haissaguerre M, Jais P, Shah DC, et al. Spontaneous initiation of atrial fibrillation by ectopic beats originating in the pulmonary veins. *N Engl J Med* 1998; 339: 659–666.

3 Gage BF, Waterman AD, Shannon W, et al. Validation of clinical classification schemes for predicting stroke: results from the National Registry of Atrial Fibrillation, *JAMA* 2001; 285: 2864–2870.

4 National Institute for Health and Clinical Excellence. Atrial Fibrillation. NICE Guidance CG36 [issued June 2006]. Available from: http://www.nice.org.uk/CG36.

5 Johnson WD, Ganjoo AK, Stone CD, et al. The left atrial appendage: our most lethal human attachment! Surgical implications. *Eur J Cardiothorac Surg* 2000; 17: 718–722.

6 Garcia-Fernandez MA, Perez-David E, Quiles J, et al. Role of left atrial appendage obliteration in stroke reduction in patients with mitral valve prosthesis: a transoesophageal echocardiographic study. *J Am Coll Cardiol* 2003; 42: 1253–1258.

7 Blackshear JL, Odell JA. Appendage obliteration to reduce stroke in cardiac surgical patients with atrial fibrillation. *Ann Thorac Surg* 1996; 61: 755–759.

8 Bonow RO, Carabello BA, Chatterjee K, et al. ACC/AHA 2006 guidelines for the management of patients with valvular heart disease: a report of the American College of Cardiology/American Heart Association Task Force on Practice Guidelines developed in collaboration with the Society of Cardiovascular Anesthesiologists endorsed by the Society for Cardiovascular Angiography and Interventions and the Society of Thoracic Surgeons. *J Am Coll Cardiol* 2006; 48: e1–148.

9 Holmes DR, Reddy VY, Turi Z, et al. Percutaneous closure of the left atrial appendage versus warfarin therapy for prevention of stroke in patients with atrial fibrillation: a randomized non-inferiority trial. *Lancet* 2009; 374: 534–542.

10 Martinez-Marcos FJ, Garcia-Garmendia JL, Ortega-Carpio A, et al. Comparison of intravenous flecainide, propafenone, and amiodarone for conversion of acute atrial fibrillation to sinus rhythm. *Am J Cardiol* 2000; 86: 950–953.

11 Galve E, Rius T, Ballester R, et al. Intravenous amiodarone in treatment of recent onset atrial fibrillation: results of a randomized, controlled study. *J Am Coll Cardiol* 1996; 27: 1079–1082.

12 Singh BN, Singh SN, Reda DJ, et al. Amiodarone versus sotalol for atrial fibrillation. *N Engl J Med* 2005; 352: 861–872.

13 Roy D, Talajic M, Dorian P, et al. Amiodarone to prevent recurrence of atrial fibrillation. *N Engl J Med* 2000; 342: 913–920.

14 Kochiadakis GE, Marketou ME, Igomenidis NE, et al. Amiodarone, sotalol or propafenone in atrial fibrillation: which is preferred to maintain normal sinus rhythm? *Pacing Clin Electrophysiol* 2000; 23: 1883–1887.

15 Gronefeld GC, Hohnloser SH. Beta-blocker therapy in atrial fibrillation. *Pacing Clin Electrophysiol* 2003; 26: 1607–1612.

16 Benditt DG, Williams JH, Jin J, et al. Maintenance of sinus rhythm with oral d,l-sotalol therapy in patients with symptomatic atrial fibrillation and/or atrial flutter. *Am J Cardiol* 1999; 84: 270–277.

17 Roden DM. Anti-arrhythmic drugs: from mechanisms to clinical practice. *Heart* 2000; 84: 339–346.

18 Crijns HJ, van Gelder IC, Lie KI. Supraventricular tachycardia mimicking ventricular tachycardia during flecainide treatment. *Am J Cardiol* 1988; 62: 1303–1306.

19 Lubitz SA, Fischer A, Fuster V. Catheter ablation of atrial fibrillation. *BMJ* 2008; 336: 819–826.

20 Bajpai A, Savelieva I, Camm AJ. Treatment of atrial fibrillation. *Br Med Bull* 2008; 88: 75–94.

21 O'Neill MD, Jais P, Hocini M, et al. Catheter ablation for atrial fibrillation. *Circulation* 2007; 116: 1515–1523.

22 Cappato R, Calkins H, Chen SA, et al. Worldwide survey on the methods, efficacy, and safety of catheter ablation for human atrial fibrillation. *Circulation* 2005; 111: 1100–1105.

23 Calkins H, Reynolds MR, Spector P, et al. Treatment of atrial fibrillation with anti-arrhythmic drugs or radiofrequency ablation: two systematic literature reviews and meta-analyses. *Circ Arrhythm Electrophysiol* 2009; 2: 349–336.

24 Le Heuzey J, De Ferrari GM, Radzik D, et al. A short-term, randomized, double-blind, parallel group study to evaluate the efficacy and safety of dronedarone versus amiodarone in patients with persistent atrial fibrillation: the DIONYYSOS study. *J Cardiovasc Electrophysiol* 2010; 21: 597–605.

25 Hohnloser SH, Crijns HJ, van Eickels M, et al. Effect of dronedarone on cardiovascular events in atrial fibrillation. *N Engl J Med* 2009; 360: 668–678.

26 Sanofi–Synthelabo Italy. Discontinuation of one of the studies (ANDROMEDA) with dronedarone [issued 17 Jan 2003]. Available from: http://www.sanofi-synthelabo.it/live/it/en/layout.jsp?cnt = F4BA0D93-F93C-408C-B594-0EF1A67DA40F.

27 The Task Force for the management of atrial fibrillation of the European Society of Cardiology. Guidelines for the management of atrial fibrillation. *Eur Heart J* 2010; 31: 2369–2429.

28 Savelieva I, Camm AJ. Anti-arrhythmic drug therapy for atrial fibrillation: current anti-arrhythmic drugs, investigational agents and innovative approaches. *Europace* 2008; 10: 647–665.

29 Connolly SJ, Ezekowitz MD, Yusuf S, et al; the RE-LY Steering Committee and Investigators. Dabigatran versus warfarin in patients with atrial fibrillation. *N Engl J Med* 2009; 361: 1139–1151.

30 Katritsis DG, Camm AJ. Catheter ablation of atrial fibrillation. Do we know what we are doing? *Europace* 2007; 9: 1002–1005.

31 Ernst S. The future of atrial fibrillation ablation: new technologies and indications: atrial fibrillation. *Heart* 2009; 95: 158–163.

32 AFFIRM First Anti-arrhythmic Drug Substudy Investigators. Maintenance of sinus rhythm in patients with atrial fibrillation: an AFFIRM substudy of the first anti-arrhythmic drug. *J Am Coll Cardiol* 2003; 42: 20–29.

17 Ventricular tachycardia in a 'normal' heart

Shouvik Haldar

ⓒ **Expert commentary** Dr Anthony Chow

Case history

A 25-year-old woman attended the Accident & Emergency (A&E) department, complaining of fast palpitations. She led a very active lifestyle and had no medical history of note. She was a non-smoker and drank 15 units of alcohol per week. She also drank a significant amount of caffeine. There was a family history of ischaemic heart disease.

She had first noticed her symptoms whilst at the gym two months earlier. Whilst training on the exercise bike, she had felt her heart suddenly start pounding quickly. She denied any associated chest pain, breathlessness, or syncope, but had felt dizzy. Having stopped exercising, the palpitations continued for ten minutes before suddenly stopping whilst drinking cold water. Similar episodes had occurred on three other occasions, all during exercise. She had also experienced numerous short bursts of palpitations, lasting for two to three minutes each time. Notably, they had occurred whilst under stressful situations at work.

By the time she was assessed, her symptoms had improved, but she was still aware of an irregular heartbeat. Examination of her cardiovascular system was unremarkable with an irregular pulse of approximately 75 beats per minute (bpm) with a blood pressure (BP) of 130/80 mmHg. Her heart sounds were normal with no murmurs on auscultation.

Her 12-lead electrocardiogram (ECG) (Figure 17.1) showed frequent ventricular ectopics and routine blood tests, including full blood count (FBC), urea and electrolytes (U&E), thyroid function, and inflammatory markers were all within normal limits. As she was a young, healthy adult, she was reassured that her symptoms were related to benign 'extra beats', possibly precipitated by stress. She was advised to reduce her caffeine intake and was discharged home.

Six weeks later, she re-presented to A&E, again with palpitations. The medical registrar who reviewed her documented the ECG as sinus rhythm interspersed with short bursts of non-sustained broad complex tachycardia, with left bundle branch block (LBBB) morphology (Figure 17.2). As the patient was young, he felt that this was most likely to represent short paroxysms of supraventricular tachycardia (SVT) with aberrant conduction. Again, her laboratory tests including FBC, U&E, and magnesium levels were normal. She was given 2.5 mg of intravenous (IV) metoprolol which settled her symptoms and was admitted overnight for observation.

Three hours later, the medical team was called to review the patient urgently. She was now in a sustained broad complex tachycardia (BCT) at 190 bpm (Figure 17.3),

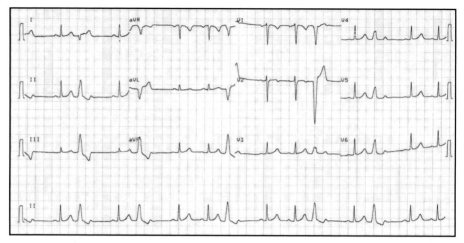

Figure 17.1 ECG on first admission.

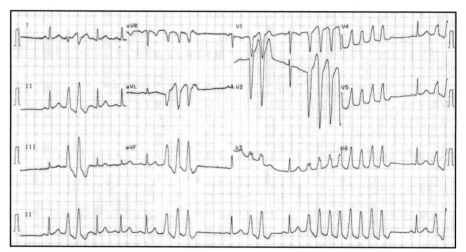

Figure 17.2 Second admission ECG showing non-sustained, repetitive bursts of monomorphic VT with LBBB morphology and an inferior axis.

with the same LBBB morphology as seen in the earlier ECG (Figure 17.2). She was symptomatic although haemodynamically stable with a BP of 115/75 mmHg. Despite being doubtful about the origin of the arrhythmia, the presumed diagnosis was one of ventricular tachycardia (VT) and the patient was started on an IV infusion of amiodarone via a central venous line.

> **⭐ Learning point** Bundle branch block patterns: features suggestive of ventricular tachycardia [1,2]
>
> BCT with bundle branch block patterns can either be SVT with aberrancy or VT. If the QRS complexes have a LBBB type pattern, features suggestive of ventricular tachycardia are (Figure 17.4):
> - QRS complexes with duration >160 ms;
> - Presence of an R wave in V1 or V2 of >30 ms in width;
> - Time from the start of the QRS wave to the nadir of the S is >70 ms in V1 or V2;
> - A slurred or notched S in V1 or V2;
>
> *continued*

- A qR complex in V6;
- Inferior axis (QRS complexes are positive in inferior leads) or right axis deviation.

If there is a right bundle branch block (RBBB) type pattern, features suggestive of VT are:
- QRS complex with duration >140 ms;
- Superior axis (negative in inferior leads);
- A QS wave or predominantly negative complex in lead V6;
- Concordance throughout the chest leads with all deflections positive;
- A single (R) or biphasic (QR or RS) R wave in lead V1;
- A triphasic R wave in lead V1, with the initial R wave taller than the secondary R wave and an S wave that passes through the isoelectric line.

⊕ **Clinical tip** Features that favour supraventricular tachycardia with aberrant conduction in broad complex tachycardia

- QRS morphology looks like 'typical' right or left bundle branch block morphology;
- QRS morphology in sinus rhythm shows bundle branch block or pre-excitation with a pattern similar to the QRS morphology during tachycardia.

⊕ **Clinical tip** Features that favour ventricular tachycardia in broad complex tachycardia

- Evidence of independent atrial activity (dissociated P waves);
- Different broad QRS morphologies during tachycardia and sinus rhythm;
- QRS concordance in leads V1 to V6 (i.e. all leads show deflections in the same direction);
- Patient has history of structural or ischaemic heart disease.

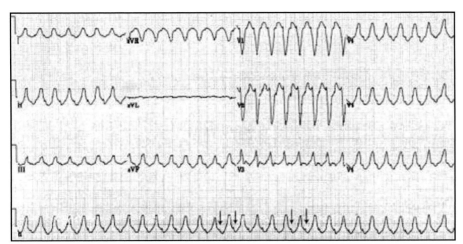

Figure 17.3 ECG showing sustained RVOT tachycardia with LBBB morphology and an inferior axis with arrows denoting dissociated P waves.

🔍 **Expert comment**

The 12-lead ECG during sustained tachycardia clearly confirms that this is a VT. The QRS morphology is exactly the same as the non-sustained VT appearance. There is clear dissociation of P waves with the QRS morphology, as can be seen on the lead II rhythm strip (black arrows on Figure 17.3); this is diagnostic of VT. The inferior axis with LBBB suggests that this is an outflow tract tachycardia, but more subtle changes can be used to distinguish a right from left ventricular outflow tract origin.

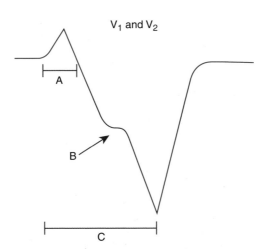

V₁ and V₂

Figure 17.4 Features suggestive of VT in QRS complexes with LBBB morphology (reproduced with permission from BMJ Publishing Group Ltd) [1].

A: > 30 ms favours VT
B: Notching, slurring favours VT
C: > 70 ms favours VT

Two hours after the amiodarone infusion had commenced, the patient remained symptomatic although the rate had slowed marginally to 180 bpm. Electrical cardioversion was, therefore, attempted under sedation and was successful with a single 100 J biphasic shock. The following day, a transthoracic echocardiogram (TTE) confirmed a structurally normal heart. Upon review by a consultant cardiologist, her arrhythmia was diagnosed as originating from the right ventricular outflow tract (RVOT). She was prescribed 2.5 mg of bisoprolol daily and discharged with arrangements for an urgent outpatient cardiac magnetic resonance imaging (MRI) and follow-up in clinic.

Learning point Key electrocardiogram features of ventricular tachycardia

In VT, atrial activity is predominantly independent of ventricular activity. P waves are, therefore, dissociated from QRS complexes; this is known as atrioventricular (AV) dissociation. This independent atrial activity may be difficult to discern due to the broad and bizarre morphology of the QRS complexes as well as its fast rate.

Evidence of independent atrial activity:

- Independent P waves which are dissociated from QRS complexes;
- More QRS complexes than P waves as atrial rates are generally slower;
- Capture beats (They represent occasional atrial impulses capturing the ventricles via the normal conduction system. These QRS complexes occur earlier and are narrow.);
- Fusion beats (They represent the simultaneous activation of the ventricles via the normal conduction system and from the ventricles themselves. The QRS complex, therefore, looks like a cross between a normal and a tachycardia complex and occurs slightly earlier than expected.).

It should be noted that some VTs conduct regularly to the atria, producing retrograde P waves seen after the QRS complex. Therefore, typical AV dissociation is not seen, but instead there is ventriculoatrial (VA) conduction which can signify VT.

Learning point What is right ventricular outflow tract tachycardia?

VT occurs predominantly in the setting of structural heart disease. However, up to 10% of patients with VT have no obvious structural abnormalities [4]. They generally have a normal baseline ECG, echocardiogram, and coronary angiogram, although subtle abnormalities may be found on MRI. These ventricular arrhythmias can be caused by RVOT VT, LVOT VT, and idiopathic left ventricular tachycardia (ILVT). These are monomorphic, not familial, and collectively termed idiopathic VT. Others types are due to inherited channelopathies such as Brugada syndrome, long QT syndrome, and catecholaminergic VT, giving rise to polymorphic VT.

RVOT VT constitutes 90% of the outflow tract tachycardias and the majority of patients have a good prognosis [5]. It is a distinctive wide QRS complex tachycardia with LBBB morphology and inferior axis, and is sensitive to adenosine. The ECG in sinus rhythm is predominantly normal although a small proportion will have RBBB. There is a female preponderance and patients present in the third to fifth decade of life [6]. Common symptoms include palpitations, dizziness, and pre-syncope. Frank syncope is unusual. Precipitants include exercise and emotional stress.

There are two distinct forms of RVOT VT: firstly a non-sustained, repetitive, monomorphic VT which is often suppressed by exercise; secondly a paroxysmal, exercise-induced sustained VT [7]. Patients may exhibit overlapping features of both forms. Symptomatic episodes may occur as rare or frequent isolated premature ventricular complexes (PVCs), bursts of non-sustained VT, or as discrete episodes of sustained tachycardia. If symptoms are frequent and left untreated, then a tachycardia-induced cardiomyopathy may result. The mechanism is thought to be due to the activation of cyclic AMP (cAMP), mediated by catecholamines, which leads to high intracellular calcium concentrations. This in turn causes delayed after-depolarizations in the action potential repolarization phase, triggering the onset of a tachycardia [4].

At her review appointment, the patient reported that her symptoms had improved, but were not completely resolved. She was able to manage gentle exercise, but more strenuous exertion brought on symptomatic palpitations. Her cardiac MRI was reported as normal, showing no evidence of an underlying cardiac muscle disease that could predispose to a rhythm disturbance. She was referred to a cardiac electrophysiologist in view of her ongoing symptoms.

After consultation with the electrophysiologist, the patient agreed to a catheter ablation procedure. Under conscious sedation, multipolar catheters were introduced percutaneously via the right femoral vein and positioned in the right side of the heart. The pace-mapping technique was used to localize the site of origin of the tachycardia. This area was then successfully ablated without complication using radiofrequency energy. The patient remained symptom-free one year post-procedure, off all medication and with an unrestricted exercise capacity.

> ⊕ **Learning point** Management of right ventricular outflow tract tachycardia
>
> Terminating RVOT VT in the acute setting can be achieved with vagal manoeuvres, IV adenosine (suppresses cAMP-mediated triggered activity), beta-blockers, verapamil, and lidocaine.
>
> Long-term management options include medical therapy or catheter ablation. Beta-blockers and calcium channel blockers are generally used as first-line drugs and are effective in 25–50% of patients. Alternative anti-arrhythmic drugs (AADs) include those in class IA and class IC whilst amiodarone and sotalol are also useful [8].
>
> Catheter ablation requires intra-cardiac mapping, using either activation or pace-mapping techniques to identify the exact origin of the tachycardia. Pace-mapping involves pacing at different sites in the RVOT tract until identifying the site that reproduced the exact QRS morphology to that of the clinical tachycardia. In contrast, activation mapping aims to identify the earliest site of ventricular activation during the clinical tachycardia. Once identified, radiofrequency energy is applied to disrupt the circuit. It is curative in 90% of cases and these high success rates can be attributed to the focal origin of the tachycardia [9]. Complications such as cardiac perforation and tamponade occur in less than 1%. In the current joint European and American guidelines, catheter ablation has a class 1C recommendation for those who are 'drug-refractory, drug-intolerant, or do not want long-term drug therapy' [10].
>
> Lastly, it is worth noting that VT of LBBB morphology is also seen in a more serious condition called ARVC (see Case 14). ARVC can cause sudden cardiac death (SCD) in young adults and is commonly associated with structural abnormalities in the right ventricle although these may be subtle and easily missed. It is important, therefore, to maintain a high index of suspicion when assessing patients with LBBB morphology VT (Table 17.1).

Discussion

VT in structurally normal hearts represents a small, but important, proportion of patients within the wide clinical spectrum of VT. Generally, these patients have a good prognosis with a benign clinical course and their risk of SCD is reassuringly very low. AADs have a modest efficacy and may be sufficient to suppress the arrhythmia in some patients. For those in whom AADs fail, catheter ablation is recommended and can provide freedom from both the troublesome arrhythmia and the side effects of long-term medical therapy. Advances in radiofrequency ablation have improved the success rates in outflow tract VT to approximately 90% with a minimal risk of complications. It is easy to understand why catheter ablation, with its favourable safety and efficacy profile, has revolutionized the management of this condition.

> ⊕ **Clinical tip** Acute management of a broad complex tachycardia
>
> Management of a BCT (even when VT is suspected, but the diagnosis is unconfirmed) is dependent on the patient's haemodynamic status. If signs of haemodynamic instability (chest pain, systolic blood pressure < 90 mmHg, heart failure, decreased level of consciousness) are present, then emergent electrical cardioversion is warranted.
>
> If the patient is stable, then intravenous amiodarone, lidocaine ± beta-blockers may be used. Don't forget to treat ischaemia if VT is in the context of an acute coronary syndrome. If pharmacological therapy fails to cardiovert VT in a haemodynamically stable patient, then electrical cardioversion should be used. It is also mandatory to ensure that electrolytes such as potassium and magnesium are adequately replaced, aiming for the upper range of normal.
>
> The use of IV adenosine as a diagnostic or therapeutic manoeuvre should be limited to those with a haemodynamically stable BCT where there is an unconfirmed diagnosis of VT vs SVT.
>
> If there is doubt about the origin of a BCT, it is best to treat as VT. For example, giving IV verapamil to a BCT mistakenly identified as SVT with aberrancy could be fatal.

> ⊕ **Expert comment**
>
> Catheter ablation is indicated in those with recurrent symptomatic RVOT arrhythmias, adverse effects from drug therapy, or tachycardia-induced cardiomyopathy, which can be reversible by ablation therapy [11]. Procedural risks are low at approximately 1–2% and are generally preferred by most patients as a definitive cure.

Table 17.1 Differentiating RVOT tachycardia from ARVC

	RVOT tachycardia	ARVC
Family history of arrhythmia or SCD	No	Often
Arrhythmias	PVCs, non-sustained VT or sustained VT at rest or with exercise	Similar
SCD	Rare	1% per year
Frontal plane QRS	Positive in leads III and AVF, negative in lead AVL	Inferior or superior
T wave morphology in sinus rhythm	T wave upright V2–V5	T wave inverted beyond V1
QRS duration in sinus rhythm	QRS duration <110 ms in V1, V2, or V3	QRS duration >110 ms
Epsilon wave V1–V3	Absent	Present 30%
Signal-averaged ECG	Normal	Usually abnormal
Echocardiogram	Normal	Increased right ventricular (RV) size and/or wall motion abnormalities
RV ventriculogram	Usually normal	Usually abnormal
MRI	Usually normal, but subtle abnormalities may be present	For example, increased signal intensity of RV free wall; wall motion abnormalities with CINE MRI, fibrofatty infiltration, focal wall thinning, and RV dilatation
Treatment	Acute: vagal manoeuvres, adenosine, beta-blockers, verapamil Chronic: beta-blockers or verapamil ± class I AAD	Sotalol Amiodarone ± beta-blockers
Radiofrequency ablation	Usually curative	Seldom curative; may modify substrate to permit AAD to be effective. However, arrhythmias of different morphology tend to occur.

Adapted and reproduced with permission from Professor H. Calkins.

A final word from the expert

The 'take home' messages from this case centre around the important principles of managing BCTs which have been covered concisely.

RVOT tachycardias are not uncommon and often occur in mid-life. Although they are not usually life-threatening arrhythmias, they can cause significant symptoms, occasional syncope, and even precipitate heart failure. Drugs are often ineffective, but should be tried first-line. Catheter mapping and ablation is very successful with very low complication rates and should be offered to all patients with ongoing symptoms.

References

1 Wellens HJ. Ventricular tachycardia: diagnosis of broad QRS complex tachycardia. *Heart* 2001; 86: 579–585.
2 Edhouse J, Morris F. ABC of clinical electrocardiography. Broad complex tachycardia–part II. *BMJ* 2002; 324: 776–779.
3 Krittayaphong R, Bhuripanyo K, Punlee K, et al. Effect of atenolol on symptomatic ventricular arrhythmia without structural heart disease: a randomized placebo-controlled study. *Am Heart J* 2002; 144: e10.

4 Farzaneh Far A, Lerman BB. Idiopathic ventricular outflow tract tachycardia. *Heart* 2005; 91: 136–138.

5 Lerman BB, Stein KM, Markowitz SM, et al. Ventricular tachycardia in patients with structurally normal hearts. In: Zipes DP and Jalife J, editors. Cardiac electrophysiology: from cell to bedside. 3rd ed. Philadelphia: WB Saunders; 2000. p. 662–673.

6 Badhwar N, Scheinman MM. Idiopathic ventricular tachycardia: diagnosis and management. *Curr Probl Cardiol* 2007; 32: 7–43.

7 Srivathsan K, Lester SJ, Appleton CP, et al. Ventricular tachycardia in the absence of structural heart disease. *Indian Pacing Electrophysiol J* 2005; 5: 106.

8 Buxton AE, Waxman HL, Marchlinski FE, et al. Right ventricular tachycardia: clinical and electrophysiologic characteristics. *Circulation* 1983; 68: 917–927.

9 Lerman BB, Stein KM, Markowitz SM, et al. Ventricular arrhythmias in normal hearts. *Cardiol Clin* 2000; 18: 265–291.

10 Zipes D, Camm AJ, Borggrefe M, et al. ACC/AHA/ESC 2006 Guidelines for management of patients with ventricular arrhythmias and the prevention of sudden cardiac death—Executive Summary: A report of the American College of Cardiology/American Heart Association Task Force and the European Society of Cardiology Committee for Practice Guidelines. *Circulation* 2006; 114: 1088–1132.

11 Yarlagadda RK, Iwai S, Stein KM, et al. Reversal of cardiomyopathy in patients with repetitive monomorphic ventricular ectopy originating from the right ventricular outflow tract. *Circulation* 2005; 112: 1092–1097.

Dual-chamber vs single-chamber pacing: the debate continues

Ali Hamaad and Shouvik Haldar

⑥ Expert commentary Dr Vias Markides

Case history

A 63-year-old man was admitted with a 6-week history of increasing breathlessness and dizziness. He had a history of treated hypertension, and was taking ramipril 5 mg once daily. On admission, his pulse rate was 34 beats per minute (bpm) with a blood pressure (BP) of 180/90 mmHg. Cannon waves were visible in the jugular venous pulse (JVP), and a 12-lead electrocardiogram (ECG) confirmed complete heart block (CHB) (Figure 18.1).

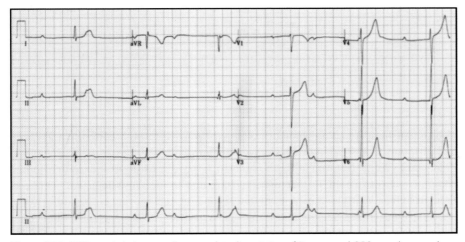

Figure 18.1 ECG on admission revealing complete dissociation of P waves and QRS complexes, and a ventricular rate of approximately 34 bpm (i.e. CHB).

> **⭐ Learning point** Investigating high-degree atrioventricular block (AVB)
>
> Causes:
> - Age-related: occurs in 5–10% of individuals over the age of 70 years with heart disease of any cause;
> - Myocardial ischaemia: particularly ischaemia involving the right coronary artery;
> - Infiltrative myocardial disease: sarcoidosis, haemochromatosis, malignancies with cardiac metastases;
> - Infective: endocarditis (particularly involving the aortic valve and root), disseminated tuberculosis with myocardial infiltration of granulomas, Lyme disease;
> - Iatrogenic: following aortic, mitral, or tricuspid valve surgery, rarely after ablation for SVT;
> - Drug-related: any drug that affects the atrioventricular (AV) conduction system e.g. cardiac glycosides, beta blockers, and calcium channel blockers.
>
> Mobitz type II AVB (i.e. constant PR interval, but intermittent non-conducting P-waves) is always pathological, and has a high risk of progressing to higher AVB, usually requiring permanent pacemaker (PPM) implantation. Mobitz type I AVB may be physiological in younger people. In Mobitz type I AVB,
> *continued*

⑥ Expert comment

Although this gentleman had treated hypertension, systolic hypertension (usually with a low diastolic BP) is a frequent presenting feature in patients with bradycardia. As it is important for the maintenance of a reasonable mean arterial pressure and often resolves with treatment of bradycardia with pacing, it should not generally be corrected acutely.

⑥ Expert comment

The need for pacing in AVB increases exponentially with age, even in patients with structurally normal hearts.

⑥ Expert comment

AV nodal re-entrant tachycardia (AVNRT or supraventricular tachycardia ['SVT']) affects some 1 in 500 of the population. As the incidence of CHB necessitating implantation of a PPM following ablation is less than 1% in experienced centres, this is now an exceedingly rare iatrogenic reason for implanting a pacemaker.

🕐 **Expert comment**

Common indications for pacing include CHB and most cases of Mobitz type II. High-grade AVB may also be intermittent and remain undiagnosed. A high index of suspicion of intermittent high-degree block must be maintained in patients with symptoms of syncope or pre-syncope and evidence of conduction tissue disease, especially left bundle branch block (LBBB), bifascicular or trifascicular block at baseline. Non-conducted P waves in isolation are not infrequently seen in fit, young individuals during sleep and are not an indication for pacing.

(i.e. progressive lengthening of PR interval until a P-wave fails to conduct and fails to produce a QRS complex) treatment with a pacemaker may be unnecessary unless symptoms occur. Third-degree AVB is associated with significant morbidity and mortality, and ultimately requires treatment with a pacemaker.

Investigations to identify the cause of AVB are often unnecessary in older people, as it is usually due to degeneration of the AV node. In younger people, transthoracic echocardiography (TTE) may help identify infiltrative causes such as granulomas in the interventricular septum. If the clinical history includes outdoor activity such as hiking or camping, then antibodies to *Borellia burgdorferi* may provide the diagnosis.

⭐ **Learning point** Indications for temporary transvenous pacing

In the absence of acute myocardial infarction (AMI):
- Second- and third-degree AVB with symptomatic bradycardia/haemodynamic compromise;
- Sinus node dysfunction (SND) with symptoms/haemodynamic compromise;
- Third-degree AVB with wide QRS escape.

In AMI:
- Mobitz type II or third-degree AVB with anterior infarction;
- New bifascicular block or alternating bundle branch block;
- Medically refractory AVB regardless of infarct size.

Prophylactic:
- New AVB or bundle branch block with acute endocarditis;
- Peri-operatively in a patient with bifasicular block and a history of syncope (although this indication remains controversial).

Treatment of tachyarrhythmias:
- Termination of recurrent ventricular tachycardia (overdrive pacing);
- Suppression of bradycardia-dependent ventricular tachyarrhythmias, including torsades des pointes.

The patient also had a degree of pulmonary congestion both clinically and radiologically, which was treated with intravenous furosemide. While in the Accident and Emergency (A&E) department, he was noted to have runs of an intermittent broad complex tachycardia (BCT) that were causing him to lose consciousness. This was thought to be a ventricular escape rhythm secondary to his severe bradycardia. Given his clinical instability, a temporary transvenous pacing wire was inserted via his right femoral vein.

The patient was stabilized on the ward. He remained dependent on the temporary pacing wire and did not regain an intrinsic sinus rhythm. The decision was made to implant a permanent dual-chamber pacemaker. Access for lead insertion was via the left cephalic vein under strict aseptic technique.

⭐ **Learning point** Basic pacing terminology

Threshold This is measured in volts (V) or milliseconds (ms), and is the smallest output voltage or the shortest pulse duration that captures the heart. A sudden rise in threshold suggests lead displacement.

Impedance This is the resistance of the electrical circuit that is formed when pacing is applied to the myocardium, and comprises the electrical resistance of the lead and tissue that is conducting the current (usually the myocardium). A rise in impedance suggests an interruption of the electrical pacing circuit due to lead displacement or lead fracture. A drop in impedance suggests damage to the electrical insulation of the pacing lead.

R wave This refers to the sensitivity of the pacing lead in detecting intrinsic myocardial depolarizations. A large R wave means the lead can detect small signals.

It became apparent during implantation that the patient had residual pulmonary oedema, as he was unable to lie flat for a prolonged period without a significant drop in oxygen saturations and tachypnoea. The procedure was abandoned following implantation of the ventricular lead in the right ventricular (RV) apex. A right atrial lead was, therefore, not inserted, and the patient was left with a single-chamber pacemaker programmed to deliver pacing in a VVIR fashion. A post-procedural pacing check was satisfactory (Table 18.1). The pulmonary oedema was treated with more intravenous furosemide, and a subsequent TTE demonstrated mild impairment of ventricular function with an ejection fraction of 45%.

> **⊕ Clinical tip** Cephalic vein access for permanent pacing
>
> Always search for a cephalic vein beneath the delto-pectoral groove when implanting a PPM system. This minimizes the chances of causing iatrogenic pneumothorax which is a risk when using a direct subclavian approach, as well as reducing the incidence of lead fracture under the clavicle.

Table 18.1 Post-procedural pacing parameters

R wave	18 mV
Impedance	760 Ω
Threshold	0.3 V at 0.50 ms

> **✪ Learning point** Pacing nomenclature (Table 18.2)
>
> The Heart Rhythm Society (HRS) and Heart Rhythm UK (HRUK) generic pacemaker codes for anti-bradyarrhythmia and adaptive-rate pacing and anti-tachyarrhythmia devices are listed below [1].
>
> For example:
> - **VVIR:** pacing and sensing in the ventricle, inhibited by spontaneous activation of the ventricle and the ability to increase the paced rate which is dependent on activity;
> - **AOO:** pacing in the atrium with no inhibition of pacing by spontaneous electrical activity in the atrium;
> - **DDDR:** pacing and sensing either atrium or ventricle or both with the ability to increase paced rate which is dependent on activity.

Table 18.2 Pacing nomenclature

Letter position	Pacing category	Letter code
1st	Chamber(s) paced	V–Ventricle A–Atrium D–Dual
2nd	Chamber(s) sensed	V–Ventricle A–Atrium D–Dual
3rd	Mode of response to spontaneous electrical activation	T–Triggered I–Inhibited D–Dual O–None
4th	Rate modulation	R-rate modulation (pacing rate can be altered dependent on activity)

On day 1 post-implantation, there was an improvement in the patient's pulmonary oedema and he was converted to oral furosemide. By day 3, however, the patient had deteriorated clinically with further tachypnoea, tachycardia, and a recurrence of fluid overload. This was accompanied by episodes of hypotension and cannon waves visible in his JVP. The pacemaker was checked and found to have satisfactory pacing parameters, that were not significantly different to those measured immediately post-implantation. However, during the pacing threshold check, it was obvious the patient did not tolerate being paced as he was visibly uncomfortable. In particular, he complained of forceful palpitations and neck pulsations. A rhythm strip recording of the patient during one of these episodes revealed retrograde P waves following pacing depolarization, indicating ventriculo-atrial (VA) conduction (Figure 18.2). Unusually, even though the patient had presented with CHB, he still had intact retrograde VA conduction. With VVI pacing, this had resulted in a phenomenon known as the pacemaker syndrome. The heart failure was treated with further doses of intravenous diuretics, and once stable, the patient had a right atrial lead implanted to encourage AV synchrony. This resulted in the resolution of his symptoms and an eventual hospital discharge.

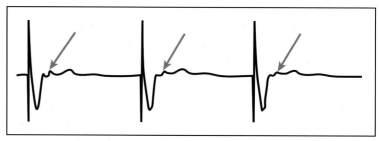

Figure 18.2 Rhythm strip taken during symptomatic episodes whilst pacing. This illustrates repetitive VA conduction as evidenced by retrograde P wave activity following pacing depolarization (arrowed).

Learning point Pacemaker syndrome (Table 18.3)

The pacemaker syndrome refers to symptoms and signs present in the pacemaker patient that are caused by inadequate timing of atrial and ventricular contractions [1]. These symptoms and signs are often relieved by restoration of AV synchrony. Although VVI pacing is the commonest culprit, other pacing modes that cause AV dyssynchrony can be implicated [1].

Clinical signs relating to the pacemaker syndrome should be carefully sought, in particular episodes of hypotension during pacing (a reduction ≥ 20 mmHg is thought to be significant), cannon waves in the JVP, and sometimes signs of cardiac failure. ECG features such as native atrial depolarization moving progressively closer to the paced ventricular depolarization, and retrograde P waves due to an intact VA conduction may also support the diagnosis [2]. Methods of overcoming the pacemaker syndrome include upgrading to a dual-chamber (DDD) system, reducing the lower pacing rate to encourage sinus rhythm, and use of hysteresis to encourage intrinsic depolarizations. Hysteresis refers to a pacing parameter which usually allows a longer escape interval after a sensed event, allowing a greater opportunity for more spontaneous depolarizations.

Although the incidence of the pacemaker syndrome is much lower in patients with a dual-chamber system, this can still occur as a result of:

- Left atrial activation delay;
- Sinus tachycardia with a long AV delay that does not shorten at higher atrial rates;
- Repetitive VA conduction;
- Pacemaker malfunction (loss of capture in the right atrial lead).

Patients with a dual-chamber system who exhibit the pacemaker syndrome may be managed by ensuring atrial capture, avoiding pacing modes that do not pace the atria (VDD), or prolonging the AV delay [1,2].

Table 18.3 Features of pacemaker syndrome

Clinical	Electrocardiographic
Dizziness, syncope, confusion	Atrial depolarization occurring in close proximity
Heart failure	to paced ventricular depolarization
Hypotension, tachycardia, desaturation	Retrograde atrial depolarization occurring as a
Fluctuating BP	consequence of intact VA conduction
Pulmonary oedema	
Cannon waves in jugular venous pulse	

Discussion

The loss of AV synchrony in those with AVB can result in atrial contraction when the mitral and tricuspid valves are closed. This in turn can lead to raised atrial pressures, impaired systolic ventricular function, and occasionally, the pacemaker syndrome, as demonstrated in this case. Re-establishing AV synchrony in these patients requires dual-chamber pacing, i.e. a more physiological mode of pacing.

The haemodynamic benefits of AV sequential pacing vs ventricular pacing have been well documented in numerous physiological studies. However, landmark clinical trials designed to test whether these benefits would translate into mortality and morbidity reductions have been disappointing. In fact, the results suggest that dual-chamber pacing offers no real clinical benefit over single chamber pacing in terms of mortality, burden of atrial fibrillation (AF), or quality of life (QoL) [3,4]. The CTOPP and MOST study, which examined pacing primarily in those with SND, found only a slight reduction in AF risk in the dual-chamber group, whereas the MOST study also found only a marginal reduction in heart failure. It should be noted, however, that two-thirds of patients recruited into CTOPP and all the MOST patients had SND which behaves in a different way when paced, compared to pacing in AVB [5,6].

After CTOPP and MOST, the logical progression was to answer the question of optimal pacing mode in elderly AVB patients. UKPACE attempted to do this, and again, results were disappointing. The trial demonstrated no difference in mortality between the single chamber and dual-chamber pacing arms, and notably did not show a reduction in AF occurrence in the dual-chamber group [7].

The QoL was not a primary outcome measure in UKPACE, but this was addressed in the PASE study which examined the effect of pacing mode on health-related QoL [8]. No significant differences were noted between treatment arms for the primary outcome measure in PASE, although there was some evidence of improvement in the cardiovascular functional status in those with dual-chamber pacing. It is, however, important to note that 26% of patients in PASE crossed over from ventricular to dual-chamber pacing, with the pacemaker syndrome cited as the main reason for a system upgrade. A similar phenomenon was also noted in the MOST study where nearly 20% of patients who were unable to tolerate single chamber pacing crossed over to dual-chamber pacing. Interestingly, after crossover, these patients reported a significant improvement in QoL measures [6].

Although there is no hard evidence to favour dual-chamber pacing over ventricular pacing patients with AVB, both national [9] and international [10] guidelines recommend implanting dual-chamber systems. In essence, modern practice aims to provide physiological pacing whenever possible (except in AF). From a cardiologist's viewpoint, dual-chamber systems may take slightly longer to implant, but the expectant benefits are a reduction in the pacemaker syndrome, a reduction in AF risk, and a potential improvement in QoL, which should outweigh most technical and time-related considerations.

Landmark trial Canadian Trial of Physiologic Pacing (CTOPP) [5]

- 2,568 patients enrolled, making it one of the largest pacing trials to date;
- Patients recruited with SND or AVB;
- Comparison made between DDDR/AAIR vs VVIR pacing;
- Primary endpoints were stroke and cardiovascular mortality;
- No difference in stroke or death between pacing modalities;
- AF less frequent in atrial-paced group.

Landmark trial Mode Selection Trial (MOST) [6]

- 2,010 patients enrolled;
- Patients with SND only;
- Comparison between DDDR and VVIR pacing modalities;
- No difference between death or stroke between pacing modalities;
- AF and heart failure lower in DDDR-paced patients.

Landmark trial United Kingdom Pacing and Cardiovascular Events Trial (UKPACE) [7]

- 2,000 patients recruited;
- Patients aged ≥70 with AVB only;
- Comparison between DDDR vs VVIR/VVI pacing modalities;
- Primary endpoint was mortality;
- No difference between groups.

Landmark trial Pacemaker Selection in the Elderly Trial (PASE) [8]

- 407 patients recruited;
- Patients with SND and/or AVB;
- Comparison between DDDR vs VVIR pacing modalities;
- Primary endpoint was QoL;
- No difference between groups;
- Better QoL outcome measures in patients with SND with DDDR pacing.

Learning point National Institute for Health and Clinical Excellence guidelines on permanent pacing [9]

Dual-chamber pacing is recommended for the management of symptomatic bradycardia due to sick sinus syndrome and/or AVB except:
- In the management of sick sinus syndrome where there is no evidence of AVB, in which case single chamber atrial pacing (AAI mode) may be appropriate;
- In the management of AVB in patients with AF, in which case single chamber ventricular pacing may be appropriate;
- In the management of AVB where factors such as age, frailty, and immobility favour the use of single chamber ventricular pacing.

Note It should be borne in mind that this guidance does not cover the more complex pacing indications. See Table 18.4 for comprehensive guidelines from Heart Rhythm Society.

Table 18.4 Recommendations for permanent pacing in acquired AVB in adults

Class I (evidence clearly in favour of pacing)

1. Third-degree and advanced second-degree AVB at any anatomic level with symptoms or ventricular arrhythmias secondary to the block.
2. Third-degree and advanced second-degree AVB associated with arrhythmias or other medical conditions requiring drug therapy that results in symptomatic bradycardia.

continued

3. Third-degree and advanced second-degree AVB at any anatomic level in awake, symptom-free patients in sinus rhythm, with documented periods of asystole greater than or equal to 3.0 seconds, or any escape rate less than 40 bpm, or with an escape rhythm that is below the AV node.
4. Third-degree and advanced second-degree AVB at any anatomic level in awake, symptom-free patients with AF and bradycardia with one or more pauses of at least 5 seconds or longer.
5. Third-degree and advanced second-degree AVB at any anatomic level after catheter ablation of the AV junction.
6. Third-degree and advanced second-degree AVB at any anatomic level associated with post-operative AVB that is not expected to resolve after cardiac surgery.
7. Third-degree and advanced second-degree AVB at any anatomic level associated with neuromuscular diseases with AVB, such as myotonic muscular dystrophy, Kearns–Sayre syndrome, Erb dystrophy (limb-girdle muscular dystrophy), and peroneal muscular atrophy with or without symptoms.
8. Second-degree AVB with associated symptomatic bradycardia regardless of type or site of block.
9. Asymptomatic persistent third-degree AVB at any anatomic site with average awake ventricular rates of 40 bpm or faster if cardiomegaly or LV dysfunction is present or if the site of block is below the AV node.
10. Second- or third-degree AVB during exercise in the absence of myocardial ischaemia.

Class IIa (reasonable to perform procedure with weight of evidence in favour of pacing)

1. Persistent third-degree AVB with an escape rate greater than 40 bpm in asymptomatic adult patients without cardiomegaly.
2. Asymptomatic second-degree AVB at intra- or infra-His levels found at electrophysiological study.
3. First- or second-degree AVB with symptoms similar to those of pacemaker syndrome or haemodynamic compromise.
4. Asymptomatic type II second-degree AVB with a narrow QRS. When type II second-degree AVB occurs with a wide QRS, including isolated right bundle branch block, pacing becomes a class I recommendation.

Class IIb (usefulness/efficacy is well established by evidence/opinion)

1. Neuromuscular diseases such as myotonic muscular dystrophy, Erb dystrophy (limb-girdle muscular dystrophy), and peroneal muscular atrophy with any degree of AVB with or without symptoms because there may be unpredictable progression of AV conduction disease.
2. AVB in the setting of drug use and/or drug toxicity when the block is expected to recur even after the drug is withdrawn.

Class III (evidence not in favour of pacing)

1. Permanent pacemaker implantation is not indicated for asymptomatic first-degree AVB.
2. Permanent pacemaker implantation is not indicated for asymptomatic type I second-degree AVB at the supra-His (AV node) level or that which is not known to be intra- or infra-Hisian.
3. Permanent pacemaker implantation is not indicated for AVB that is expected to resolve and is unlikely to recur (e.g. drug toxicity, Lyme disease, or transient increases in vagal tone or during hypoxia in sleep apnoea syndrome in the absence of symptoms).

Adapted with permission, copyright 2008, from the American College of Cardiology/American Heart Association/ North American Society for Pacing and Electrophysiology [now known as the Heart Rhythm Society] 2002 Guideline Update for Implantation of Cardiac Pacemakers and Antiarrhythmia Devices.

A final word from the expert

This case demonstrates the importance of providing physiological (AV synchronous) pacing in virtually all patients who have, or are likely to have, and maintain, regular atrial contraction (i.e. excluding patients with persistent/permanent AF). It also highlights the importance of getting this decision right when first implanting a device rather than having to revise the procedure. Re-intervention inevitably results in increased morbidity for the patient, prolonging the hospital stay and greatly increasing the risk of infection.

References

1 Travill CM, Sutton R. Pacemaker syndrome: an iatrogenic condition. *Br Heart J* 1992; 68: 163–166.

2 McComb JM, Gribbin GM. Effect of pacing mode on morbidity and mortality: update of clinical pacing trials. *Am J Cardiol* 1999; 83: 211D–213D.

3 Lamas GA, Ellenbogen KA. Evidence base for pacemaker mode selection: from physiology to randomized trials. *Circulation* 2004; 109: 443–451.

4 Montanez A, Hennekens CH, Zebede J, et al. Pacemaker mode selection: the evidence from randomized trials. *Pacing Clin Electrophysiol* 2003; 26: 1270–1282.

5 Connolly SJ, Kerr CR, Gent M, et al. Effects of physiologic pacing versus ventricular pacing on the risk of stroke and death due to cardiovascular causes. *N Engl J Med* 2000; 342: 1385–1391.

6 Lamas GA, Lee KL, Sweeney MO, et al. Ventricular pacing or dual-chamber pacing for sinus node dysfunction. *N Engl J Med* 2002; 346: 1854–1862.

7 Toff WD, Camm AJ, Skehan JD. United Kingdom Pacing: Cardiovascular Events Trial Investigators. *Single chamber versus dual-chamber pacing for high-grade atrioventricular block. N Engl J Med* 2005; 353: 145–155.

8 Lamas GA, Orav EJ, Stambler BS, et al. Quality of life and clinical outcomes in elderly patients treated with ventricular pacing as compared with dual-chamber pacing. *N Engl J Med* 1998; 338: 1097–1104.

9 National Institute for Health and Clinical Excellence. Dual-chamber pacemakers for symptomatic bradycardia due to sick sinus syndrome and/or atrioventricular block. Final Appraisal Determination [issued October 2004]. Available from: http://www.nice.org.uk.

10 Epstein AE, DiMarco JP, Ellenbogen KA, et al. A report of the American College of Cardiology/American Heart Association Task Force on Practice Guidelines (Writing Committee to Revise the ACC/AHA/NASPE 2002 Guideline Update for Implantation of Cardiac Pacemakers and Antiarrhythmia Devices): developed in collaboration with the American Association for Thoracic Surgery and Society of Thoracic Surgeons. *Circulation* 2008; 117: e350–408.

19 Reflex syncope: to pace or not to pace?

Pipin Kojodjojo

Expert commentary Professor Richard Sutton

Case history I

A 54-year-old man was referred to cardiology by a neurologist following an episode of syncope. Whilst on holiday in Thailand, he had lost consciousness without any warning. His wife, who had witnessed the event, reported that he had suddenly appeared pale, lost consciousness and then became rigid with his eyes rolling up. He then made a few jerks, let out a scream, and his lips looked blue. He did not develop any sustained clonic jerking, and there was no urinary incontinence or lateral tongue-biting. He recovered consciousness two minutes later, but was disorientated for an hour afterwards. As a result of the collapse, he sustained a wedge compression fracture of his fifth thoracic vertebra, necessitating vertebroplasty.

Expert comment

The key to determining the aetiology of syncope is a careful medical history with a collateral history from eye witnesses, and physical examinations or investigations to exclude structural heart disease. Structural heart disease predicts a cardiac cause of syncope with a sensitivity of 95% and specificity of 45% [1].

> **Learning point** Definition and classification of syncope
>
> Syncope is defined as a transient loss of consciousness due to **transient** global cerebral hypoperfusion, characterized by a **rapid onset**, **short duration**, and **spontaneous complete recovery** [2]. Based on this definition, the principal causes of syncope can be divided into three groups according to the pathophysiology, all with a common presentation, but associated with different risk profiles (Table 19.1).

Table 19.1 Classification of syncope [2]

Reflex (neurally mediated) syncope	Syncope due to orthostatic hypotension	Cardiovascular syncope
Vasovagal:	**Primary autonomic failure:**	**Primary arrhythmia:**
• Mediated by emotional distress, fear, pain, instrumentation	• Pure autonomic failure	• Bradycardia
	• Multiple system atrophy	• Tachycardia (supraventricular and ventricular)
	• Parkinson's disease with autonomic failure	• Drug-induced
• Mediated by orthostatic stress	• Lewy body dementia	**Structural disease:**
Situational:	**Secondary autonomic failure:**	• Severe aortic stenosis
• Cough, sneeze	• Diabetes	• Cardiomyopathy, e.g. hypertrophic cardiomyopathy
• Gastrointestinal stimulation	• Amyloidosis	• Cardiac masses, e.g. myxoma
	• Uraemia	• Ischaemic heart disease
• Micturition	• Spinal cord injuries	• Pericardial disease/tamponade
• Post-exercise	**Drug-induced orthostatic hypotension:**	**Others:**
• Post-prandial		• Pulmonary embolus
• Carotid sinus syncope	• Alcohol, vasodilators, diuretics, phenothiazines, antidepressants	• Pulmonary hypertension
• Atypical forms	• Volume depletion, e.g. haemorrhage	• Acute aortic dissection

His background history included frequent fainting episodes as a child, particularly with immunizations or prolonged standing. Eight years prior to this episode, his wife had witnessed another syncopal event with similar characteristics to this episode. At that time, he had regained consciousness within a few minutes and had not suffered any persistent neurological deficit. In addition, he had experienced many pre-syncopal episodes in which he would become pale and sweaty, but was able to abort the event by sitting or lying down quickly.

There was no family history of syncope or sudden cardiac death. He was not taking regular medications and did not smoke, but reported an alcohol intake of 40 units per week. Physical examination was unremarkable, with no postural drop in blood pressure (BP) on prolonged standing. Subsequent investigations including cerebral magnetic resonance imaging (MRI), electroencephalogram (EEG), 12-lead electrocardiogram (ECG), and transthoracic echocardiography (TTE) were normal. As the history had some suggestive features of reflex syncope, a tilt table test was performed.

Five minutes after head-up tilt, there was a sharp fall in BP (from 130/80 to 55/30 mmHg), followed by bradycardia of lower than 40 beats per minute (bpm) (see red arrows in Figure 19.1). This haemodynamic collapse resulted in the patient nearly losing consciousness, reproducing his symptoms of pre-syncope. Carotid sinus massage (CSM) performed on both sides, in the supine and erect positions was negative.

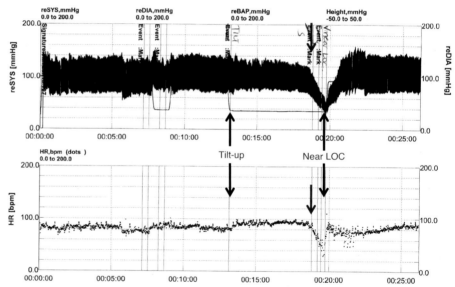

Figure 19.1 Simultaneous BP, using the photo-plethysmographic method (upper tracing), and heart rate (lower tracing) recordings during tilt testing. Tilt-up is illustrated by the first pair of black arrows. After six minutes of tilt, BP and heart rate begin to fall simultaneously (red arrows). At the nadir of BP and heart rate, there is near loss of consciousness (LOC) (second pair of black arrows).

⊕ **Learning point** Conditions that may mimic syncope [1]

There are several conditions that may resemble and hence, be mistakenly diagnosed as syncope:

Disorders with partial or complete loss of consciousness without global cerebral hypoperfusion
- Epilepsy (Table 19.2);
- Metabolic disorders, including hypoglycaemia and hyperventilation with hypocapnia;
- Intoxication;
- Vertebrobasilar transient ischaemic attack (TIA).

continued

Disorders without impairment of consciousness
- Cataplexy;
- Drop attacks;
- Falls;
- Functional (psychogenic pseudosyncope);
- Carotid TIA.

⭐ **Learning point** Summary guide to tilt table testing

Indications
- Patients with recurrent syncope without structural heart disease;
- Patients with a single episode of syncope and at high risk of serious consequences on further recurrence (e.g. airline pilot);
- To distinguish reflex syncope from orthostatic hypotension and epilepsy when abnormal movements have been observed in an attack;
- Patients with recurrent unexplained falls;
- Patients with very frequent syncope when attacks may be psychogenic;
- To demonstrate and hence reassure a patient regarding the nature of syncope.

Methodology
- Patient lies supine for 5 minutes, then tilted head up at 60–70 degrees for 20 minutes. If no haemodynamic change is noted, then sublingual glyceryl trinitrate (GTN) can be administered with an additional 15 minutes of tilt. Alternatively, an isoprotenerol infusion (commencing at 1 mcg/minute on tilt-up and progressive increase to 3 mcg/minute sufficient to raise the heart rate by 20–25% over baseline) can be used.
- If syncope is reproduced, the protocol is terminated and the test is considered positive. Conclusion of protocol without syncope is considered a negative test.
- Reflex syncope may be diagnosed in the presence of hypotension with or without bradycardia after 3 minutes of tilt whilst simultaneously reproducing the patient's usual symptoms.
- CSM is also performed in all subjects >40 years of age, serially on both sides in the supine and erect positions. It is considered positive if massage causes >3 s of asystole or a fall in BP greater than 50 mmHg with reproduction of symptoms.

Limitations
- Repeated tilt testing is not recommended for the assessment of treatment efficacy;
- Variable reproducibility (typically <67%);
- In patients with structural heart disease, cardiovascular causes of syncope must be excluded before a diagnosis of reflex syncope is made (Table 19.3).

Table 19.2 Distinguishing syncope from epilepsy

Features suggestive of syncope	Features suggestive of epilepsy
• Preceding symptoms of nausea, vomiting, abdominal discomfort, feeling cold, blurring of vision, light-headedness	• Preceding aura
• Typically associated with a trigger such as venepuncture	• Generalized or hemilateral tonic-clonic movements of whole limbs (typically coarse, rhythmic, and synchronous)
• If present, tonic-clonic movements of distal parts of limbs are always of short duration, lasting less than 15 seconds, typically starting after the loss of consciousness	• Lateral tongue biting
	• Blue face
• Complete flaccidity during unconsciousness is more likely	• Prolonged confusion, muscle aches, somnolence, and headaches after the event
• Recovery is swift after the event, but can be associated with nausea, vomiting, and pallor	• Elevation of creatinine kinase and prolactin more frequent

This mixed pattern of hypotension and bradycardia with the reproduction of symptoms confirmed the diagnosis of reflex syncope. The patient was advised to increase fluid intake to three litres per day, increase salt intake, and was educated in the use of isometric manoeuvres to abort impending syncope. He was also advised to avoid prolonged standing, and to be aware of symptoms which may herald syncope in order to allow abortive action to be taken as necessary.

Despite confirming the diagnosis of reflex syncope, the possibility that spontaneous syncopal episodes could involve more profound bradycardia remained. It was felt necessary to investigate this further as if this were proven, symptoms could be abolished by permanent pacing. In order to document the severity of bradycardia and in view of the infrequency of syncopal episodes, an implantable loop recorder (ILR) was implanted electively.

In the following 12 months, the patient experienced three further episodes of syncope or near syncope. Interrogation of the ILR revealed three episodes of regular tachycardia at a rate of approximately 180 bpm. The QRS morphology of the tachycardia was identical to his sinus rhythm morphology, in keeping with a narrow complex tachycardia. The patient underwent electrophysiological studies during which a focal atrial tachycardia was induced, but could not be sustained sufficiently to allow ablation. Therefore, oral flecainide was commenced and the patient has remained asymptomatic since.

Discussion

It appears that these short-lived episodes of atrial tachycardia were triggering episodes of reflex syncope. This phenomenon has been described in a study looking at patients with atrial fibrillation (AF) and syncope [3]. The induction of AF in the upright position elicited syncope in 42% of subjects and in some patients, syncope occurred at a heart rate of < 130 bpm. These observations suggest that these subjects are predisposed to an abnormal neural response which can be triggered by the onset of atrial tachyarrhythmias, and the resultant syncope is not solely due to rapid ventricular rates.

Table 19.3 Distinguishing reflex syncope from cardiovascular and orthostatic causes of syncope

Features suggestive of reflex syncope
- Long history of symptoms with first faint usually between 10 to 30 years of age
- Triggered by noxious stimuli, pain, prolonged standing
- Prodrome with symptoms such as nausea, sweating, vomiting, weakness, light-headedness
- During or after a meal
- After exertion
- Brief loss of consciousness lasting minutes
- Recovery accompanied by almost immediate restoration of appropriate behaviour and orientation

Features suggestive of syncope secondary to cardiovascular disease
- History of structural heart or coronary artery disease
- Family history of sudden cardiac death
- During exertion or supine
- Palpitations or chest pain at the time of syncope
- ECG abnormalities (e.g. pre-excitation, QT abnormalities, right chest leads changes suggestive of Brugada syndrome or ARVC)
- Documented broad complex tachycardia or advanced degrees of bradycardia

Features suggestive of syncope due to orthostatic hypotension
- Presence of autonomic neuropathy or Parkinson's disease
- Close correlation with use or change in dosages of vasodilators
- Occurs within three minutes of standing up

Case history II

A 71-year-old lady presented with a 20-year history of recurrent syncope, leading to hospitalization on at least four occasions. She described her episodes as of sudden onset, without warning, and associated with pallor, nausea, and loss of consciousness for several minutes. On one occasion, she was unconscious for several hours. These episodes were not associated with urinary incontinence or convulsions. She had a history of hypertension and had undergone hysterectomy and oophorectomy for endometriosis at the age of 41. Her regular medication included aspirin, simvastatin, thiazide, bisoprolol, citalopram, and hormone replacement therapy. She had undergone tilt testing five years ago, which had resulted in transient severe bradycardia (cardio-inhibitory pattern), and the reproduction of her symptoms. She was conservatively managed at that time. Despite lifestyle modifications such as reducing caffeine, increasing fluid intake, and an awareness of abortive isometric manoeuvres, she continued to be symptomatic. As a severely cardio-inhibitory tilt test result has a > 80% predictive value for asystole during spontaneous attacks, it was likely that she would benefit from permanent pacing. A dual-chamber pacemaker with rate drop response (pacing at faster rates when there is a sudden drop in heart rate) was implanted, with subsequent complete resolution of her symptoms.

> **Expert comment**
>
> A negative tilt test does not exclude reflex syncope. An asystolic response to tilt testing predicts a high probability of spontaneous asystolic episodes. In addition, the presence of a positive vasodepressor or mixed response does not exclude the presence of asystole during spontaneous syncope in patients older than 40 years of age.

> **Clinical tip** Be patient when assessing orthostatic hypotension
>
> - Measure BP repeatedly with a cuff for at least 3 minutes.
> - Orthostatic hypotension is diagnosed when systolic BP falls >20 mmHg or to <90 mmHg or diastolic BP falls >10 mmHg from baseline, associated with symptoms.

> **Learning point** Management of reflex syncope
>
> Reflex syncope occurs when there is an abnormal or exaggerated autonomic response of the cardiovascular reflexes that regulate the circulatory system. This is often in response to a trigger such as standing or emotion, and results in vasodilatation and an increase in vagal tone. This in turn results in reduced cardiac filling and bradycardia, with a subsequent fall in arterial BP and global cerebral hypoperfusion.
>
> The term 'vasodepressor' is commonly used if hypotension due to a loss of upright vasoconstrictor tone predominates; 'cardio-inhibitory' is used when bradycardia or asystole predominates (Case II) and 'mixed' is used if both mechanisms are present (Case I).
>
> Reflex syncope can also be classified according to the nature of its trigger, e.g. micturition or cough, although the triggers do not predict the nature of the haemodynamic response. However, recognition of the various triggers is important both in diagnosis and in the education of patients to be vigilant for recurring symptoms. Amongst triggers, CSS deserves a special mention as it is commonly diagnosed in subjects aged over 40 by CSM. From a therapeutic perspective, it is highly responsive to permanent pacing [4].
>
> The number of episodes of syncope during life is the strongest predictor of recurrence. For instance, in patients with an uncertain diagnosis, low risk of sudden cardiac death, and age >40 years, a history of one to two episodes of syncope during life can predict a recurrence of 15% and 20% after one and two years, respectively. Those with a history of three episodes of syncope during their lifetime can predict a recurrence of 36% and 42% after one and two years, respectively [5].
>
> The goal of therapy is to prevent recurrence and its associated injuries, along with improving the quality of life. Treatment of reflex syncope should include appropriate explanation and reassurance, avoidance of triggers and situations which may induce syncope, modification of any hypotensive drug regimen, adjustment of fluid and/or salt intake, and the use of isometric manoeuvres as physical countermeasures (PCM) to combat falling BP during a prodrome. PCM can significantly increase BP during the phase of impending reflex syncope, and allows the patient to avoid or delay losing consciousness in most cases. Their efficacy has been confirmed in a multicentre prospective trial which randomized 223 patients to either conventional therapy alone vs conventional therapy plus training in PCM [6]. Fifty-one percent of patients with conventional treatment and 32% of patients trained in PCM experienced recurrence of syncope during follow-up (p<0.005, relative risk reduction of 39%).

continued

Expert comment

PCMs are useful in aborting impending reflex syncope in patients with warning symptoms. These exercises include leg crossing (crossing of legs with tensing of leg, abdominal and buttock muscles), handgrip (maximal voluntary contraction of any available object taken in the dominant hand), or arm tensing (gripping one hand with the other and simultaneously abducting both arms).

Expert comment Ongoing trials to clarify the role of pacing

It remains to be proven whether pacing would be beneficial when applied only to patients with documented asystole during spontaneous syncope by ILR. The ISSUE 2 study hypothesized that spontaneous asystole, and not tilt test results should form the basis for patient selection for pacemaker therapy [12]. This study followed 392 patients with presumed reflex syncope with an ILR. Of the 102 patients with symptom–rhythm correlation, 53 underwent loop recorder-guided therapy and pacing. These patients experienced a striking reduction in the recurrence of syncope compared with the remainder who had non-loop recorder-guided therapy (10% vs 41%, p = 0.002). It must be stressed that ISSUE 2 was not a randomized trial, but provided the basis for the ongoing ISSUE 3 which is a randomized controlled trial. This study is randomizing patients with ILR-documented asystole to implantation of a dual-chamber pacemaker, but with pacing turned on in the study group and off in the control group. The subject in Case I is a participant in the ISSUE 3 study and unexpectedly, his ILR documented episodes of narrow complex tachycardia rather than bradycardia.

Expansion of extracellular volume is also an important goal to treat orthostatic intolerance. In the absence of hypertension, patients increase salt and water intake, aiming for two to three litres of fluid and 10 g of sodium chloride per day. Most patients seen in specialist syncope clinics are managed successfully with these conservative measures.

Midodrine, an alpha-agonist vasoconstrictor with predominant venoconstrictive action, may be helpful in reducing reflex syncope, although evidence of its benefit is greater in the treatment of orthostatic hypotension [7,8]. It should be used cautiously in older males due to potential adverse effects on urinary outflow. No other drug, including beta-blockers, fludrocortisone, and selective serotonin reuptake inhibitors, has clinical evidence in its favour for use in reflex syncope.

Syncope is very frequent in the general population and as a result, has significant socio-economic implications via direct clinical and indirect social costs. Approximately 1% of referrals to Accident and Emergency (A&E) is for syncope and of these, 40% of patients are hospitalized with a median in-hospital stay of 5.5 days [9]. The use of a standardized care pathway can result in considerable improvement in diagnostic yield and cost-effectiveness [1].

Discussion

Syncope is common in the general population, but only a small proportion of patients with syncope seek medical attention. Structural heart disease is a major risk factor for sudden cardiac death and the onset of syncope in the context of underlying cardiovascular disease, such as severe aortic stenosis or hypertrophic cardiomyopathy, often predicts an increased risk of mortality. Reflex syncope is not associated with a reduced life expectancy, but can have a very detrimental effect on the quality of life. The causes of syncope differ according to age. Reflex syncope is most common in those under 40 years, whereas orthostatic hypotension is more common in those over 40 years of age. Syncope due to cardiovascular disease is more prevalent in those over 75 years [10].

The benefits of dual-chamber pacing in CSS are well established, but its use in reflex syncope remains controversial. Pacing has been evaluated in several randomized controlled trials, whereby patients were selected based on their pre-implant tilt test response. Based on a meta-analysis, a non-significant 17% reduction in syncope was seen from double-blinded studies (all patients receiving pacemakers, but randomized to pacing either being switched on or off), whereas an 84% reduction was seen in studies where the control group did not receive a pacemaker [11]. This observation implies a potentially strong placebo effect in subjects being treated with pacing for reflex syncope.

Learning point Syncope and driving

The Driving and Vehicles Licensing Authority (DVLA) in the United Kingdom (UK) categorizes syncope into several risk categories, each with varying restrictions on driving entitlements [13]. Patients in the UK have a legal duty to inform the DVLA about any condition likely to affect their ability to drive safely. The doctor's duty is to advise the patient when they should cease to drive, and ask them to notify the DVLA (Table 19.4) in a prompt fashion.

Table 19.4 Syncope and the DVLA

	Group 1 entitlement (ordinary driving licence for cars or motorcycles)	Group 2 entitlement (vocational, e.g. heavy goods vehicles, taxis)
Simple faint Definite **provocational** factors with associated **prodromal** symptoms and which are unlikely to occur whilst sitting or lying **(postural)**. If recurrent, need to check that the '3 Ps' apply on each occasion.	No driving restrictions DVLA need not be notified	No driving restrictions DVLA need not be notified
Loss of consciousness/loss of or altered awareness likely to be unexplained syncope and low risk of recurrence Low risk is determined by absence of structural heart disease and a normal ECG.	Can drive four weeks after event	Can drive three months after the event
Loss of consciousness/loss of or altered awareness likely to be unexplained syncope and high risk of recurrence Factors indicating high risk: (a) Abnormal ECG (b) Clinical evidence of structural heart disease (c) Syncope causing injury, occurring at the wheel or whilst sitting or lying (d) More than one episode in previous six months	Can drive four weeks after the event if the cause has been identified and treated. If no cause identified, licence revoked for six months.	Can drive three months after the event if the cause has been identified and treated. If no cause identified, licence revoked for one year.
Loss of consciousness with no clinical pointers Had appropriate cardiac and neurological investigations, but with no abnormalities detected	Licence revoked for six months	Licence revoked for one year
Carotid sinus sensitivity treated by pacemaker implantation	Cease driving for one week	Disqualified from driving for six weeks

---

💬 A final word from the expert

In conclusion, pacing occupies a small niche in the therapeutic options for reflex syncope, and should be considered only when symptoms occur in those over the age of 40 with documented severe bradycardia or asystole during a spontaneous attack (or on tilt testing). Education and the avoidance of predisposing triggers remains the mainstay of treatment, whilst interventional therapy plays a minor role due to the paucity of evidence for its efficacy.

References

1 Alboni P, Brignole M, Menozzi C, et al. Diagnostic value of history in patients with syncope with or without heart disease. *J Am Coll Cardiol* 2001; 37: 1921–1928.

2 The Task Force for the Diagnosis and Management of Syncope of the European Society of Cardiology (ESC). Guidelines for the diagnosis and management of syncope (version 2009). *Eur Heart J* 2009; 30: 2631–2671.

3 Brignole M, Gianfranchi L, Menozzi C, et al. Role of autonomic reflexes in syncope associated with paroxysmal atrial fibrillation. *J Am Coll Cardiol* 1993; 22: 1123–1120.

4 Brignole M, Menozzi C, Lolli G, et al. Long-term outcome of paced and non-paced patients with severe carotid sinus syndrome. *Am J Cardiol* 1992; 69: 1039–1043.

5 Brignole M, Vardas P, Hoffman E, et al. Indications for the use of diagnostic implantable and external ECG loop recorders. *Europace* 2009; 11: 671–687.

6 van Dijk N, Quartieri F, Blanc JJ, et al. Effectiveness of physical counterpressure manoeuvres in preventing vasovagal syncope: the Physical Counterpressure Manoeuvres Trial (PC-Trial). *J Am Coll Cardiol* 2006; 48: 1652–1657.

7 Perez-Lugones A, Schweikert R, Pavia S, et al. Usefulness of midodrine in patients with severely symptomatic neurocardiogenic syncope: a randomized control study. *J Cardiovasc Electrophysiol* 2001; 12: 935–938.

8 Low PA, Gilden JL, Freeman R, et al. Efficacy of midodrine vs placebo in neurogenic orthostatic hypotension. A randomized double-blind multicentre study. Midodrine Study Group. *JAMA* 1997; 277: 1046–1051.

9 Brignole M, Menozzi C, Bartoletti A, et al. A new management of syncope: prospective systematic guideline-based evaluation of patients referred urgently to general hospitals. *Eur Heart J* 2006; 27: 76–82.

10 Soteriades ES, Evans JC, Larson MG, et al. Incidence and prognosis of syncope. *N Engl J Med* 2002; 347: 878–885.

11 Sud S, Massel D, Klein GJ, et al. The expectation effect and cardiac pacing for refractory vasovagal syncope. *Am J Med* 2007; 120: 54–62.

12 Brignole M, Sutton R, Menozzi C, et al. Early application of an implantable loop recorder allows effective specific therapy in patients with recurrent suspected neurally mediated syncope. *Eur Heart J* 2006; 27: 1085–1092.

13 Driver and Vehicle Licensing Agency. Guide to current medical standards of fitness to drive. Available from: http://www.dft.gov.uk/dvla/medical/ataglance.aspx.

Cryptogenic stroke

Arif Anis Khan

⊕ Expert commentary Dr Michael Mullen

Case history

A 38-year-old woman developed sudden onset slurred speech one afternoon whilst working in her office. She noticed simultaneous weakness of her right arm and hand. There was no associated headache and her symptoms persisted for one hour. She was taken to the local hospital. Her only past medical history was of migraine with visual aura which had been treated with ergonovine. She did not take any other medication, did not drink alcohol, but was a long-term smoker.

On arrival at the hospital, the patient had a pulse of 72 beats per minute (bpm), blood pressure (BP) of 128/76 mmHg, and oxygen saturations of 96% on room air. Her body mass index (BMI) was 32. Routine blood tests were unremarkable (Table 20.1).

Cardiovascular and respiratory system examinations were unremarkable. Neurological examination revealed mild dysarthria and moderate weakness of her right arm, particularly of elbow extension, wrist dorsiflexion, and the intrinsic hand muscles. A 12-lead electrocardiogram (ECG) confirmed normal sinus rhythm. No other objective abnormalities were found. She was admitted to hospital and underwent cerebral magnetic resonance angiography (MRA). This suggested thrombosis of the left middle cerebral artery. A duplex ultrasound of her carotid arteries was normal.

An inpatient transthoracic echocardiogram (TTE) was undertaken, although due to the patient's body habitus, suboptimal echocardiographic images were obtained. Despite this, the echo was able to confirm normal biventricular size and systolic function and normal right and left atrial size. There was no valvular dysfunction. No vegetations were seen and there was no visible inter-atrial communication. In view of the patient's age and presentation, an agitated saline contrast study (ASCS) was performed. The study was negative at rest, and inconclusive on Valsalva due to suboptimal images.

Table 20.1 Blood test results on arrival to hospital

Hb	14.1 g/dL (13.0–17.0)
Haematocrit/PCV	40% (36–46)
MCV	88 fL (83–99)
Platelet count	399 x 10⁹/L (150–400)
Na	139 mmol/L (134–145)
K	4.2 mmol/L (3.5–5.2)
Creatinine	86 micromol/L (50–104)
Blood urea nitrogen	4.0 mmol/L (2.5–6.5)
Clotting screen	Normal

⊕ Expert comment

This history is already highly suggestive of cardiac thromboembolism secondary to a patent foramen ovale (PFO). Both cryptogenic stroke and migraine with aura are associated with an increased incidence of PFO, and when present in the same patient, a PFO is likely to be found. Other causes such as vascular disease should be excluded, but her young age and absence of atherosclerotic disease in her carotid arteries make this an unlikely aetiology. Early diagnosis and thrombolytic therapy should be considered in patients presenting with embolic stroke.

✚ Clinical tip Aetiology of ischaemic stroke in a young person

A 12-lead ECG is important to look for possible causes of a cerebral embolus, such as atrial fibrillation (AF) or a recent myocardial infarction.

✚ Clinical tip Assessment of cryptogenic stroke

A neurological assessment and haematological thrombophilia work-up are essential components in investigating cryptogenic stroke or transient ischaemic attack (TIA). Thrombophilia screening includes protein C, protein S, anti-thrombin, activated protein C resistance (APCR) assay, factor V Leiden, prothrombin gene mutation, and lupus anticoagulant. It is not possible to carry out a thrombophilia screen after warfarin therapy is commenced, as proteins C and S are both vitamin K-dependent and therefore, will be reduced after starting treatment.

Expert comment

When considering a PFO, it is important to assess not just the presence of a shunt, but also its magnitude. PFOs are present in 25–35% of the population, but large PFOs that are likely to cause disease are less common, typically around 10%. Excess mobility of the intra-atrial septum (often termed an aneurysm although this is a misnomer), should also be considered as this has been independently associated with a risk of stroke. Whether the aneurysm itself is the cause of stroke, perhaps by promoting *in situ* thrombus formation or AF, or whether it simply reflects a larger defect, is not yet known.

TTE is highly sensitive for detecting and quantifying shunts. The heart is imaged in the apical 4-chamber view and should be optimized to enhance the endocardial borders. Agitated saline contrast is injected via an antecubital vein. The first run should be at rest during normal breathing and it is important to image the contrast entering the right atrium, and wait until it has started to disappear. The shunt, if present, is usually best visualized in the left ventricle. Shunt capacity is assessed in a semi-quantitative fashion. Bubble counting is not possible on TTE and if necessary, the shunt is probably small. Subsequent injections can be evaluated during provocative manoeuvres, including Valsalva, coughing, or sniffing to increase right atrial pressure. Again, care should be taken to maintain the image throughout the study, as large bubbles can pass through the left heart and disappear within a few heartbeats. This often requires the echocardiographer and patient to practise these techniques a few times before injecting the contrast.

Expert comment

Clinical trials have not demonstrated a benefit of warfarin therapy over aspirin in patients with cryptogenic stroke. Warfarin is associated with an increased risk of bleeding. In general, therefore, patients are normally treated with aspirin in the first instance unless a specific thrombophilic disorder requiring anticoagulation is identified.

Learning point Right-to-left shunts in patent foramen ovale

PFOs are covered by a flap of tissue so that under normal circumstances, there is often no shunt between the atria. However, if the right atrial pressure is increased (e.g. during a Valsalva manoeuvre), the flap may be displaced and right-to-left shunting may occur.

Clinical tip Agitated saline contrast study to diagnose intracardiac shunts

- A positive bubble contrast study is diagnostic of a PFO.
- Agitated saline is injected at rest via a peripheral vein whilst in the apical 4-chamber view on TTE.
- A cardiac shunt is suggested by the appearance of bubbles in the left heart within four cycles of their presence in the right heart.
- If there is no evidence of shunt during normal respiration, the Valsalva manoeuvre should be performed. This is useful because at the end of a Valsalva manoeuvre, when the strain is released, venous return increases, transiently increasing right atrial pressure above left atrial pressure (and thus the apparent size of the shunt). This technique increases the sensitivity for the diagnosis of PFO, and can unmask those PFOs not apparent during quiet breathing.
- Injection of agitated saline should occur during the strain phase of the Valsalva whilst in the release phase, bubbles should be looked for in the left heart. It is essential to time the Valsalva manoeuvres accurately in relation to the bubble injection whilst obtaining good quality echo images.
- The sensitivity and specificity for the detection of large shunts, which are more clinically relevant, are surprisingly better with TTE compared to transoesophageal echocardiography (TOE) [1].

In view of the patient's young age and the fact that no obvious origin of the thrombus was detected, it was felt that warfarin would be the most appropriate anticoagulant to prevent future thromboembolic events. Daily physiotherapy gradually improved the right arm weakness and she was discharged home with further outpatient physiotherapy and medical follow-up.

Unfortunately, the patient presented one month later with a further episode of TIA. She was admitted for further investigations to try and elicit the source of her embolic events. As her previous bubble contrast study was inconclusive, a transcranial Doppler (TCD) study was performed to search for an intracardiac shunt. This was strongly suggestive of a PFO (Figure 20.1), although a further MRA of her brain did not show any new changes. In view of her recurrent neurological symptoms, the patient was referred for a percutaneous PFO closure.

The patient was subsequently admitted and underwent a successful closure of her PFO with a 23 mm STARFlex® device (Figures 20.3 and 20.4). There were no complications, and the patient was discharged the following day. She was advised to continue six months of low-dose aspirin and clopidogrel for six weeks [11]. Two years following the deployment of the device, the patient had not experienced any further neurological events.

⭐ **Learning point** What is the best technique to diagnose an intracardiac shunt?

TCD can detect the presence of right-to-left shunts such as PFO with similar sensitivity and specificity compared to TOE, particularly for those who have poor echo windows [1]. This investigation requires the administration of agitated saline via a peripheral vein, after which the patient performs a Valsalva manoeuvre. The test is positive for a right-to-left shunt if a shower of high signal material (air) is detected (Figure 20.1) in the middle cerebral artery (MCA) by TCD, five to ten seconds after the intravenous injection of 10 mL of agitated saline [2]. TOE is considered the method of choice for the diagnosis of PFO [3,4], however, colour flow Doppler is less sensitive at detecting atrial shunts compared to bubble contrast in both TTE and TOE techniques.

⭐ **Learning point** The association between stroke and patent foramen ovale

PFO is defined as the failure of the flap valve of the oval fossa to fuse with the rim of the atrial septum. It is the most frequent inter-atrial communication and is found in up to 25% of the general population. Decompression sickness and platypnoea-orthodeoxia syndrome (postural hypoxaemia accompanied by breathlessness induced by the upright position), are well recognized associations although the latter condition is extremely rare.

PFO has been increasingly recognized as a possible mediator of paradoxical embolism, allowing the passage of air, thrombus, and fat. The larger the size of the PFO and the presence of an atrial septal aneurysm (ASA) have been identified as morphological characteristics associated with a greater risk of paradoxical embolism [5]. When other causes of stroke have been excluded (such as cerebral aneurysms or carotid disease), the presence of a PFO or other shunt makes a paradoxical embolus the most likely aetiology, even if no identifiable source of distal thrombus such as a deep venous thrombosis is found. The association of PFO and cryptogenic stroke (odds ratio of stroke with PFO 3:1, 95% confidence interval 2.3–4.2) has been consistently reported in patients less than 55 years of age. Interestingly, migraine is also more common (35% vs 12%) in cryptogenic stroke patients with PFO although the literature now contains a range of results [6].

Normal

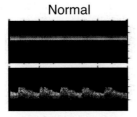

Doppler signals of normal blood flow in the middle cerebral artery.

PFO

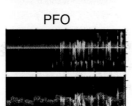

Series of high signals corresponding to air bubbles in the middle cerebral artery, five seconds after post-intravenous injection, consistent with the diagnosis of intracardiac shunt.

Figure 20.1 Transcranial Doppler study consistent with an intracardiac shunt.

The evidence and clinical argument for closure are greatest in patients with stroke rather than TIA. Nevertheless, TIA is associated with a high recurrence rate in the short term, and should still be considered for closure. CLOSURE-1 is a randomized trial of PFO closure vs medical therapy for the treatment of cryptogenic stroke and TIA. Its results have shown that PFO closure is not superior to best medical but other trials are also nearing completion and will be awaited before a final decision can be reached regarding the indications for PFO closure.

⭐ **Learning point** The risk of recurrent stroke in patients with patent foramen ovale

Patients with PFO and ASA have an average annual risk of recurrent stroke of 4.4%, and similar stroke rates on medical treatment have been reported from the Lausanne stroke registry [7]. The percentage of cryptogenic strokes among ischaemic strokes (about 75% of all strokes) varies from 8% to 44% with a mean of 31% [8]. A pooled analysis suggests that the presence of a PFO alone increased the risk for recurrent events 5-fold, with an even greater risk in the presence of an ASA [9]. This relationship remains controversial in the absence of prospective, randomized controlled clinical trials [10]. Determinants of risk for stroke in patients with a PFO include:

- ASA;
- Presence of an Eustachian valve directed towards the PFO;
- The gap diameter (approximate size) of the PFO;
- The number of micro-bubbles present in the left heart during the first four seconds after release of a Valsalva during a bubble test.

⭐ **Learning point** The evidence for percutaneous patent foramen ovale closure

Results from the first randomized controlled trial of PFO closure versus best medical therapy for stroke/TIA have recently been published. It showed no differences in the primary endpoint of stroke, or TIA at 2 years, all-cause mortality at 30 days, or neurological mortality between 31 days and 2 years. Despite this outcome, lower recurrence rates have been observed following percutaneous closure. The ease of device closure and the low procedural risks have currently made percutaneous closure the treatment of choice in some centres for appropriately selected patients. There are a number of devices currently in use for percutaneous PFO closure (Figure 20.2).

Currently, approved indications for device closure are in patients with recurrent stroke, orthodeoxia syndrome, and scuba divers with decompression syndrome. All other uses, including patients with a single occurrence of a cryptogenic stroke, are currently not approved by the US Food and Drug Administration.

⭐ **Learning point** Percutaneous closure of patent foramen ovale

Devices are positioned using a combination of fluoroscopy, TOE, or intra-cardiac echocardiography. Access for closure is almost always via the femoral vein. Defects can be sized in two ways. Firstly, a preoperative TOE should provide sufficient information about the atrial septum to allow the selection of an appropriate device, in addition to guiding measurement and deployment of the device (Figure 20.3). Often the inflation of a static balloon within the defect is required to allow a correct measurement of the PFO (Figure 20.4). This method of balloon sizing is not always recommended as it can damage the thin atrial septum.

Major peri-procedural complications occur in 0.9% of patients. Complications may include wire fracture, air embolism, tension pneumothorax, retroperitoneal haemorrhage, perforation of the atrial wall, and allergic reactions to the device.

A recent advance in technology includes the BioSTAR device (Figure 20.2). This is a bioabsorbable device specifically designed for the closure of PFOs and atrial septal defects (ASDs). The device uses a layer of collagen matrix, mounted on a 'double umbrella' framework. The device is coated with a heparin complex (to reduce thrombus formation), and is mounted on a nitinol spring frame connected between the left and right atrial umbrellas. The collagen matrix incorporates into the atrial septum, which results in early sealing of the defect. Gradual remodelling occurs over a period of 24 months during which the collagen is absorbed and replaced by host tissue [12]. Another innovative product is the Sutura® Superstitch EL. This is a novel bidirectional suture device which allows direct suturing of the PFO without the need for an open surgical approach [13].

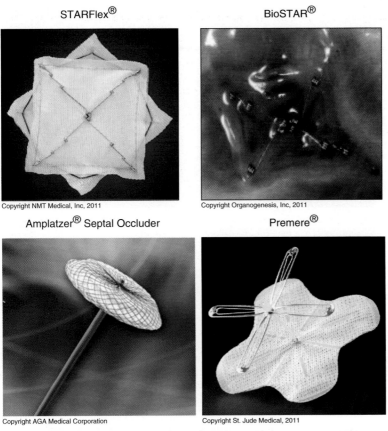

STARFlex®

BioSTAR®

Copyright NMT Medical, Inc, 2011

Copyright Organogenesis, Inc, 2011

Amplatzer® Septal Occluder

Premere®

Copyright AGA Medical Corporation

Copyright St. Jude Medical, 2011

Figure 20.2 Examples of percutaneous PFO closure devices currently in use.

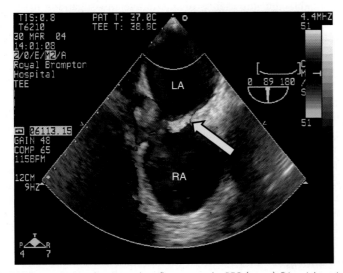

Figure 20.3 TOE long axis view showing colour flow across the PFO (arrow). RA = right atrium; LA = left atrium.

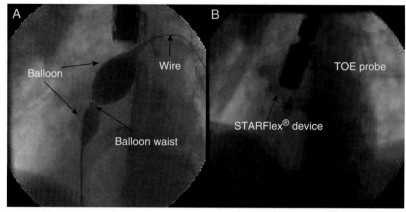

Figure 20.4 Fluoroscopy during closure of the PFO with a STARFlex® device. A balloon mounted on an exchange wire inflates across the PFO. The balloon waist correlates to the diameter of the PFO and is used for device sizing.

⭐ Learning point The risk of stroke following percutaneous patent foramen ovale closure

The probability of recurrence of stroke or TIA following device closure of a PFO is around 7.8% after four years [14,15]. In a reported comparison of device closure vs medical therapy (aspirin or warfarin), the recurrence rate of embolic events was significantly lower at 0.5% per year in patients with device closure as opposed to 2.9% per year for patients treated with medical therapy [15]. Patients are generally advised to take six months of low-dose aspirin and six weeks of clopidogrel after PFO device closure, although it is important to note that this duration of antiplatelet therapy is recommended on the basis of observational data, rather than randomized control data.

Discussion

Patients with PFOs can present numerous diagnostic and management challenges. This case highlights the importance of alternative investigations in those patients where there is a high clinical suspicion of an intra-cardiac shunt, but who have poor echocardiographic windows.

There are a number of conflicting studies regarding the best approach for the secondary prevention of embolic events. Warfarin is thought to be the gold standard for medical management although some studies have shown that aspirin may be just as efficacious [16].

Percutaneous closure of a PFO is now a reasonably well-established therapeutic option in those with recurrent embolic events and has a favourable safety to efficacy ratio. It has largely superseded the traditional open-heart surgical approach which came with its attendant risks of cardiopulmonary bypass, and it seems to be equivalent in clinical efficacy to medical therapy [17,18].

Two further randomized controlled trials comparing medical therapy vs percutaneous closure in this subset of patients (PC-trial and RESPECT) are currently in progress and their results are eagerly awaited after the negative results (with regard to device closure) from CLOSURE-1 to help define the best management strategy in patients with cryptogenic stroke.

A final word from the expert

Stroke and TIA are very common disorders, particularly in the elderly. In up to 20%, the cause is unknown, so-called cryptogenic stroke and this rate is even higher in younger patients below the age of 65 years. In those with cryptogenic stroke, the prevalence of PFO has been shown to be higher both in young and older patients. Very rarely, a thrombus has been identified within the PFO, or patients have presented with deep venous thrombosis and simultaneous pulmonary embolism, and the diagnosis of paradoxical embolization is relatively straightforward. However, in the majority of cases, the aetiology of the stroke is less clear, and based largely on a process of elimination. Many of these patients also suffer from migraine with aura and interestingly, following closure of the PFO, many observational studies have reported an improvement in migraine, suggesting both conditions are mediated by paradoxical embolism. However, migraine itself is associated with stroke, and in many studies, the differentiation between complex migrainous aura and a TIA has not been clear.

While cryptogenic stroke in the elderly is proportionally less common, the actual number of cases is larger. However, the role of PFO in these patients has not been well studied and is poorly understood.

With modern echocardiographic technology, PFO can usually be diagnosed non-invasively by transthoracic imaging if performed carefully following a standardized protocol. Invasive TOE is more specific, but not more sensitive and rarely necessary. The maximum capacity of the shunt is an important factor in deciding whether closure is warranted, and should be assessed and reported.

PFO closure is a low-risk and usually effective procedure, and can be achieved using any one of the numerous commercially available devices. Variability in the anatomy means that some devices may be better suited to individual patient characteristics. At this time, the benefit of PFO closure over and above medical therapy is not established, and hence, the indications for this procedure are controversial. Randomized controlled trials are underway and due to be reported in the near future. In the meantime, it is important that patients understand the lack of hard data supporting closure before consenting for this procedure.

References

1 Nemec JJ, Marwick TH, Lorig RJ, et al. Comparison of transcranial Doppler ultrasound and transoesophageal contrast echocardiography in the detection of inter-atrial right-to-left shunts. *Am J Cardiol* 1991; 68: 1498–1502.

2 Droste DW, Kriete JU, Stypmann J, et al. Contrast transcranial Doppler ultrasound in the detection of right-to-left shunts: comparison of different procedures and different contrast agents. *Stroke* 1999; 30: 1827–1832.

3 de Belder MA, Tourikis L, Griffith M, et al. Transoesophageal contrast echocardiography and colour flow mapping: methods of choice for the detection of shunts at the atrial level? *Am Heart J* 1992; 124: 1545–1550.

4 Caputi L, Carriero MR, Falcone C, et al. Transcranial Doppler and transoesophageal echocardiography: comparison of both techniques and prospective clinical relevance of transcranial Doppler in patent foramen ovale detection. *J Stroke Cerebrovasc Dis* 2009; 18: 343–348.

5 Agmon Y, Khandheria BK, Meissner I, et al. Frequency of atrial septal aneurysms in patients with cerebral ischaemic events. *Circulation* 1999; 99: 1942–1944.

6 Reisman M, Christofferson RD, Jesurum J, et al. Migraine headache relief after transcatheter closure of patent foramen ovale. *J Am Coll Cardiol* 2005; 45: 493–495.

7 Lamy C, Giannesini C, Zuber M, et al. Clinical and imaging findings in cryptogenic stroke patients with and without patent foramen ovale: the PFO-ASA Study. *Atrial Septal Aneurysm. Stroke* 2002; 33: 706–711.

8 Meier B, Lock JE. Contemporary management of patent foramen ovale. *Circulation* 2003; 107: 5–9.

9 Overell JR, Bone I, Lees KR. Inter-atrial septal abnormalities and stroke: a meta-analysis of case-control studies. *Neurology* 2000; 55: 1172–1179.

10 Almekhlafi MA, Wilton SB, Rabi DM, et al. Recurrent cerebral ischaemia in medically treated patent foramen ovale: a meta-analysis. *Neurology* 2009; 73: 89–97.

11 Franke A, Kuhl HP. The role of antiplatelet agents in the management of patients receiving intra-cardiac closure devices. *Curr Pharm Des* 2006; 12: 1287–1291.

12 Mullen MJ, Hildick–Smith D, De Giovanni JV, et al. BioSTAR Evaluation STudy (BEST): a prospective, multicentre, phase I clinical trial to evaluate the feasibility, efficacy, and safety of the BioSTAR bioabsorbable septal repair implant for the closure of atrial level shunts. *Circulation* 2006; 114: 1962–1967.

13 Anita W, Asgar NW, Khan AA, Mullen MJ. A novel transcatheter suture technique for PFO closure: the Superstitch EL, ACC i2, 2009.

14 Windecker S, Wahl A, Nedeltchev K, et al. Comparison of medical treatment with percutaneous closure of patent foramen ovale in patients with cryptogenic stroke. *J Am Coll Cardiol* 2004; 44: 750–758.

15 Mas JL, Arquizan C, Lamy C, et al. Recurrent cerebrovascular events associated with patent foramen ovale, atrial septal aneurysm, or both. *N Engl J Med* 2001; 345: 1740–1746.

16 Homma S, Sacco RL, DiTullio MR, et al. Effect of medical treatment in stroke patients with patent foramen ovale. *The Patent Foramen Ovale in Cryptogenic Stroke Study. Circulation* 2002; 105: 2625–2631.

17 Khairy P, O'Donnell CP, Landzberg MJ. Transcatheter closure versus medical therapy of patent foramen ovale and presumed paradoxical thromboemboli: a systematic review. *Ann Intern Med* 2003; 139: 753–760.

18 Windecker S, Wahl A, Nedeltchev K, et al. Comparison of medical treatment with percutaneous closure of patent foramen ovale in patients with cryptogenic stroke. *J Am Coll Cardiol* 2004; 44: 750–758.

Surgically-corrected tetralogy of Fallot and associated arrhythmias

Sarah Bowater

❝ **Expert commentary** Professor Michael A Gatzoulis

Case history

A 60-year-old man was admitted with a short history of palpitations and pre-syncope. He was known to have tetralogy of Fallot (ToF) (Figure 21.1) and was under the follow-up of the adult congenital heart disease (ACHD) clinic. He had had a radical repair of his ToF in 1989 at the age of 40 years. He had infective endocarditis in 1991 with a subsequent tissue aortic valve replacement (AVR). In 2001, he developed an atrial tachyarrhythmia and had a successful catheter ablation to a low right atrial focus. In 2003, he had had an episode of ventricular tachycardia (VT) whilst on holiday in Austria, requiring emergency electrical cardioversion and later had an ablation to an inferobasal segment at the edge of the patch overlying his intraventricular septum. Following a recent clinic attendance at which time he had complained of palpitations, a 24-hour Holter monitor had shown frequent ventricular ectopics. He was taking metoprolol, lisinopril, furosemide, and aspirin.

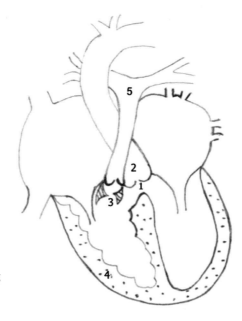

Figure 21.1 Features of tetralogy of Fallot. RA = right atrium; Ao = aorta; PA = pulmonary artery; LA = left atrium; LV = left ventricle; RV = right ventricle; 1. subaortic VSD; 2. overriding aorta; 3. subpulmonary stenosis; 4. right ventricular hypertrophy.

Expert comment

A transannular patch was extensively used to repair ToF in the 1960s and 1970s, but less so nowadays that the adverse long-term effect of pulmonary regurgitation (PR) has been appreciated. Instead, surgeons now relieve the right ventricular outflow tract (RVOT) obstruction with infundibular resection and fine valvuloplasty (or when necessary, with subvalvular or supravalvar patches), thus avoiding transannular incisions and limiting the extent of PR. Furthermore, most patients with ToF would undergo primary repair in early childhood, thus preventing longstanding RV hypertrophy and cyanosis with all the late problems associated with them.

Clinical tip ECG in tetralogy of Fallot

- More than 99% patients who have undergone radical repair will have a right bundle branch block (RBBB).
- The right bundle runs in the floor of the VSD and is damaged during surgical repair.

Learning point Radical surgical repair of tetralogy of Fallot

- Patch closure of the ventricular septal defect (VSD);
- Resection of infundibular stenosis;
- Transannular patch to enlarge the pulmonary valve annulus.

On admission, he was talking, but appeared confused and was clammy with cool peripheries. Heart rate was 160 beats per minute (bpm) and blood pressure (BP) 80/50 mmHg. A 12-lead electrocardiogram (ECG) demonstrated a broad complex tachycardia with a left bundle morphology and an inferior axis (Figure 21.2). A diagnosis of ventricular tachycardia (VT) with evidence of haemodynamic compromise was made and as a result, he was urgently electrically cardioverted under sedation. A single 150 J shock cardioverted him back to sinus rhythm (Figure 21.3) with a rate of 75 bpm and BP 100/70 mmHg. On auscultation, he had a 4/6 ejection systolic murmur at the lower left sternal edge and normal heart sounds. There was no clinical evidence of cardiac failure. Chest X-ray (CXR) confirmed significant cardiomegaly, but clear lung fields (Figure 21.4). Routine blood tests were normal.

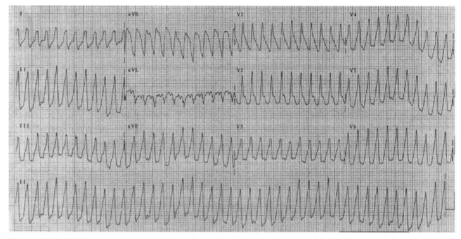

Figure 21.2 ECG on admission showing ventricular tachycardia with left bundle morphology.

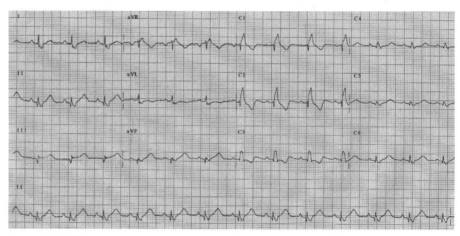

Figure 21.3 ECG post-emergency cardioversion confirming sinus rhythm with right bundle branch block (courtesy of Jonas de Jong).

Expert comment

There is further prolongation of the QRS duration with time, reflecting progressive RV dilatation, usually with significant PR. This dynamic QRS change is predictive of VT and subsequent sudden cardiac death (SCD) as discussed below.

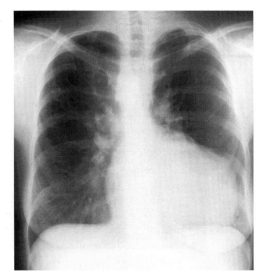

Figure 21.4 Chest radiograph on admission.

ⓘ Expert comment

The characteristic 'boot-shaped' heart (coeur-en-sabot) is the result of an elevated cardiac apex (as a result of RV hypertrophy), pulmonary artery 'bay' (i.e. a relatively small pulmonary trunk), and right aortic arch.

He was admitted to the coronary care unit and commenced on an intravenous loading dose of amiodarone that was converted to oral therapy after 24 hours. No further VT was recorded. The following day, he had a transthoracic echocardiogram (TTE). This showed good left ventricular (LV) function, but the right ventricle was markedly dilated with severely impaired function (tricuspic annulus plane systolic excursion [TAPSE] 7 mm, RV free wall Sm 6 cm/s). There was laminar flow from the right ventricular outflow tract into the right ventricle consistent with severe PR (Figures 21.5 and 21.6). There was no residual VSD.

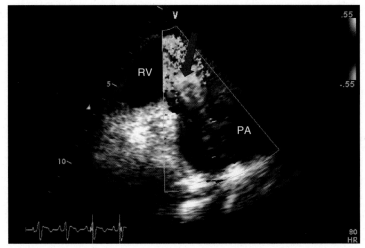

Figure 21.5 Parasternal short axis view showing severe PR (arrow) and dilated right ventricle. RV = right ventricle; PA = pulmonary artery.

✪ Learning point Echocardiographic assessment of the right ventricle (normal values)

- TAPSE >14 mm;
- Myocardial performance index ≤0.4;
- Tissue Doppler imaging of free wall ≥12 cm/s.

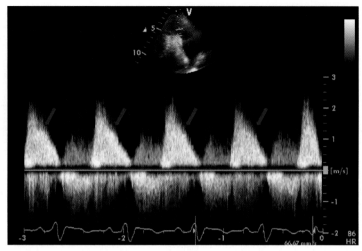

Figure 21.6 Continuous wave Doppler through the pulmonary valve demonstrating severe regurgitation (arrows).

He was reviewed by an electrophysiologist who felt that in view of his haemodynamic compromise at presentation and the severely impaired right ventricle, he should receive an implantable cardioverter-defibrillator (ICD). A left arm venogram was performed prior to implantation, which excluded the presence of a left superior vena cava (LSVC). Implantation was via the left subclavian vein and was uncomplicated. Prior to discharge, he underwent a right and left heart catheter with a view to pulmonary valve replacement (see Table 21.1).

> **★ Learning point** Pacing in complex congenital heart disease
>
> Pacing in complex congenital heart disease has its own unique set of problems and should only be performed by a specialist with an understanding of the underlying anatomy and physiology. Problems include abnormal venous access such as a persistent LSVC and no direct venous access to the heart as seen in the Fontan circulation requiring extracardiac lead placement, scar tissue from previous surgery, tricuspid or pulmonary regurgitation, making lead implantation difficult, and the presence of an intra-atrial baffle in repaired transposition of the great arteries.

Table 21.1 Right and left heart catheter procedure notes

Pressures (mmHg)	Right atrium 8 mmHg
	Right ventricle 31/10 mmHg
	Pulmonary artery 34/10, mean 17 mmHg
	PCWP 13 mmHg
RV angiogram	Dilated right ventricle, poor function
	Dilated, pulsatile pulmonary arteries
	Free PR
Left heart catheter	Good LV function
	No VSD
	No obstructive coronary disease

He was discharged home after being reviewed by the congenital cardiac surgeons and was listed for pulmonary valve replacement plus surgical ablation and excision of the portion of right ventricle responsible for the VT.

⭐ **Learning point** Atrial tachyarrhythmias in tetralogy of Fallot

Atrial tachyarrhythmias have been reported in up to 34% of patients after repair of ToF and contribute significantly to morbidity [2]. They are most commonly macro-re-entrant and originate around scars or incision lines from previous surgery. Rapid conduction is poorly tolerated and should be urgently cardioverted. Risk factors for atrial tachyarrhythmias are increased atrial size, ventricular dysfunction, and valvular regurgitation. Gatzoulis et al. also demonstrated that atrial tachyarrhythmias were more likely in those patients who underwent repair at a later age, had previous palliation with a Potts or Waterston shunt, or re-operation before 1985 [3]. Macro-re-entrant pathways may be suitable for catheter ablation although recurrence is common, occurring in up to 20% [4].

⭐ **Learning point** Ventricular tachycardia in tetralogy of Fallot

Repaired ToF is the commonest group of all ACHD to have VT with an incidence of 11.9% in long-term follow-up [3]. It is the commonest cause for SCD in these patients. The VT is usually macro-re-entrant, originating around a scar, patch, or ventriculotomy site and usually has RVOT morphology (LBBB and inferior axis). Pharmacological treatment is often unsatisfactory and treatment should be focused towards ablation and/or ICD therapy. There are no large published trials looking at catheter ablation with significant recurrence rates being reported in small studies [4]. Reported difficulties include poorly tolerated induced arrhythmias, complex anatomy, and the induced arrhythmia not matching the morphology of the one at clinical presentation.

⭐ **Learning point** Risk factors for ventricular tachycardia and sudden cardiac death in tetralogy of Fallot

The incidence of SCD in repaired ToF is 6% at 30 years' follow-up [5] with the commonest underlying cause being VT. It is therefore important to identify and intervene on those patients deemed high-risk at an early stage. Identified risk factors for VT and SCD include a QRS duration of >180 ms on a resting ECG [6] and lengthening of the QRS duration late after surgery [3]. Khairy et al. demonstrated a prognostic significance in risk, stratifying patients with programmed ventricular stimulation, inducible sustained VT being an independent risk factor for subsequent events (relative risk 4.7, 95% confidence interval 1.2–18.5) [7]. Moderate to severe PR is the main underlying haemodynamic lesion for VT. Long-term PR leads to progressive RV dilatation and functional deterioration. Severe RV dilatation and dysfunction are associated with adverse clinical outcomes, including sustained VT [8]. RV fibrosis, as detected by late gadolinium enhancement on MRI, has also recently been shown to be a positive predictor of arrhythmias [9]. Other reported risk factors include later age at repair, frequent ventricular ectopics [4], prior palliative shunts, and left ventricular dysfunction [8,10]. However, these factors have poor specificity for identifying patients at risk of VT or SCD and the optimal model for risk stratification is still unclear.

⭐ **Learning point** Implantable cardioverter-defibrillators in tetralogy of Fallot and congenital heart disease

ICDs are widely used in both primary and secondary prevention of SCD in high risk, mainly ischaemic heart disease, patients. Their benefit in congenital heart disease, however, is less well defined with no large outcome studies. The National Institute of Health and Clinical Excellence guidelines are broad and recommend consideration of ICD therapy in all patients with surgically repaired ToF. Joint guidelines from the European Society of Cardiology, American College of Cardiology, and American Heart Association give class I indications to survivors of cardiac arrest or spontaneous VT that are not successfully ablated [11]. ToF patients are the commonest recipients of ICDs in ACHD due to their relatively high risk of late SCD. Cohort studies looking at recipients of ICDs show appropriate shocks were given in 23–30% of patients. However, up to 41% received at least one inappropriate shock [12–14] with some patients receiving up to 22 [12]. The commonest reasons for inappropriate shocks were supraventricular or sinus tachycardia. Late lead-related complications, including dislodgement, lead failure or fracture, endocarditis, under- or over-sensing, and thrombosis are also more common in ACHD [12,13,15].

🔹 **Expert comment**

In parallel, treatment for arrhythmia should be matched with haemodynamic intervention when a haemodynamic target is present, as with this case. Improving haemodynamics in this setting may modulate arrhythmic burden and/or improve its clinical tolerance.

Many patients with ACHD will be young people who are physically active, in employment, and may participate in sports. The psychological burden of ICD therapy may be greater in younger patients and they may be more prone to anxiety or depression, especially if they receive inappropriate shocks. They will also be committed to numerous battery changes and possible lead replacements throughout their life. It is therefore vital to ensure they receive appropriate counselling on these issues as well as education regarding legal issues such as driving.

> ⭐ **Learning point** Pulmonary valve replacement and arrhythmias
>
> PR is a common finding in surgically repaired ToF and inevitable if a transannular patch was used to relieve the RVOT obstruction initially. Over time, PR leads to progressive RV dilatation and dysfunction. This may be tolerated for many years, but will, over time, lead to progressive exercise intolerance, heart failure, tachyarrhythmias and in some patients, SCD. Pulmonary valve replacement has a low operative morbidity and mortality and good mid- to long-term results. It is associated with a reduction in RV volume, improvement in RV function, and symptomatic benefit. The benefits on long-term outcome are less clear. Therrien et al. demonstrated that PVR leads to stabilization of the QRS duration and when done in conjunction with cryoablation, leads to a reduction in pre-existing atrial and ventricular arrhythmias [16]. However, Harrild et al. failed to show any reduction in death or VT post-pulmonary valve replacement when performed for symptomatic PR and RV dilatation and suggests that there is a 'window of opportunity' for intervention beyond which there is irreversible damage to the RV myocardium and reverse remodelling does not occur [17]. The optimal timing for pulmonary valve replacement remains unclear and requires a balance of risks between RV dysfunction and arrhythmias and the finite lifespan of the bioprosthetic valves [16].

Discussion

Atrial and ventricular arrhythmias are common in surgically repaired ToF. They are often poorly tolerated, especially on a background of poor ventricular function and hence, urgent cardioversion should be performed. These patients have a significant risk of SCD, usually due to VT. Regular assessment of the patient's risk of a life-threatening arrhythmia is imperative although the optimal method for risk stratification is still unclear. Factors, including QRS duration > 180 ms and RV dilatation and dysfunction secondary to PR, are known to increase the risk of VT and SCD. ICD therapy is being increasingly used in patients with ToF; however, large studies looking at the long-term mortality benefit from ICDs are still needed in this particular cohort.

Severe PR is the commonest haemodynamic lesion contributing to arrhythmias. There is currently no consensus as to the optimal timing of pulmonary valve replacement with a narrow window of opportunity before irreversible damage occurs. Patients should undergo serial testing to evaluate exercise capacity and RV volume and function in order to detect any deterioration at an early stage.

Patients with ToF and other forms of ACHD are frequently young and active and in employment and females may wish to consider pregnancy. These factors must be considered when assessing the patient and appropriate counselling and education given.

A final word from the expert

Primary prevention of sustained VT and SCD late after repair of ToF remains challenging. However, progress has been made on risk stratification in recent years in this group of patients and a number of non-invasive and invasive risk markers have been identified for periodic use. Right, left and/or biventricular dysfunction, QRS prolongation, progressive exercise intolerance, and the presence of ventricular fibrosis on cardiac MR (as shown with gadolinium enhancement) identify patients at risk. Such patients together with patients assessed for suspected VT should be considered for invasive electrophysiological assessment where inducible sustained VT has been shown to be predictive of recurrent VT and/or SCD. While VT ablation may have a role in these patients, many should be referred for ICD implantation, particularly if extensive RV fibrosis is present. Target haemodynamic lesions such as pulmonary regurgitation should be addressed at the same time as per our case.

References

1 Niwa K, Siu SC, Webb GD, et al. Progressive aortic root dilatation in adults late after repair of tetralogy of Fallot. *Circulation* 2002; 106: 1374–1378.
2 Harrison DA, Siu SC, Hussain F, et al. Sustained atrial arrhythmias in adults late after repair of tetralogy of fallot. *Am J Cardiol* 2001; 87: 584–588.
3 Gatzoulis MA, Balaji S, Webber SA, et al. Risk factors for arrhythmia and sudden cardiac death late after repair of tetralogy of Fallot: a multicentre study. *Lancet* 2000; 356: 975–981.
4 Walsh EP. Interventional electrophysiology in patients with congenital heart disease. *Circulation* 2007; 115: 3224–3234.
5 Silka M, Hardy B, Menashe V, Morris C. A population-based prospective evaluation of risk of sudden cardiac death after operation from common congenital heart defects. *J Am Coll Cardiol* 1998; 32: 245–251.
6 Gatzoulis MA, Till J, Somerville J, Redington AN. Mechano-electrical interaction in tetralogy of Fallot: QRS prolongation relates to right ventricular size and predicts malignant ventricular arrhythmias and sudden death. *Circulation* 1995; 92: 231–237.
7 Khairy P, Landzberg MJ, Gatzoulis MA, et al. Value of programmed ventricular stimulation after tetralogy of Fallot repair: a multicentre study. *Circulation* 2004; 109: 1994–2000.
8 Knauth AL, Gauvreau K, Powell AJ, et al. Ventricular size and function assessed by cardiac MRI predict major adverse clinical outcomes late after tetralogy of Fallot repair. *Heart* 2008; 94: 211–216.
9 Babu-Narayan SV, Kilner PJ, Li W, et al. Ventricular fibrosis suggested by cardiovascular magnetic resonance in adults with repaired tetralogy of Fallot and its relationship to adverse markers of clinical outcome. *Circulation* 2006; 113: 405–413.
10 Ghai A, Silversides C, Harris L, et al. Left ventricular dysfunction is a risk factor for sudden cardiac death in adults late after repair of tetralogy of Fallot. *J Am Coll Cardiol* 2002; 40: 1675–1680.
11 Task FM, Zipes DP, Camm AJ, et al. ACC/AHA/ESC 2006 guidelines for management of patients with ventricular arrhythmias and the prevention of sudden cardiac death—executive summary: a report of the American College of Cardiology/American Heart Association Task Force and the European Society of Cardiology Committee for Practice Guidelines (Writing Committee to Develop Guidelines for Management of Patients with Ventricular Arrhythmias and the Prevention of Sudden Cardiac Death): developed in collaboration with the European Heart Rhythm Association and the Heart Rhythm Society. *Eur Heart J* 2006; 27: 2099–2140.
12 Yap SC, Roos-Hesselink JW, Hoendermis ES, et al. Outcome of implantable cardioverter-defibrillators in adults with congenital heart disease: a multicentre study. *Eur Heart J* 2007; 28: 1854–1861.

13 Khairy P, Harris L, Landzberg MJ, et al. Implantable cardioverter-defibrillators in tetralogy of Fallot. *Circulation* 2008; 117: 363–370.

14 Berul CI, Van Hare GF, Kertesz NJ, et al. Results of a multicentre retrospective implantable cardioverter-defibrillator registry of paediatric and congenital heart disease patients. *J Am Coll Cardiol* 2008; 51: 1685–1691.

15 Tomaske M, Buersfeld U. Experience with implantable cardioverter-defibrillator therapy in grown-ups with congenital heart disease. *Pacing Clin Electrophysiol* 2008; 31: S35–S37.

16 Therrien J, Siu SC, Harris L, et al. Impact of pulmonary valve replacement and arrhythmia propensity late after repair of tetralogy of Fallot. *Circulation* 2001; 103: 2489–2494.

17 Harrild DM, Berul CI, Cecchin F, et al. Pulmonary valve replacement in tetralogy of Fallot: impact on survival and ventricular tachycardia. *Circulation* 2009; 119: 445–451.

22 A case of refractory systemic hypertension

Lynne Williams

Expert commentary Professor Gareth Beevers

Case history

A 61-year-old Afro-Caribbean man was referred to the specialist hypertension clinic with a 10-year history of hypertension which had been difficult to control despite treatment with multiple anti-hypertensive agents and persistent hypokalaemia despite potassium supplementation. He was known to be sickle trait-positive and to have chronic renal impairment, but the past medical history was otherwise unremarkable. There was a family history of non-insulin-dependent diabetes mellitus and hypertension. His medication at the time of referral included lisinopril 20 mg once daily (od), atenolol 100 mg od, furosemide 40 mg od, amlodipine 10 mg od, terazosin 10 mg od, and Sando-K three tablets daily.

On examination, he was in sinus rhythm at a rate of 90 beats per minute (bpm) with a blood pressure (BP) of 205/115 mmHg (with no significant difference between the left and right arms). His jugular venous pressure (JVP) was not raised and there was no evidence of peripheral oedema. All peripheral pulses were present and equal with no radio-femoral or radio-radial delay. His apex beat was not displaced; heart sounds revealed a normal S1 and S2 with the presence of a fourth heart sound with no murmurs. Examination of the chest was unremarkable and his abdomen was soft and non-tender with no audible renal bruits. His electrocardiogram (ECG) revealed normal sinus rhythm with evidence of left ventricular hypertrophy (LVH) and strain. Chest X-ray was unremarkable. Blood results are shown in Table 22.1.

An isotope renogram excluded renal artery stenosis, but showed evidence of bilateral impairment of renal function. In view of the hypernatraemia and persistent hypokalaemia despite potassium supplementation, the patient was admitted electively for investigation of possible Conn's syndrome or primary hyperaldosteronism. Renin and aldosterone levels were taken in the recumbent, sitting, and erect position (Table 22.2).

> **⊕ Clinical tip** Electrocardiogram criteria for left ventricular hypertrophy
>
> There are several sets of criteria used to diagnose LVH via electrocardiography. None of these are perfect though by using multiple criteria, the sensitivity and specificity are increased.
>
> The Sokolow–Lyon index:
> - S in V1 + R in V5 or V6 ≥35 mm;
> - R in AVL ≥11 mm.
>
> The Cornell voltage criteria:
> - S in V3 + R in AVL >28 mm (men);
> - S in V3 + R in AVL >20 mm (women).

> **❻ Expert comment**
>
> As a test for LVH, the ECG is very insensitive, but fairly specific. False negatives do occur commonly, particularly in obese patients. False positives are seen in thin athletic people. However, if there is LVH by either of the above criteria and repolarization abnormalities in leads V4 to V6 (the so-called 'strain' pattern), then LVH is definitely present and paradoxically, there is little to be gained from doing an echocardiogram; it will merely confirm the LVH. If the ECG shows a surprising lack of LVH, then an echocardiogram may show LVH. When ECG LVH is present, the risk of a heart attack or stroke is up to four times higher than in a patient with the same level of BP and no LVH.

Table 22.1 Blood results on admission

Full blood count	Renal function	Liver function
Hb 12.9 g/dL	Na **149 mmol/L**	Albumin 43 g/L
WCC 7.0 × 10⁹/L	K **2.9 mmol/L**	Bilirubin 9 micromol/L
Platelets 190 × 10⁹/L	Urea 8.9 mmol/L	ALP 132 IU/L
	Creatinine **169 micromol/L**	ALT 14 IU/L

Table 22.2 Renin and aldosterone levels (normal values in parentheses)

	Renin	Aldosterone
Recumbent	**0.03** (0.3–2.03)	**2474** (28–445)
Sitting	0.07	2904
Erect	**0.08** (0.7–3.20)	**3065** (110–860)

⭐ **Learning point** Secondary hypertension

Secondary hypertension accounts for 5–10% of all cases and represents a potentially curable disease. Testing for secondary hypertension can be expensive and requires a high index of suspicion. Patient groups in whom a secondary cause for hypertension should be considered include those with a new onset of hypertension below the age of 30. patients with medically refractory hypertension, and those patients with clinical or laboratory features typical of an underlying disease.

Causes	Investigation
Renal	
Parenchymal disease	Creatinine clearance
Renovascular disease	Duplex ultrasound
	Magnetic resonance angiography
Renin-secreting tumours	Plasma renin levels
Endocrine	
Conn's syndrome (primary hyperaldosteronism)	Plasma renin and aldosterone levels/CT adrenals
Congenital adrenal hyperplasia	
Cushing's syndrome	24-hour urinary free cortisol
	Low-dose dexamethasone suppression test
	CT or MRI pituitary gland
Phaeochromocytoma	Plasma/24-hour urine metanephrine levels
	CT or MRI/MIBG scintigraphy
Hyperparathyroidism	Calcium and parathyroid hormone levels
Acromegaly	Growth hormone and IGF levels
	Oral glucose tolerance test
	MRI pituitary
Miscellaneous	
Pregnancy-induced	
Coarctation of the aorta	Echocardiography/CT angiography
Obstructive sleep apnoea	Sleep study
Drug-induced	
Oral contraceptives	History and drug-screening
Non-steroidal anti-inflammatory agents	
Cyclosporine	
Glucocorticoids	
Mineralocorticoids (including liquorice)	
Erythropoietin	
Antidepressants	
Phenothiazines	

The results confirmed the presence of primary hyperaldosteronism, as evidenced by a suppressed plasma renin activity and an increase in circulating aldosterone levels. In view of these findings, the patient underwent an abdominal computed tomography (CT) scan which demonstrated a possible low-density adrenal mass measuring 2.2 x 1.7 cm (Figure 22.1).

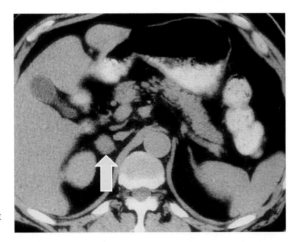

Figure 22.1 Computed tomography of the abdomen demonstrating a right adrenal adenoma (arrow).

① Expert comment

Adrenal vein catheterization is a highly skilled procedure which should only be undertaken by an experienced radiologist. There are frequently problems catheterizing the right adrenal vein which drains directly into the inferior vena cava. It is crucial to take blood for plasma cortisol as well as aldosterone concentrations. If the plasma cortisol is roughly the same in both adrenal veins, then any disparity in plasma aldosterone is probably genuine and not due to problems locating the catheter. Adrenal vein catheterization is less often performed now that we have high resolution CT and magnetic resonance scanners.

✪ Learning point Primary hyperaldosteronism

Classic hyperaldosteronism (with hypokalaemia) accounts for about 0.7% of cases of hypertension. Milder hyperaldosteronism without hypokalaemia is more common with a prevalence of 5–14% among hypertensive patients. Clinical findings include hypertension, muscular weakness, headache, polyuria and polydypsia, and paraesthesiae with frank tetany. Biochemistry results include a high normal sodium, hypokalaemia (may be normal in 40% of cases), and metabolic acidosis. All anti-hypertensive agents should be discontinued prior to the measurement of renin and aldosterone activity, with particular attention to the avoidance of angiotensin-converting enzyme (ACE) inhibitors, angiotensin receptor blockers, spironolactone, eplerenone, and diuretics. Importantly, calcium channel blockers may normalize aldosterone secretion and beta-blockers suppress renin activity and should be withheld prior to biochemical testing. The diagnosis is confirmed by demonstrating a low plasma renin activity and an increase in plasma or urine aldosterone levels. Additionally, aldosterone can be measured while the patient is supine after overnight recumbency and again in the erect position. Localization of the source of excess aldosterone production can be achieved using a thin section CT scan of the adrenal glands. A discrete adrenal adenoma (>1 cm in diameter with a normal contralateral adrenal) is found in 60–80% of patients (Conn's syndrome) whereas 20–30% of patients have evidence of bilateral adrenal hyperplasia. However, 20% of adrenal adenomas are found to have hyperplasia at the time of surgery. Adrenal vein sampling may be used to supplement CT localization of the site of excess production, but is frequently unsuccessful even in the best hands.

Despite multiple anti-hypertensive agents, the patient's BP control was suboptimal. His atenolol was gradually reduced and his furosemide was stopped. The lisinopril was changed to a valsartan/hydrochlorothiazide combination at a dose of 160/25 mg and he was commenced on spironolactone. His amlodipine was changed to diltiazem in view of peripheral oedema at a dose of 240 mg. His spironolactone was changed to eplerenone as a result of painful gynaecomastia and the dose uptitrated to 100 mg.

✪ Learning point Guidelines for the management of hypertension

The British Hypertension Society (BHS), along with the National Institute of Health and Clinical Excellence (NICE), have published guidelines for the management of hypertension as well as targets at which anti-hypertensive therapy should be initiated [1,2]. The use of ambulatory BP monitoring is indicated in cases of possible white coat hypertension, in the evaluation of medically refractory hypertension, for the evaluation of symptomatic hypotension, and for the diagnosis and treatment of hypertension in pregnancy.

continued

All patients should ideally have a urine dipstick performed for blood and protein, a serum creatinine and electrolytes, fasting blood glucose and lipid profile, and an ECG.

Treatment should be commenced based on a BP of >140/90 mmHg and in the presence of evidence of target organ damage, cardiovascular complications, or diabetes. If there are no associated complications or risk factors, the patient may be reassessed yearly. In cases of a BP >160/100 mmHg, anti-hypertensive therapy should be commenced immediately. Optimal BP control should aim to maintain BP at a value <140/85 mmHg in non-diabetic patients and <130/80 mmHg in diabetic patients.

Lifestyle modification plays an important role in the management of hypertension and patients should aim to maintain a normal weight (aiming for a body mass index [BMI] of 20–25). Sodium intake should be reduced to <100 mmol (2.3 g)/day which is roughly equivalent to 6 g of salt/day and alcohol consumption should be restricted to less than three units per day for men and less than two units per day for women. Patients should take regular aerobic exercise for 30 minutes at least three times per week and should reduce their daily intake of total and saturated fats.

The approach to anti-hypertensive therapy depends on both patient age and ethnic group. For patients under the age of 55 years, first-line therapy should be with an ACE inhibitor (A) with the addition of either a diuretic or calcium channel blocker (A+C or A+D). In those over the age of 55 years or Afro-Caribbean patients of any age, first-line therapy should be either a calcium channel blocker or diuretic (C or D) with the addition of an ACE inhibitor, if necessary. For both groups, inadequate BP control requires the use of all three agents (A+C+D) with the addition of further diuretic therapy (spironolactone, eplerenone, or amiloride), an alpha-blocker, or a beta-blocker, if necessary.

Despite multiple anti-hypertensive agents, his BP control remained poor with clinic readings of 191/106 mmHg and home BP readings averaging 172/80 mmHg. For this reason, doxazosin was added at a dose of 16 mg od. His serum potassium remained low despite eplerenone at a dose of 100 mg per day and potassium supplementation. His renal function deteriorated slowly to the point of grade 3 chronic kidney disease with a serum creatinine of 203 micromol/L. A repeat CT scan of the adrenal glands again showed a low attenuation lesion between the two limbs of the right adrenal gland, measuring 2.2 x 1.5 cm, with no significant change from the previous scan.

⭐ **Learning point** Hypertension and ethnic group

Afro-Caribbean patients tend to develop hypertension at an earlier age and target organ damage differs from Caucasian patients. Several studies have confirmed that renin activity is lower in both normotensive and hypertensive Afro-Caribbean subjects than in the Caucasian population [3,4]. Afro-Caribbean patients demonstrate a lower nephron mass as well as an amino acid substitution in the epithelial sodium ion channel, contributing to low-renin hypertension [5]. This difference in renin activity explains in part the difference in response pattern to therapy between Caucasian and Afro-Caribbean patients. Low-renin hypertension predicts a better response to calcium channel blockers and diuretics (C and D group) than to ACE inhibitors and beta-blockers (A and B group). Afro-Caribbean patients demonstrate a poorer response to treatment with ACE inhibitors compared to white people, as demonstrated in ALLHAT [6]. The evidence of beta-blockers being less effective is also clear-cut [7]. Diuretics, however, are more effective in young Afro-Caribbean patients, both because of the role of salt in causing hypertension and because there is less of a compensatory increase in renin than in Caucasian patients. This is reflected in the current NICE guidelines which specify first-line therapy based both on age and ethnicity.

In view of the persistent hypokalaemia and suboptimal BP control, it was felt that the patient was at significant risk of developing a stroke and at great risk of developing atrial fibrillation (AF), which would greatly increase his risk of stroke and would necessitate the addition of warfarin. For these reasons, the patient was referred for consideration of a laparoscopic adrenalectomy.

⊗ **Learning point** Risk of stroke in hypertension

Hypertension is a major risk factor for stroke with epidemiological studies demonstrating a 3-fold increased risk. This risk is greater in patients with AF. Lowering of BP is effective in reducing the risk of stroke. However, the strongest evidence for stroke reduction is associated with the use of an ACE inhibitor for BP control. In PROGRESS, the use of perindopril in combination with indapamide reduced stroke risk by 43%, compared with a 32% reduction in stroke with ramipril in the HOPE study [9,10]. In the ALLHAT study, prevention of stroke was the secondary focus of the study, hence results should be interpreted with some caution [6]. The finding that diuretics were superior to the other classes of anti-hypertensive agents was driven mainly by the benefits in Afro-Caribbean patients.

⊗ **Learning point** Risk of atrial fibrillation

In general population studies, hypertension is an independent risk factor for AF with an increased risk of between 1.4 and 1.9 times. Age, left ventricular mass, and left atrial dilatation have been shown to be independent predictors of AF development in essential hypertension. The role of ACE inhibitors in the prevention of morbidity and mortality in patients with hypertensive heart disease is well accepted. Vasodilators potentially slow the progression of left ventricular diastolic dysfunction and potentially result in beneficial effects on left atrial remodelling. However, drugs that modify the activity of the renin-angiotensin-aldosterone system appear to have effects over and above load reduction. In animal studies of LVH, ACE inhibitor therapy has been shown to reduce cardiac fibrosis (in particular, atrial fibrosis) and AF episode duration. ACE inhibition also has beneficial effects on atrial stretch, interstitial fibrosis, and electrical remodelling, and has been shown to delay or defer first and recurrent episodes of AF in patients with hypertension.

In patients with primary hyperaldosteronism, hypokalaemia is often associated with cardiac arrhythmias in those patients who also have cardiac ischaemia, heart failure, or LVH. Several case reports describe the development of symptomatic paroxysmal AF coinciding with episodes of hypokalaemia in such patients with resolution of the arrhythmia upon correction of the serum potassium level. In this group of patients, it is important to frequently monitor and correct serum potassium levels, particularly before commencing anti-arrhythmic therapy.

Discussion

Hypertension affects approximately 28% of women and 31% of men in the United Kingdom (UK) with an increase in prevalence with age. Cardiovascular morbidity and mortality increase as both systolic and diastolic BP rise, but in individuals over the age of 50 years, the systolic pressure and pulse pressure are better predictors of complications than diastolic pressure. Since BP readings in many individuals are highly variable (especially in the hospital setting), the diagnosis of hypertension should be made only after noting a mean elevation on two or more readings on two or more visits, unless the elevation is severe and associated with comorbid conditions such as diabetes mellitus, chronic kidney disease, heart failure, stroke, or a high risk of coronary artery disease. Ambulatory BP monitoring may be helpful in patients with borderline or variable readings as well as in assessing resistant hypertension. Although only 5–10% of patients will have an underlying cause for their hypertension, this represents a potentially curable condition. In these cases, the history, examination, and laboratory investigations may identify patients who warrant further investigation for secondary hypertension.

✦ **Expert comment**

The target BP laid down by BHS and other guideline committees of around 140/80 mmHg is mainly based on the results of the Hypertension Optimal Treatment (HOT) trial [8]. The main problem is that this trial was based on reducing the diastolic BP. The systolic target is therefore less certain. There is now, however, a general consensus that 'systolic BP is all that matters'.

Examination of the in-trial BP in large numbers of hypertensive patients randomized into the many anti-hypertensive treatment trials reveals that the optimum systolic BP in the long term is around 120 mmHg. The weakness of this observation is that it is not based on a dedicated trial of differing targets.

There is now increasing awareness that the most important predictor of cardiovascular events is the BP measured at home, either by self-monitoring or with 24-hour ambulatory monitoring. A single one-off BP reading by a harassed clinician in a busy clinic is almost useless information. Patients should be encouraged to purchase their own automatic BP machine and they need instructions on how to monitor their pressure, i.e. three readings 60 seconds apart in a silent room with the arm supported and all readings recorded. With home monitoring, many patients will be shown to have good BP control at all times except when they are visiting their doctor. In some patients, it may be possible to reduce the number of tablets they need to take.

> **A final word from the expert**
>
> Primary aldosteronism, whether due to an aldosterone-producing adenoma (APA) or to idiopathic hyperaldosteronism (IHA), is much commoner than phaeochromocytoma. The average general practitioner (GP) in the UK should expect to have two or three such patients on his or her list. Unfortunately, the diagnosis is often missed. Almost all published series report long delays between the patient being detected as hypertensive and underlying APA or IHA being diagnosed. There is an inverse correlation between the duration of known hypertension and the response to adrenalectomy or the use of aldosterone receptor antagonists (usually spironolactone). A late diagnosis leads to a poorer response to treatment. This may be due to structural damage to the peripheral arterioles as a consequence of a longstanding high BP.
>
> Clinicians should respond to serum potassium being persistently in the lower part of the normal range in the absence of diuretic therapy when it is associated with a serum sodium in the upper part of the normal range. Don't wait until there is overt hypokalaemia.
>
> Patients with primary aldosterone excess have a greatly increased risk of heart attack and stroke as well as AF when compared to patients with essential hypertension and similar BP levels. If a clinician encounters a hypertensive patient with AF, but with evidence of structural changes on echocardiography, then a diagnosis of aldosterone excess should be considered. A critical look at the plasma electrolyte profile as above is all that is necessary.
>
> Management of hypertension should take into account the patient's age and ethnic group, particularly when considering first-line anti-hypertensive therapy. This is reflected in the guidelines from BHS (2004) [2] and NICE (2006) [1] which advocate the use of a diuretic or calcium channel blocker as first-line therapy in Afro-Caribbean patients and older patients. In contrast to previous guidelines, beta-blockers are no longer included for first-line therapy based on the evidence that they perform less well than other drugs, particularly in the elderly, along with increasing evidence for an unacceptably high risk of provoking type 2 diabetes when these agents are used at usual doses.
>
> Several trials have assessed the effects of different anti-hypertensive agents on cardiovascular morbidity and mortality. The HOT trial demonstrated a low rate of cardiovascular events with intensive BP lowering [8]. Trials of ACE inhibitor therapy such as HOPE, EUROPA, and PROGRESS have shown substantial reductions in cardiovascular disease events, accompanied by reductions in BP [9-11]. The benefits of BP lowering in the elderly have recently been established with the publication of the HYVET trial which demonstrated a significant reduction in stroke, heart failure, and total mortality [12].
>
> When comparing individual anti-hypertensive agents, very little difference in cardiovascular outcomes was observed when comparing older regimes (diuretic- or beta-blocker-based) with newer regimes (based on ACE inhibitor and calcium channel blocker therapy). In the ALLHAT series of trials, four different anti-hypertensive agents were compared to assess their effect on both non-fatal and fatal myocardial infarction. The alpha-blocker limb was stopped prematurely due to an excess of combined cardiovascular events (primarily an increase in heart failure), but the remaining three limbs showed no significant difference in primary outcome or all-cause mortality after an average of 5 years' follow-up [6].
>
> In terms of other medications for hypertensive patients, two trials (ALLHAT and ASCOT) have recently reported cardiovascular outcomes associated with the use of statins in hypertensive patients [13,14]. In ALLHAT, statin therapy was associated with a non-significant reduction in cardiovascular events with no impact on all-cause mortality whereas ASCOT, in contrast, showed highly significant cardiovascular benefits independent of BP control. The Heart Protection Study (HPS) and the PROSPER study showed that the benefits of lipid lowering with statins in terms of preventing major coronary events were similar for hypertensive and normotensive patients [15,16]. However, the overall stroke risk was reduced by 15–30% with the use of statins in HPS, which is of particular importance in hypertensive patients. Since the 1999 guidelines, no new evidence regarding the use of aspirin in hypertensive patients has been produced, hence the guidelines remain unchanged. Aspirin should only be used in hypertensive patients for primary prevention in those older than 50 years whose BP is controlled and who have a baseline cardiovascular disease risk >20% over ten years [2].

References

1 National Institute for Health and Clinical Excellence. Management of hypertension in adults in primary care. NICE CG34 [issued 2006]. Available from: http://www.nice.org.uk.

2 Williams B, Poulter NR, Brown MJ, et al. Guidelines for management of hypertension: report of the fourth working party of the British Hypertension Society, 2004-BHS IV. *J Hum Hypertens* 2004; 18: 139–185.

3 Falkner B. Differences in blacks and whites with essential hypertension: biochemistry and endocrine. State of the art lecture. *Hypertension* 1990; 15: 681–686.

4 James GD, Sealey JE, Muller F, et al. Renin relationship to sex, race and age in a normotensive population. *J Hypertens Suppl* 1986; 4: S387–S389.

5 Baker EH, Dong YB, Sagnella GA, et al. Association of hypertension with T594M mutation in beta subunit of epithelial sodium channels in black people resident in London. *Lancet* 1998; 351: 1388–1392.

6 The ALLHAT Officers and Coordinators for the ALLHAT Collaborative Research Group: major outcomes in high-risk hypertensive patients randomized to angiotensin-converting enzyme inhibitor or calcium channel blocker vs diuretic: the Antihypertensive and Lipid-Lowering Treatment to Prevent Heart Attack Trial (ALLHAT). *JAMA* 2002; 288: 2981–2997.

7 Materson BJ, Reda DJ, Cushman WC, et al. Single-drug therapy for hypertension in men. A comparison of six anti-hypertensive agents with placebo. The Department of Veterans Affairs Cooperative Study Group on Anti-hypertensive Agents. *N Engl J Med* 1993; 328: 914–921.

8 Hansson L, Zanchetti A, Carruthers SG, et al. Effects of intensive blood pressure lowering and low-dose aspirin in patients with hypertension: principal results of the Hypertension Optimal Treatment (HOT) randomized trial. HOT Study Group. *Lancet* 1998; 351: 1755–1762.

9 PROGRESS Collaborative Group. Randomized trial of a perindopril-based blood pressure lowering regimen among 6,105 individuals with previous stroke or transient ischaemic attack. *Lancet* 2001; 358: 1033–1041.

10 Yusuf S, Sleight P, Pogue J, et al. Effects of an angiotensin-converting enzyme inhibitor, ramipril, on cardiovascular events in high-risk patients. The Heart Outcomes Prevention Evaluation Study Investigators. *N Engl J Med* 2000; 342: 145–153.

11 Fox KM. Efficacy of perindopril in reduction of cardiovascular events among patients with stable coronary artery disease: randomized, double-blind, placebo-controlled, multicentre trial (the EUROPA study). *Lancet* 2003; 362: 782–788.

12 Bloch MJ, Basile JN. Treating hypertension in the oldest of the old reduces total mortality: results of the Hypertension in the Very Elderly Trial (HYVET). *J Clin Hypertens (Greenwich)* 2008; 10: 501–503.

13 ALLHAT Officers and Coordinators for the ALLHAT Collaborative Research Group. The Antihypertensive and Lipid-Lowering Treatment to Prevent Heart Attack Trial. Major outcomes in moderately hypercholesterolemic, hypertensive patients randomized to pravastatin vs usual care: the Antihypertensive and Lipid-Lowering Treatment to Prevent Heart Attack Trial (ALLHAT-LLT). *JAMA* 2002; 288: 2998–3007.

14 Sever PS, Dahlof B, Poulter NR, et al. Prevention of coronary and stroke events with atorvastatin in hypertensive patients who have average or lower-than-average cholesterol concentrations, in the Anglo-Scandinavian Cardiac Outcomes Trial-Lipid Lowering Arm (ASCOT-LLA): a multicentre randomized controlled trial. *Lancet* 2003; 361: 1149–1158.

15 Heart Protection Study Collaborative Group. MRC/BHF Heart Protection Study of cholesterol lowering with simvastatin in 20,536 high-risk individuals: a randomized placebo-controlled trial. *Lancet* 2002; 360: 7–22.

16 Shepherd J, Blauw GJ, Murphy MB, et al. Pravastatin in elderly individuals at risk of vascular disease (PROSPER): a randomized controlled trial. *Lancet* 2002; 360: 1623–1630.

23 Syncope secondary to pulmonary arterial hypertension: an ominous sign?

Bejal Pandya and Shouvik Haldar

⊕ Expert commentary Dr Gerry Coghlan

Case history

A 32-year-old woman was referred to her local cardiologist having experienced three syncopal episodes in the preceding 12 months. She also complained of increasing breathlessness, such that she was breathless after one flight of stairs, and had been forced to reduce her dance classes from four sessions to one session per week. There was no other past medical or family history of note.

On examination, she was warm and well perfused. Her saturations at rest were 94% on air. She was tachypnoeic. Her heart rate was 124 beats per minute (bpm) and blood pressure (BP) 119/77 mmHg. The jugular venous pressure (JVP) was raised 3 cm above the sternal angle. There was a right ventricular (RV) heave in addition to a loud pulmonary component to the second heart sound (P2). There was no hepatomegaly or signs of peripheral oedema.

Her 12-lead electrocardiogram (ECG) showed normal sinus rhythm and evidence of RV hypertrophy (Figure 23.1). Her chest X-ray (CXR) revealed a ground glass appearance of both hemithoraces and enlarged pulmonary arteries (PA) (Figure 23.2).

> **⊕ Clinical tip** Examination findings in pulmonary hypertension
>
> - Loud pulmonary component to S2, palpable S2;
> - RV heave;
> - Pitting oedema or ascites;
> - Elevated JVP;
> - Pulmonary regurgitation murmur (Graham Steel).

Figure 23.1 ECG on admission (courtesy of Jonas de Jong).

✦ Expert comment

The clinical signs of pulmonary hypertension are often quite subtle and in some patients, absent. Unless specifically looked for in breathless patients, they are easily missed. Surveys show that patients are symptomatic for an average of over two years and see four or more doctors before a diagnosis of pulmonary hypertension is made.

✦ Expert comment

In idiopathic PAH (iPAH), the ECG is usually abnormal by the time of diagnosis. For some other types of PAH such as PAH associated with systemic sclerosis, ECG abnormalities are less common. The lung fields are usually clear in iPAH; the presence of ground glass abnormalities strongly suggests pulmonary hypertension secondary to lung disease.

✪ Learning point Definition of pulmonary arterial hypertension (PAH)

PAH is a disorder of pulmonary vessels that results in a progressive rise in pulmonary vascular resistance (PVR). It is haemodynamically defined by a mean pulmonary artery pressure (PAP) at rest ≥25 mmHg in the presence of a pulmonary capillary wedge pressure (PCWP) ≤15 mmHg.

✪ Learning point The electrocardiogram in pulmonary arterial hypertension

- Tall P waves suggesting atrial enlargement;
- Prominent R wave in precordial leads;
- Deep S waves in V5 and V6;
- Rightward axis;
- Right bundle branch block;
- RV strain (a pattern of asymmetric ST-segment depression and T wave inversion, typically seen in inferior and/or anterior leads).

Note: The ECG may be normal in early pulmonary hypertension.

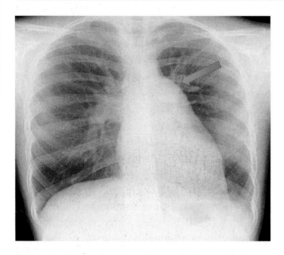

Figure 23.2 CXR on admission revealing a ground glass appearance in the lung fields and enlarged pulmonary arteries (arrow).

✦ Expert comment

Echocardiography is an important test in breathless patients, but can never be used as a diagnostic test. While some prognostic parameters have been identified, current two-dimensional techniques correlate very poorly with changes in RV function and thus provide very limited information on the tolerance of the right ventricle to increased workload in individual cases.

Transthoracic echocardiography (TTE) (Figure 23.3a-c) revealed normal intra-cardiac vascular connections with a dilated right atrium and an intact inter-atrial septum that bulged to the left. The right ventricle was dilated and reduced in systolic function. There was severe tricuspid regurgitation (TR), giving rise to an estimated PAP of 95 mmHg + right atrial pressure. The PA were dilated and there was mild pulmonary regurgitation. The four pulmonary veins returned unobstructed to the left atrium. The left ventricle was squashed and 'D'-shaped with good function. The aortic valve and aortic arch were normal.

✪ Learning point Echocardiographic findings in pulmonary arterial hypertension 2D

- Enlarged right-sided chambers (assessment of RA area should be made);
- RV hypertrophy and reduced RV function;
- Systolic flattening of the interventricular septum;
- 'D'-shaped left ventricle with reduced diastolic and systolic volumes, but often preserved function;
- Pericardial effusion;
- Mitral valve prolapse;
- Echocardiography may be normal in early PAH.

Colour Doppler
- Accurate assessment of PAP as TR peak velocity and right ventricular outflow tract (RVOT) acceleration times have linear correlations with PAP [1].

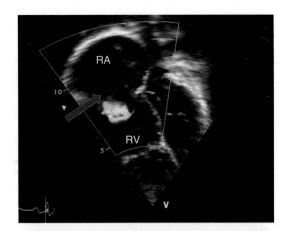

Figure 23.3a Transthoracic echocardiogram demonstrating a large jet of tricuspid regurgitation (arrow) between grossly dilated right atrium (RA) and ventricle (RV).

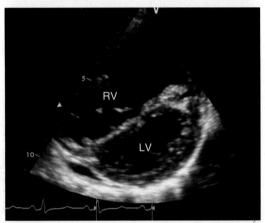

Figure 23.3b Characteristic D-shaped left ventricle (LV) as a result of a grossly dilated and pressure-overloaded RV.

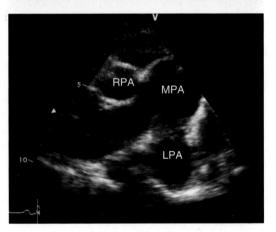

Figure 23.3c Grossly dilated right (RPA) and left (LPA) pulmonary arteries. MPA = main pulmonary artery.

- Tricuspid annular displacement (tricuspid annular plane systolic excursion [TAPSE]) of less than 1.8 cm is associated with greater RV systolic dysfunction [2]. For every 1 mm decrease in TAPSE, the unadjusted risk of death increases by 17%. Baseline TAPSE powerfully reflects RV function and prognosis in PAH.
- The right atrial volume index (RAVI) is a determinant of right-sided systolic dysfunction. This quantitative and reproducible echocardiographic marker provides an independent risk prediction of long-term adverse clinical sequelae [3].
- The LV eccentricity index and RV Doppler index also contribute prognostic information.
- The estimated PAP from TR velocity, however, does not provide prognostic information.

➕ **Clinical tip** The 6-minute walk test

- Used to measure functional capacity, but can predict morbidity and mortality;
- Variables measured include distance, oxygen saturations, and evidence of fatigue;
- Widely used to measure response to therapeutic interventions.

🔖 **Expert comment**

This patient will also have undergone further assessments, including a history of anorexogen or stimulant consumption, abdominal ultrasonography (cirrhosis of the liver or portal hypertension), blood testing for HIV, antibody profile, including extractable nuclear antigens, and for antiphospholipid syndrome, in addition to lung function testing, before making a firm diagnosis. A three-generation family history for premature death would have been taken. If positive, this would lead to a genetic assessment for hereditable pulmonary hypertension.

To assess functional status, the patient underwent a 6-minute walk test (6MWT). She managed 450 metres with saturations remaining unchanged at 94%. Her heart rate increased from 71 to 121 bpm.

She was admitted to a specialist tertiary centre for further imaging and investigations in order to identify the cause of her elevated PAP. Interestingly, although presenting with class II exercise limitation, her functional capacity was deemed to be class IV in view of the recent history of syncope (Table 23.1).

⭐ **Learning point** Mechanism of syncope in pulmonary arterial hypertension

- In essence, this reflects acute right heart failure.
- The mechanism of syncope is related to diastolic pressure rising in the right ventricle under exertion. This in turn results in a reduced pulse pressure of the right heart, which leads to an overall reduction in systemic pressure. This can ultimately lead to cerebral hypoperfusion and hence syncope.

The patient underwent a series of routine haematological, biochemical, and serological investigations to help classify her disease (Table 23.2). These ruled out connective tissue disease, human immunodeficiency virus (HIV) infection, and metabolic disorders. The echocardiogram had already eliminated significant left heart disease and valvular disorders. Pulmonary function tests did not show evidence of restrictive or obstructive lung disease. A collateral history excluded the use of drugs that could have led to pulmonary hypertension such as 'diet' pills and appetite suppressants (e.g. fenfluramine).

Table 23.1 Functional assessment of patients with pulmonary arterial hypertension [4]

Class I
Patients with pulmonary hypertension, but without resulting limitation of physical activity. Ordinary physical activity does not cause undue dyspnoea or fatigue, chest pain or near syncope.

Class II
Patients with pulmonary hypertension, resulting in slight limitation of physical activity. These patients are comfortable at rest, but ordinary physical activity causes undue dyspnoea or fatigue, chest pain or near syncope.

Class III
Patients with pulmonary hypertension, resulting in marked limitation of physical activity. These patients are comfortable at rest, but less than ordinary physical activity causes undue dyspnoea or fatigue, chest pain or near syncope.

Class IV
Patients with pulmonary hypertension, resulting in inability to perform any physical activity without symptoms. These patients manifest signs of right heart failure. Dyspnoea and/or fatigue may be present at rest and discomfort is increased by any physical activity. Syncope may occur.

Modified from the New York Heart Association classification of patients with cardiac disease.

Case 23 Syncope secondary to pulmonary arterial hypertension: an ominous sign?

227

Table 23.2 Classification of pulmonary arterial hypertension [5]

Type	Specific disorders
PAH	Hereditable
	Idiopathic
	Associated with connective tissue/HIV/congenital heart disease/ metabolic disorders/drugs/haemoglobinopathies
PAH with left heart disease	LA or LV disorders
	Valvular heart disorders
PAH associated with lung disorders	Chronic obstructive pulmonary disease, high altitude, interstitial lung disease, sleep disordered breathing
PAH due to chronic thrombotic/embolic disease	Pulmonary thromboembolism, tumours, parasites, foreign body
Miscellaneous	Fibrosing mediastinitis
	Lymphangiomatosis
	Pulmonary Langerhans' cell granulomatosis (histiocytosis)

Adapted from the Updated Clinical Classification of Pulmonary Hypertension (Dana Point, 2008)

The patient proceeded to a computed tomography (CT) scan of her thorax. This confirmed central pulmonary arterial dilatation with peripheral pruning of the pulmonary arteries in keeping with established PAH. The lung parenchyma exhibited a marked nodular ground glass appearance within the vicinity of the enlarged centri-lobular pulmonary arteries. No thrombus was seen within the central or peripheral pulmonary vessels. The scan confirmed PAH, but did not reveal any further information as to its aetiology (Figure 23.4a-b).

Right and left heart catheterization were performed with pressures recorded at baseline and after the administration of oxygen and nitric oxide (Table 23.3). Measurements were taken from the right atrium and ventricle, pulmonary arteries, and

Expert comment

A nodular ground glass abnormality is not usually a finding in iPAH, but appears in this patient to be localized. If pulmonary function testing shows no significant abnormality, one can exclude severe lung disease-associated PAH. An expert review of the scans may then reveal whether these changes simply reflect mosaic perfusion. High resolution CT abnormalities due to pulmonary veno-occlusive disease or pulmonary capillary haemangiosis must also be considered (thickened septal lines with fissural thickening) as these conditions have a very different prognosis and response to therapy.

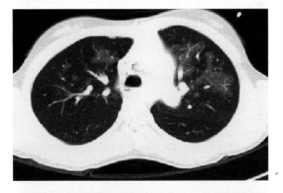

Figure 23.4a CT thorax demonstrating ground glass appearance in both lung fields.

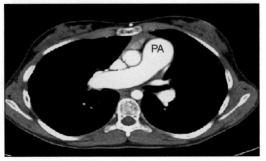

Figure 23.4b CT thorax demonstrating a grossly dilated main pulmonary artery (PA).

Expert comment

This patient meets the criteria for a positive acute responder. The mean PAP has fallen by more than 10 mmHg (23 mmHg) to reach a post-vasodilation mean PAP (mPAP) of <40 mmHg (36 mmHg) with preservation of cardiac output (as evidenced by the increase in PA saturation). The PCWP of 11 mmHg excludes significant left heart disease.

The near normalization of mPAP to 23 mmHg is typical of a classical acute responder. In rare cases such as this, a trial of a high-dose calcium channel blocker (CCB) (increasing doses of diltiazem up to 720 mg/day) over 6–12 weeks should be tried. Repeat catheterization on a CCB is essential as only 50% of patients with an acute response have a persistent response and the prognosis remains poor if CCB therapy is continued, unless the PAP falls dramatically on treatment.

Table 23.3 Cardiac catheterization data

Condition	Site	Pressure (mmHg)	Oxygen saturations (%)
Baseline	RV	85 (EDP 15)	73
Baseline	RA	17	
Baseline	mPAP	59	68
Baseline	PCW	11 (mean)	
Baseline	LV	87 (EDP 14)	96
Baseline	PVR	4.1 MPa·s/m³	
Baseline	Cardiac index	3.2	
PVR O₂/NO	RV	53 (EDP 9)	
PVR O₂/NO	mPAP	36	73
PVR O₂/NO	LV	91 (EDP 8)	99
PVR O₂/NO	PVR	2.9 MPa·s/m³	
PVR O₂/NO	Cardiac index	2.2	

Normal PAP is 25/15 mmHg. The mean value ranges from 12 to 16 mmHg.

left ventricle, and a mean PCWP was obtained. The cardiac output and index were calculated. The RV systolic pressures were near systemic (85 mmHg compared to LV pressure of 87 mmHg), suggesting that there was evidence of high PVR. The mean pressures dropped significantly (from 59 to 36 mmHg) with vasodilatation. Vasodilatation also improved the patient's oxygen saturations from 68 to 73% in the PA whilst dropping PVR from a baseline of 4.1 to 2.9. The cardiac index also reduced from 3.2 to 2.2 post-vasodilation. These results confirmed a diagnosis of iPAH.

Learning point Wood units explained

- Standard units for measuring vascular resistance are dyn·s·cm⁵ or pascal seconds per cubic metre (Pa·s/m³);
- Cardiologists use hybrid reference units (HRU) called Wood units to simplify the measurement of PVR using pressures instead of more complicated units;
- To convert from Wood units to Pa·s/m³, you must multiply by 8 or to dyn·s·cm⁵, you must multiply by 80.

Learning point Calculation of pulmonary vascular resistance

- 80 x (mPAP – PCWP)
- Cardiac output
- The pressures are measured in mmHg and the cardiac output is measured in L/min. The PCWP approximates to the left atrial pressure.
- Therefore, the numerator of the above equation is the pressure difference between the input to pulmonary blood circuit (where the right ventricle connects to the pulmonary trunk) and the output of the circuit (which is the input to the left atrium of the heart).

A transeptal puncture and balloon atrial septostomy (Figure 23.5) was conducted after the vasodilator testing to offload the right heart. Although this procedure is generally reserved as a bridge to lung transplantation, it was conducted at this early stage in view of the patient's syncope and right heart pressures.

Learning point Balloon atrial septostomy

- Generally reserved as a palliative procedure or as a bridge to transplantation;
- Benefits patients with deteriorating conditions or those in extremis;
- It allows inter-atrial right-to-left shunting to help decompress the right heart;
- Increases LV preload and cardiac output.

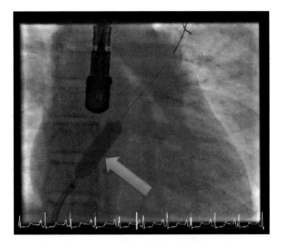

Figure 23.5 Right coronary angiogram illustrating inflated atrial septostomy balloon (arrow).

❝ Expert comment

Atrial septostomy is regarded as a particularly effective intervention for preventing syncope in PAH as it helps to maintain cardiac output even when the flow through the lungs is critically embarrassed. The increased shunting leads to worsening of cyanosis, but as long as the systemic saturations are kept in the 80s or above, the increase in cardiac output has been shown to compensate more than adequately with increased tissue oxygen delivery.

With the confirmation of iPAH and a positive vasodilator response, a central venous (Hickman) line was implanted. Prostacyclin therapy was commenced through this with a continuous infusion of epoprostenol which was uptitrated accordingly. The patient started to feel more energetic although a repeat TTE still revealed impaired RV function with a TR velocity of 4 m/s. She was discharged home a week after commencing epoprostenol on long-term oral anticoagulation and a CCB (amlodipine).

⊕ Clinical tip 'Responders'

- Patients are subjected to vasodilator testing with substances such as nitric oxide or adenosine and those who demonstrate vasodilatation to this challenge are shown to have long-term benefits and better prognosis on vasodilator therapy.
- A positive acute responder is defined as those demonstrating a reduction in mPAP of >10 mmHg to reach an absolute mean of <40 mmHg with increased or unchanged cardiac output.
- Only up to 10% of patients with PAH demonstrate significant pulmonary vasoreactivity and of these responders, up to 50% do not demonstrate sustained vasodilation and require repeat catheterization.

✪ Learning point

Standard medical therapy for pulmonary arterial hypertension

Diuretics and oxygen
- Diuretic treatment and supplemental oxygen are indicated in cases of fluid retention and hypoxaemia, respectively. Oxygen should be used to maintain saturations above 90% [6].
- There is no evidence for either of these, but they remain important.
- Monitor potassium levels when using loop diuretics; patients may require supplementation or conversion to potassium-sparing diuretics.

Calcium channel blockers
- CCBs act on the vascular smooth muscle to dilate the pulmonary resistance vessels and lower the PAP.
- They have both clinical and haemodynamic benefits [7].
- CCBs improve the quality of life and mortality in patients who are proven to respond to them.
- CCBs can be potentially deleterious in the absence of a positive sustained vasodilator response and should not be used in these cases.
- Commonly used CCBs are nifedipine, diltiazem, and amlodipine with particular emphasis on the first two.
- High doses are required, i.e. up to 120–240 mg/day for nifedipine, 240–720 mg/day for diltiazem, and up to 20 mg of amlodipine.
- Start with low doses (i.e. 30 mg of extended-release nifedipine bd, or 60 mg of diltiazem tds, or 5 mg of amlodipine od) and then uptitrate cautiously and progressively in the subsequent weeks to the maximal tolerated dose.

Oral anticoagulation
- Oral anticoagulation is proposed for all patients since several retrospective studies have shown a mortality benefit.
- No randomized controlled trials of oral anticoagulation in PAH exist; thus the data are mostly consensus-driven rather than based on prospective evidence-based medicine.

Digoxin
- Digoxin produces a modest increase in cardiac output in patients with PAH and RV failure as well as a significant reduction in circulating norepinephrine.
- No detectable effects of digoxin on baroreceptor responsiveness are apparent.
- It does not reduce PAP [8].
- There are no randomized trial data evaluating the use of digoxin.

Over the next few months, the patient's breathlessness worsened and became associated with chest discomfort on exertion, but no further syncopal episodes were reported. Repeat TTE and CT scanning showed no deterioration of RV systolic pressure. Her PAH treatment was intensified with the addition of bosentan and sildenafil to her ongoing therapy of epoprostenol.

Learning point

Disease-targeted medical therapy [10]

Prostacyclin analogue; epoprostenol
- Has potent vasodilatory properties, an immediate onset of action, and a half-life of approximately five minutes;
- Also inhibits platelet aggregation and smooth muscle proliferation, which may be beneficial in favourably remodelling the pulmonary vasculature;
- Administered as a continuous intravenous infusion because of its short half-life [11].

Prostacyclin analogue; treprostinil
- Structurally very similar to epoprostenol, but has a much longer half-life;
- Therefore, can be given as a subcutaneous infusion via a much smaller pump;
- Elicits direct vasodilation of the pulmonary and systemic arterial vessels and inhibits platelet aggregation;
- Vasodilation reduces RV and LV afterload and increases cardiac output and stroke volume.

Phosphodiesterase inhibitor; sildenafil
- Promotes selective smooth muscle relaxation in lung vasculature by inhibiting phosphodiesterase type-5;
- Results in subsequent reduction of PAP and increases cardiac output;
- Adult dose is 20 mg tds [12].

Phosphodiesterase inhibitor; tadalafil
- Type-5 inhibitor, increases cyclic GMP, the final mediator in the nitric oxide pathway;
- Well tolerated, improves exercise capacity and quality of life measures, and reduces clinical worsening [13].

Inhaled vasodilators; iloprost
- Inhaled synthetic prostacyclin analogue that dilates systemic and pulmonary arterial vascular beds;
- Indicated for PAH World Health Organization (WHO) class I patients with New York Heart Association (NYHA) class III or IV symptoms to improve exercise tolerance and symptoms and delay clinical deterioration [14].

Endothelin receptor antagonists; bosentan
- Mixed endothelin A and endothelin B receptor antagonist that improves exercise capacity, decreases the rate of clinical deterioration, improves functional class and haemodynamics;
- Increases cardiac index with significant reduction in PAP and PVR, resulting in improved exercise capacity (as measured by the 6MWT) and symptoms;
- Evidence suggests that initial treatment with oral bosentan, followed by or with the addition of other treatments, does not adversely affect the long-term outcome compared with initial intravenous epoprostenol in patients with class III iPAH [15];
- There is also evidence to suggest that first-line bosentan therapy, followed by the addition of other disease-specific therapies as required, improves survival in patients with advanced PAH [16].

Endothelin receptor antagonists; ambrisentan
- Endothelin receptor antagonist indicated for PAH patients with WHO class II or III symptoms;
- Improves exercise capacity and decreases progression of clinical symptoms;
- Inhibits vessel constriction and elevation of BP by competitively binding to endothelin-1 A and B receptors (ET_A and ET_B, respectively) in endothelial and vascular smooth muscle;
- This leads to a significant increase in cardiac index associated with a significant reduction in PAP, PVR, and mean RA pressure [17].

Having intensified her disease-modifying therapy, a magnetic resonance imaging (MRI) scan was performed (Figure 23.6). This demonstrated a small atrial septal communication shunting right to left as expected post-septostomy. The right atrium and right ventricle were dilated and severely hypertrophied with global systolic

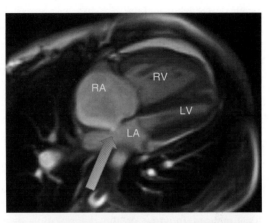

Figure 23.6a Cardiac MR scan demonstrating an inter-atrial communication (arrow) and dilated right atria and ventricle which is also significantly hypertrophied. LA = left atrium; LV = left ventricle; RV = right ventricle; RA = right atrium.

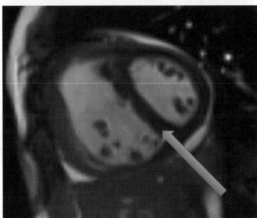

Figure 23.6b Flattened interventricular septum in diastole (arrow).

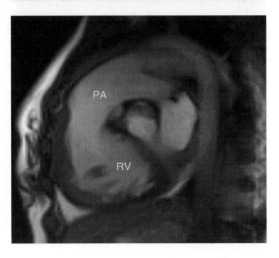

Figure 23.6c Cardiac MR revealing a grossly dilated main pulmonary artery. PA = pulmonary artery; RV = right ventricle.

dysfunction with a grossly dilated main pulmonary artery. There was paradoxical bowing of the IVS during systole and flattening in diastole. The MRI findings were consistent with progressive disease status and concurred with the patient's clinical status.

> ⭐ **Learning point** Lifestyle advice
>
> - **Physical activity**: Strenuous exercise is not recommended and weightlifting is contraindicated. Gentle exercise, however, should be encouraged. Rehabilitation has been shown to improve effort tolerance substantially.
> - **Smoking and diet**: Patients should maintain a healthy low-salt diet and stop smoking.
> - **Pregnancy and contraception**: Pregnancy should be avoided. Oestrogen-free contraception should be used.
> - **Fitness to fly**: High-altitude destinations should be avoided. Supplemental oxygen may be required if patient is deemed fit to fly.
> - **Saunas/steam rooms**: May cause dehydration and lower BP, leading to syncope and so should be avoided.

ℹ️ **Expert comment**

The 6MWT is an important test to monitor patient progress. Most patients who can walk more than 380 metres in six minutes have a good functional status and prognosis; however, as with all tests, it should never be judged in isolation.

At outpatient review six months later, the patient described reducing exercise tolerance and continued to be in NYHA class IV. She walked 430 metres during the 6MWT during which her saturations dropped from 96 to 80%. Repeat TTE showed worsening RV function. In view of the deterioration despite maximal medical therapy, she was referred to the cardiothoracic transplant team for consideration of bilateral lung transplantation vs heart–lung transplantation and currently remains on the transplant waiting list.

> ⭐ **Learning point** Transplantation
>
> - A single- or double-lung transplant is indicated for patients who do not respond to medical therapy.
> - Simultaneous cardiac transplantation may not be necessary even with severe RV dysfunction [18].
> - Prostacyclin therapy is an effective means of delaying the need for lung transplantation in patients with PAH and excellent results can be obtained when lung transplantation is performed after prostacyclin therapy [19].

Discussion

This case highlights the complexities of managing PAH. Patients with PAH can present with a variety of cardiorespiratory symptoms. Chest pain and syncope, as in this case, are ominous symptoms, suggesting significant disease progression.

The investigation of these patients is complex. Echocardiography can often raise the suspicion of PAH and provide aetiological and prognostic data. Additional investigations such as CT scanning, cardiac catheterization, and cardiac MRI provide additional diagnostic or prognostic information. Functional capacity assessment allows the patient to be classified prior to the commencement of medical therapy. Once treatment is commenced, these tests can also be used to monitor disease progression.

Pulmonary hypertension remains a difficult disease to treat. Medical therapy remains non-curative, but has reduced the morbidity dramatically and delayed progression to surgical transplantation. The mortality rate for untreated PAH is approximately 50% at three years. With the introduction of prostacyclin therapy, this has reduced to 35% at five years. Long-term results of the other medical therapies are still being evaluated.

Case 23 Syncope secondary to pulmonary arterial hypertension: an ominous sign?

233

As understanding of the molecular mechanisms in PAH increases, more and more novel treatments are being evaluated. These include anti-proliferative agents, stem cell therapy, and targeted RV treatments.

Sitaxentan, another endothelin receptor antagonist with a higher affinity for the ET_A receptor, has proven efficacy in the management of moderate to severe PAH in the STRIDE trials. The beneficial effects of sitaxentan therapy on exercise capacity and NYHA/WHO functional class were maintained up to two years after treatment [20].

In experimental and clinical PAH, tyrosine kinase inhibitors have been shown to reduce PAP. One study using the novel multikinase inhibitor, sorafenib, found beneficial effects with regard to reduced pulmonary remodelling with improved cardiac and pulmonary function in experimental PAH. Its effects are mediated via inhibition of the Raf kinase pathway in male rats, leading to direct myocardial anti-hypertrophic effects [21].

Rho-kinases (ROCKs) are effectors of the small G-protein RhoA and are involved in a variety of cellular functions, including muscle cell contraction and proliferation, and vascular inflammation. There is increasing evidence in animal models that suggests that heightened RhoA/ROCK signalling is important in the pathogenesis of PAH and ROCK inhibitors may be a promising new class of drug [22].

Deletion of the vasoactive intestinal peptide (VIP) gene leads to spontaneous expression of moderately severe PAH in mice. Although not an exact model of iPAH, the VIP$^{-/-}$ mouse could prove useful in studying the molecular mechanisms of PAH and evaluating potential therapeutic agents. VIP replacement therapy holds promise for the treatment of PAH and mutations of the VIP gene may be a factor in the pathogenesis of iPAH [23].

☻ A final word from the expert

Pulmonary hypertension is not a single diagnosis, rather a range of conditions that may be difficult to diagnose. Breathlessness is the dominant symptom that should lead to consideration of pulmonary hypertension and echocardiography is the most useful screening tool. Precise diagnosis requires extensive investigation and must include right heart catheterization. PAH is a progressive condition, associated with a poor prognosis. The designation of national referral centres has ensured seamless comprehensive investigation of patients with suspected PAH, followed by immediate treatment with the highly effective therapies that are currently available.

References

1 Stojnic BB, Brecker SJ, Xiao HB, et al. Left ventricular filling characteristic in pulmonary hypertension: a new mode of ventricular interaction. *Br Heart J* 1992; 68: 16–20.

2 Forfia PR, Fisher MR, Mathai SC, et al. Tricuspid annular displacement predicts survival in pulmonary hypertension. *Am J Respir Crit Care Med* 2006; 174: 1034–1041.

3 Sallach JA, Tang WH, Borowski AG, et al. Right atrial volume index in chronic systolic heart failure and prognosis. *JACC Cardiovasc Imaging* 2009; 2: 527–534.

4 Rich S, ed. Executive summary from the World Symposium on Primary Pulmonary Hypertension; 1998 Sep 6–10; Evian, France.

5 Simonneau G, Robbins IM, Beghetti M, et al. Updated clinical classification of pulmonary hypertension. *J Am Coll Cardiol* 2009; 54(1 Suppl): S43–S54.

6 Galiè N, Seeger W, Naeije R, et al. Comparative analysis of clinical trials and evidence-based treatment algorithm in pulmonary arterial hypertension. J Am Coll Cardiol 2004; 43: 81S–88S.

7 Rich S, Kaufmann E, Levy PS. The effect of high doses of calcium channel blockers on survival in primary pulmonary hypertension. *N Engl J Med* 1992; 327: 76–81.

8 Rich S, Seidlitz M, Dodin E, et al. The short-term effects of digoxin in patients with right ventricular dysfunction from pulmonary hypertension. *Chest* 1998; 114: 787–792.

9 Simonneau G, Rubin LJ, Galie N, et al. Safety and efficacy of sildenafil-epoprostenol combination therapy in patients with pulmonary arterial hypertension [abstract]. *Am J Respir Crit Care Med* 2007; 175: A300.

10 Badesch DB, Abman SH, Simonneau G, et al. Medical therapy for pulmonary arterial hypertension: updated ACCP evidence-based clinical practice guidelines. *Chest* 2007; 131: 1917–1928.

11 Sitbon O, Humbert M, Nunes H, et al. Long-term intravenous epoprostenol infusion in primary pulmonary hypertension: prognostic factors and survival. *J Am Coll Cardiol* 2002; 40: 780–788.

12 Simonneau G, Rubin LJ, Galiè N, et al; PACES Study Group. Addition of sildenafil to long-term intravenous epoprostenol therapy in patients with pulmonary arterial hypertension: a randomized trial. *Ann Intern Med* 2008; 149: 521–530.

13 Galiè N, Brundage BH, Ghofrani HA, Oudiz RJ, et al. Pulmonary Arterial Hypertension and Response to Tadalafil (PHIRST) Study Group. Circulation 2009; 119: 2894–2903.

14 Seybert A, Mathier MA. Evidence-based pharmacologic management of pulmonary arterial hypertension. *Clin Ther* 2007; 29: 2134–2153

15 Sitbon O, McLaughlin VV, Badesch DB, et al. Survival in patients with class III idiopathic pulmonary arterial hypertension treated with first-line oral bosentan compared with a historical cohort of patients started on intravenous epoprostenol. Thorax 2005; 60: 1025–1030.

16 McLaughlin VV. Survival in patients with pulmonary arterial hypertension treated with first-line bosentan. *Eur J Clin Invest* 2006; 36(Suppl 3): 10–15.

17 Liu C, Chen J. Endothelin receptor antagonists for pulmonary arterial hypertension. *Cochrane Database Syst Rev* 2006; 3: CD004434.

18 Manes A, Marinelli A, Palazzini M, et al. Pulmonary arterial hypertension. *G Ital Cardiol (Rome)* 2009; 10: 366–381.

19 Conte JV, Gaine SP, Orens JB, et al. The influence of continuous intravenous prostacyclin therapy for primary pulmonary hypertension on the timing and outcome of transplantation. *J Heart Lung Transplant* 1998; 17: 679–685.

20 Scott LJ. Sitaxentan *in pulmonary arterial hypertension. Drugs* 2007; 67: 761–770.

21 Klein M, Schermuly RT, Ellinghaus P, et al. Combined tyrosine and serine/threonine kinase inhibition by sorafenib prevents progression of experimental pulmonary hypertension and myocardial remodelling. *Circulation* 2008; 118: 2081–2090.

22 Barman SA, Zhu S, White RE. RhoA/Rho-kinase signalling: a therapeutic target in pulmonary hypertension. *Vasc Health Risk Manag* 2009; 5: 663–671.

23 Said SI, Hamidi SA, Dickman KG, et al. Moderate pulmonary arterial hypertension in male mice lacking the vasoactive intestinal peptide gene. *Circulation* 2007; 115: 1260–1268.

24 Cardiovascular preoperative risk assessment: a calculated gamble?

Joseph Tomson and Aung Myat

❝ **Expert commentary** Dr Derek Chin

Case history

The colorectal surgeons referred a 74-year-old male inpatient to cardiology for a preoperative cardiovascular assessment. The patient had presented with a 6-week history of abdominal pain and altered bowel habit. He had also noticed blood in his stools. On admission, his blood results showed a normocytic normochromic anaemia, but no other abnormalities (Table 24.1). His chest X-ray and electrocardiogram (ECG) were normal. He was diagnosed with a caecal tumour. Subsequent staging by computed tomography (CT) showed a T3N1M0 tumour. He was found to have an incidental infrarenal aortic aneurysm measuring 5.5 cm. An elective right hemicolectomy was planned.

> ✪ **Learning point** Cardiovascular risk estimation for non-cardiac surgery
>
> - Surgical risk varies with the length of procedure and potential haemodynamic imbalance;
> - Laparoscopic procedures can involve as much cardiac stress as open procedures;
> - **Low risk**: eye, dental, endocrine, gynaecology, reconstructive, minor urological and orthopaedic procedures;
> - **Intermediate risk**: ear/nose/throat, carotid, neurologic, pulmonary, abdominal, renal/liver transplant, major urological and orthopaedic procedures, percutaneous aortic/arterial procedures;
> - **High risk**: aortic and major vascular surgery, peripheral vascular surgery.

A day before surgery, the patient complained of central chest discomfort with radiation to the jaw. The episode lasted for 20 minutes at rest. It was relieved by two puffs of glyceryl trinitrate (GTN) spray. An ECG conducted at the time did not show any acute ischaemia. Troponin T levels were not elevated.

Table 24.1 Blood results on admission

Blood tests	Results
Hb	**10.0 g/dL**
MCV	84.0 fL
WCC	10.49 x 10^9/L
Platelets	**49 x 10^9/L**
Na	**133 mmol/L**
K	4.7 mmol/L
Urea	7.3 mmol/L
Creatinine	72 micromol/L
C reactive protein	9 mg/L
Liver function tests	Within normal range

✪ **Learning point** Active cardiac conditions

- Unstable angina;
- Acute heart failure;
- Significant cardiac arrhythmia;
- Symptomatic valvular disease;
- Myocardial infarction (MI) within 30 days and residual myocardial ischaemia.

✪ **Learning point** Clinical risk factors

- Angina pectoris;
- Prior MI;
- Heart failure;
- Stroke/transient ischaemic attack;
- Renal dysfunction (serum creatinine >170 micromol/L or creatinine clearance <60 mL/min);
- Insulin dependent diabetes mellitus.

On further assessment, the patient reported a history of stable angina, Canadian Cardiovascular Society (CCS) class I to II. Since his admission, his use of GTN spray had become more frequent. There was no history of palpitations, shortness of breath, orthopnoea, or paroxysmal nocturnal dyspnoea. He was found to be diabetic by his family doctor. He had a stroke ten years ago and was left with very limited hemiparesis. He smoked for 25 pack years and had quit ten years ago. He had a moderate alcohol intake of 20 units per week. He lived with his wife and normally kept himself busy with gardening at home. His functional capacity was deemed to be at least four metabolic equivalents (METs).

✪ **Learning point** Estimation of exercise and physical capacity: a simplified guide

- 1 MET: walking indoors, light house work;
- 4 METs: walking 100 m on the flat, climbing a flight of stairs;
- 7 METs: walking up 2 flights of stairs, playing a round of golf, lifting furniture;
- >10 METs: running while playing tennis or football, swimming.

✪ **Learning point** The Canadian Cardiovascular Society functional classification of angina [5]

A grading system that affords the clinician a quick and easy-to-remember method of categorizing patients according to the severity of their angina symptoms.

- **Class I: no limitation of ordinary activity**

Ordinary physical activity (e.g. walking or climbing stairs) does not cause angina. Angina may occur with strenuous rapid or prolonged exertion at work or recreation.

Exercise tolerance = 7–8 METs.

- **Class II: slight limitation of ordinary activity**

Angina may occur with:

  - Walking or climbing stairs rapidly;
  - Walking uphill;
  - Walking or stair-climbing after meals, in the cold, in windy conditions, or under emotional stress;

Exercise tolerance = 5–6 METs.

- **Class III: marked limitation of ordinary physical activity**

Angina may occur after:

  - Walking 1–2 blocks on the level or;
  - Climbing one flight of stairs in normal conditions at a normal pace.

Exercise tolerance = 3–4 METs.

- **Class IV: unable to carry out any physical activity without discomfort**

Angina may be present at rest.

Exercise tolerance = 1–2 METs.

His general examination revealed a right carotid bruit. His cardiovascular examination was unremarkable. His blood pressure (BP) was 130/70 mmHg and the pulse was regular at a rate of 74 beats per minute (bpm).

In view of the troponin-negative unstable angina, the patient underwent an exercise treadmill test. He completed three minutes and 15 seconds of the Bruce protocol. There was an appropriate increase in BP and heart rate, the latter to a peak of 95% maximum predicted for age. The test was stopped as it induced ischaemic ST-segment depression in the inferior leads. The patient had no angina, but complained of fatigue in his legs. An echocardiogram was performed and demonstrated good left ventricular function and no valvular defects. A subsequent diagnostic coronary angiogram (Figures 24.1 & 24.2) revealed severe triple-vessel coronary artery disease (CAD).

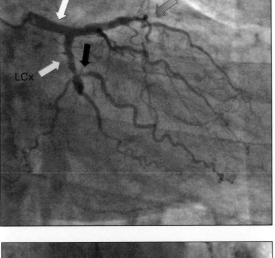

Figure 24.1 Coronary angiogram of the left coronary artery revealing an essentially normal left main stem (LMS) with slight tapering of its distal segment (white arrow), moderate diffuse disease of the left circumflex (LCx) artery (yellow arrow) with a tight ostial stenosis of its first obtuse marginal branch (red arrow), and an occluded left anterior descending (LAD) artery at its mid-segment (blue arrow).

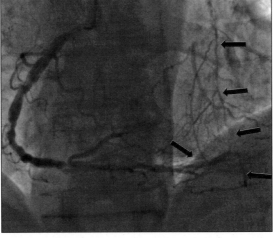

Figure 24.2 Coronary angiogram of the dominant right coronary artery demonstrating extensive diffuse disease along its entire length and branching collaterals from the distal segment to the occluded LAD (arrows).

This patient is scheduled to undergo intermediate-risk abdominal surgery. He developed unstable angina, an active cardiac condition. The algorithm (no to step 1, yes to step 2) directs us towards the investigation of coronary disease and discussion of its treatment in the context of a surgical delay. If the patient remained stable, his functional capacity of 4 METS would have allowed medical prophylaxis and surgery (no to steps 1–3, yes to step 4). There is no need for preoperative stress testing, even in the presence of three potential clinical risk factors.

ⓖ Expert comment

Peri-operative MI may be precipitated by coronary plaque rupture caused by operative stress. The culprit plaque may not be flow-limiting until it ruptures and is therefore undetectable by functional tests. The pathophysiology may be the reason why prophylactic revascularization directed at flow-limiting stenoses does not reduce peri-operative infarction in stable CAD.

✪ Learning point Utility of non-invasive stress testing

- Indications for non-invasive stress tests are generally the same when risk-stratifying a patient for a primary cardiac problem or non-cardiac surgery.
- Exercise tolerance testing helps to assess functional capacity, but may not be useful when activity is limited by frailty or non-cardiac disease.
- In those who are unsuitable for exercise treadmill testing, echocardiography, magnetic resonance, or radionuclide myocardial perfusion scans with pharmacological stress should be considered. There is some evidence to suggest that dobutamine stress echocardiography is superior to other imaging modalities; it has a high negative predictive value and a moderately positive predictive value in this setting [6,7]. Radionuclide scanning has a high sensitivity, but a lower specificity for the prediction of cardiac complications. Local facilities and expertise will determine the choice of non-invasive testing.

The case was discussed in an MDT meeting. Although the CAD was amenable to percutaneous coronary intervention (PCI), the impending elective hemicolectomy weighed against this approach. Drug-eluting stents (DES) were deemed necessary in view of the extensive disease on a background of diabetes and with that the need for a protracted course of dual antiplatelet therapy (DAPT) for at least 12 months. Surgical revascularization was therefore thought to be the best option. However, as this would also potentially delay the planned surgery, it was decided to treat the patient medically in the short term and consider surgical revascularization of his coronary arteries on an outpatient basis after the hemicolectomy.

✪ Learning point Cardiac interventions: when and what to do?

- Prophylactic coronary revascularization with coronary artery bypass grafting (CABG) or PCI in patients with stable CAD may not reduce cardiac events during non-cardiac surgery [8,9]. European and American guidelines, therefore, do not recommend routine revascularization in stable CAD patients prior to surgery. Preoperative interventions should be limited to the subset of high-risk unstable acute coronary syndrome patients.
- Bare metal coronary stenting: surgery should be deferred for ideally three months after implantation to allow adequate re-endothelialization. Clopidogrel can be discontinued after this period.
- Drug-eluting stents: DAPT cannot be discontinued for 12 months due to the risk of stent thrombosis [10]. DAPT will therefore prohibit some types of surgery for this period.
- Second- or third-degree atrioventricular block and trifascicular block merit prophylactic ventricular pacing during non-cardiac surgery.
- Cardiovascular risk associated with severe aortic stenosis is estimated to be around 10%. This risk is further increased by factors such as left ventricular dysfunction, diabetes, a raised creatinine, and the presence of unstable arrhythmias. If indicated, severe valve disease may be treated prior to non-urgent non-cardiac surgery.
- Patients with grown-up congenital heart (GUCH) disease or heart disease during pregnancy should ideally be operated upon in a specialist centre with a dedicated cardiac anaesthetist and input from the GUCH/cardiac specialist.
- Patients with implantable cardiac defibrillators (ICD) or pacemakers require device interrogation and programming in the peri-operative period. ICDs may need to be 'turned off' during surgery. Due care should be taken by theatre staff whilst using cautery/diathermy.
- Patients on warfarin for prosthetic valves or ventricular assist devices need to discontinue oral anticoagulation three days before surgery. They need to be pre-admitted for a 'bridging' intravenous infusion of unfractionated heparin (UFH) with the dose titrated to achieve the target activated partial thromboplastin time ratio. The UFH infusion can be stopped four hours before surgery and then restarted when deemed haemostatically safe by the surgeon. Low molecular weight heparin protocols have also been published. Warfarin is re-introduced at the earliest opportunity.
- Warfarin for atrial fibrillation patients can be omitted for three to five days prior to the planned procedure without a need for heparin bridging. It is restarted (at the normal daily dose) once post-operative bleeding risks have resolved.

His medications were reviewed. He was on aspirin, a statin, metformin, and an angiotensin-converting enzyme (ACE) inhibitor. A beta-blocker was initiated, aiming for a resting heart rate of around 60 bpm to reduce his angina burden, optimize the cardiac function, and prevent infarction. He then underwent a hemicolectomy which confirmed the diagnosis of caecal carcinoma. After a period of convalescence, he was listed for CABG.

⊘ **Learning point** Risk factor modification: medical prophylaxis

- **Beta-blockade:** protective mechanisms include plaque stabilization during catecholamine stress, preventing oxygen supply/demand mismatch, and anti-inflammatory effects. A large meta-analysis of studies involving more than 1,000 patients showed a beneficial reduction in peri-operative MI [12]. The POISE study which initiated short-acting beta-blockade two or four hours before surgery showed protection against MI, but an increased risk for hypotension, stroke, and overall mortality [13]. A long-acting beta-blocker should therefore be initiated a few weeks prior to surgery, aiming for a target heart rate of 60 bpm and target systolic BP >100 mmHg. The greatest benefit of beta-blockade is gained by the highest-risk surgical patients [14]. Beta-blockade should be maintained for several months after surgery to avoid late events. They should be used long-term in patients with CAD, hypertension, arrhythmia, and left ventricular dysfunction.
- **Statins**: reduce peri-operative cardiovascular risk. Studies have demonstrated up to 4-fold significant reduction in all-cause mortality [15,16]. Proposed mechanisms include atherosclerotic plaque stabilization, oxidative stress reduction, and a decrease in vascular inflammation. The benefit of reducing peri-operative cardiovascular risk outweighs the risk of side effects from statin therapy, i.e. myositis and hepatitis. Similar to patients with CAD, a sudden withdrawal of statin therapy is thought to be harmful [17]. Current recommendations suggest the initiation of a statin at least a week (ideally 30 days) prior to surgery and continuing this peri-operatively.
- **Aspirin:** the protective benefit of aspirin is unclear. However, peri-operative withdrawal of aspirin in CAD patients is associated with a 3-fold increase in cardiac events [18]. This must be balanced against a 1.5-fold increase in the risk of bleeding complications during surgery.

ℹ **Expert comment**

The DECREASE-V study showed that prophylactic revascularization did not improve peri-operative outcomes in drug-stabilized patients with multivessel obstruction, high ischaemic burden, and left ventricular dysfunction [11]. In such patients, revascularization decisions should be based on coronary factors and delayed till after non-cardiac surgery. Preoperative revascularization should be performed for drug-refractory unstable CAD and intervention should be directed at a culprit lesion. Most cases of unstable CAD will receive balloon angioplasty alone or bare metal stenting to avoid inappropriate delay of the non-cardiac surgery. Cardiac intervention should also be considered when the coronary, valvular, electrophysiologic, or cardiomyopathic prognosis takes precedence over that of the surgical condition and the delayed treatment of it. Intra-aortic balloon pumping, valvuloplasty, transcatheter aortic valve implantation, ablation, or resynchronization pacing can be used to reduce peri-operative risk.

Discussion

The frequency of post-operative cardiac complications after non-cardiac surgery is estimated at 0.5–2.5%; this is higher for patients undergoing vascular surgery (around 6%). In addition, most post-operative cardiac events are not heralded by symptoms. The pathophysiology of the increased cardiovascular risk is unclear, but plaque desta-bilization and a prothrombotic state have been postulated [19]. Urgency of surgery and the presence and stability of cardiac risk factors strongly determine what decisions are taken to modify risk. Medical therapy in the form of beta-blockade, statin therapy, and aspirin play an important role. Prophylactic coronary revascularization strategies are best reserved for those at very high risk, though the evidence is sparse.

💬 **A final word from the expert**

The American guidelines state that 'the goal of the consultation is to identify the most appropriate testing and treatment strategies to optimize care of the patient, provide assessment of short- and long-term cardiac risk, and avoid unnecessary and costly testing ... ' [3]. The published algorithms therefore focus the cardiologist on the surgical and clinical factors that determine which patients should undergo risk stratification with cardiac tests or proceed directly to cardiac intervention, or surgical treatment with cardiac prophylaxis. The ultimate aim of such an exercise should be to transfer a patient, having had the appropriate risk modification, in the best possible physical state to your anaesthetic and surgical colleagues.

References

1 Campeau L. Grading of angina pectoris (letter to the editor). *Circulation* 1976; 54: 522–523.

2 Poldermans D, Bax JJ, Boersma E, et al. Guidelines for preoperative cardiac risk assessment and peri-operative cardiac management in non-cardiac surgery: the Task Force for Preoperative Cardiac Risk Assessment and Peri-operative Cardiac Management in Non-cardiac Surgery of the European Society of Cardiology (ESC) and endorsed by the European Society of Anaesthesiology (ESA). *Eur Heart J* 2009; 30: 2769–2812.

3 Fleisher LA, Beckman JA, Brown KA, et al. ACC/AHA 2007 guidelines on peri-operative cardiovascular evaluation and care for non-cardiac surgery. A report of the American College of Cardiology/American Heart Association Task Force on Practice Guidelines (Writing Committee to Revise the 2002 Guidelines on Peri-operative Cardiovascular Evaluation for Non-Cardiac Surgery). *J Am Coll Cardiol* 2007; 50: e159–e241.

4 Detsky AS, Abrams HB, Forbath N, et al. Cardiac assessment for patients undergoing non-cardiac surgery. A multifactorial clinical risk index. *Arch Intern Med* 1986; 146: 2131–2134.

5 Lee TH, Marcantonio ER, Mangione CM, et al. Derivation and prospective validation of a simple index for prediction of cardiac risk of major non-cardiac surgery. *Circulation* 1999; 100: 1043–1049.

6 Kertai MD, Boersma E, Bax JJ, et al. A meta-analysis comparing the prognostic accuracy of six diagnostic tests for predicting peri-operative cardiac risk in patients undergoing major vascular surgery. *Heart* 2003; 89: 1327–1334.

7 Beattie WS, Abdelnaem E, Wijeysundera DN, et al. A meta-analytic comparison of preoperative stress echocardiography and nuclear scintigraphy imaging. *Anesth Analg* 2006; 102: 8–16.

8 McFalls EO, Ward HB, Moritz TE, et al. Coronary artery revascularization before elective major vascular surgery. *N Engl J Med* 2004; 351: 2795–2804.

9 Schouten O, van Kuijk JP, Flu WJ, et al. for the DECREASE Study Group. Long-term outcome of prophylactic coronary revascularization in cardiac high-risk patients undergoing major vascular surgery (from the randomized DECREASE-V Pilot Study). *Am J Cardiol* 2009; 103: 897–901.

10 Poldermans D, Hoeks SE, Feringa HH. Preoperative risk assessment and risk reduction before surgery. *J Am Coll Cardiol* 2008; 51: 1913–1924.

11 Poldermans D, Schouten O, Vidakovic R, et al. A clinical randomized trial to evaluate the safety of a non-invasive approach in high-risk patients undergoing major vascular surgery: the DECREASE-V pilot study. *J Am Coll Cardiol* 2007; 49: 1763–1769.

12 Schouten O, Shaw LJ, Boersma E, et al. A meta-analysis of safety and effectiveness of peri-operative beta-blocker use for the prevention of cardiac events in different types of non-cardiac surgery. *Coron Artery Dis* 2006; 17: 173–179.

13 Devereaux PJ, Yang H, Guyatt GH, et al. Rationale, design, and organization of the Peri-operative Ischaemic Evaluation (POISE) trial: a randomized controlled trial of metoprolol versus placebo in patients undergoing non-cardiac surgery. *Am Heart J* 2006; 152: 223–230.

14 Lindenauer PK, Pekow P, Wang K, et al. Peri-operative beta-blocker therapy and mortality after major non-cardiac surgery. *N Engl J Med* 2005; 353: 349–361.

15 Poldermans D, Bax JJ, Kertai MD, et al. Statins are associated with a reduced incidence of peri-operative mortality in patients undergoing major non-cardiac vascular surgery. *Circulation* 2003; 107: 1848–1851.

16 Dunkelgrun M, Boersma E, Schouten O, et al. for the Dutch Echocardiographic Cardiac Risk Evaluation Applying Stress Echocardiography Study Group. Bisoprolol and fluvastatin for the reduction of peri-operative cardiac mortality and myocardial infarction in intermediate-risk patients undergoing non-cardiovascular surgery: a randomized controlled trial (DECREASE-IV). *Ann Surg* 2009; 249: 921–926.

17 Le Manach Y, Godet G, Coriat P, et al. The impact of post-operative discontinuation or continuation of chronic statin therapy on cardiac outcome after major vascular surgery. *Anaesth Analg* 2007; 104: 1326–1333.

18 Biondi–Zoccai GG, Lotrionte M, Agostoni P, et al. A systematic review and meta-analysis on the hazards of discontinuing or not adhering to aspirin among 50,279 patients at risk for coronary artery disease. *Eur Heart J* 2006; 27: 2667–2674.

19 Mangano DT. Adverse outcomes after surgery in the year 2001—a continuing odyssey. *Anaesthesiology* 1998; 88: 561–564.

25 The role of cardiac rehabilitation following cardiac surgery

Imogen Clarke and Aung Myat

🎓 **Expert commentary** Dr Jane Flint

Case history

A 77-year-old gentleman presented to the Rapid Access Chest Pain Clinic with a month-long history of exertional central chest pain which had progressed to pain at rest in the last two weeks. He had a history of rheumatic fever as a child and stopped smoking ten years previously. On examination, the patient was pain-free and the chest was clear on auscultation. Both heart sounds were present as was a loud pansystolic murmur heard best at the lower left sternal edge. The patient was in rate-controlled atrial fibrillation (AF) confirmed by an electrocardiogram (ECG) which also revealed antero-lateral ST-segment depression. Given the classical history of unstable angina and corresponding ECG changes, he was admitted directly to the ward for further investigation and commenced on a standard acute coronary syndrome (ACS) treatment protocol. A 12-hour troponin T was found to be raised at 1.2 ng/mL.

Subsequent transthoracic echocardiogram (TTE) revealed mild to moderately impaired systolic function with mid and apical anterior and anteroseptal akinesia, giving rise to an aneurysmal apex. Ejection fraction (EF) was estimated at 50%. The TTE also demonstrated mild to moderate mitral stenosis (MS) with moderate to severe mitral regurgitation (MR) and a grossly dilated left atrium. The mitral valve was thickened and calcified with a virtually immobile posterior leaflet. The tricuspid valve was also mildly thickened and calcified with moderate tricuspid regurgitation (TR) and an estimated pulmonary artery pressure of 60 mmHg. Subsequent transoesophageal echocardiography (TOE) confirmed gross thickening of both mitral valve leaflets with flecks of calcium in a fixed posterior leaflet and in the chordae. The anterior leaflet was mobile with a severe central jet of MR. The left ventricular size was normal, but the septum and apex were akinetic.

The patient proceeded to an inpatient coronary angiography which revealed a normal left main stem, a 95% proximal left anterior descending (LAD) artery stenosis with a 60% lesion in the mid-segment, mild irregularities in a dominant left circumflex artery, and a recessive right coronary artery with significant disease in the proximal segment. Left ventriculogram confirmed anteroapical akinesis with an aneurysmal appearance and severe MR.

On the basis of these findings, the patient proceeded to an inpatient mitral valve repair, tricuspid valve annuloplasty, and coronary artery bypass graft (CABG) surgery with a left internal mammary artery (LIMA) graft to the LAD artery. The operation was performed without complication and the post-operative period remained uneventful. He was discharged home on the eighth post-operative day, having been commenced on long-term warfarin therapy given his age (i.e. > 65 years), persistent AF, and known ischaemic and valvular heart disease. It was also deemed prudent that the patient

Expert comment

The combined aetiology of the patient's heart disease needs especially careful explanation to him and clear patient understanding of the need to prevent both heart failure recurring and progression of coronary heart disease. He would be placed on both the coronary heart disease (CHD) and heart failure registers in primary care.

Cardiac rehabilitation programmes have concentrated to a greater extent on patients with ischaemic heart disease; education programmes must ensure they include appropriate coverage of heart failure and valve disease also. Patients with dual aetiology of heart disease need to understand their components in appropriate proportion.

Expert comment

A degree of heart failure in the post-operative recovery period would not be unexpected here, particularly given the demonstrated left ventricular systolic dysfunction preoperatively and the combined pathology of ischaemic and valvular heart disease.

continues on a year's course of clopidogrel following his preoperative non-ST-elevation myocardial infarction (NSTEMI).

He was referred to the community cardiac rehabilitation (CR) service and was first seen a month after discharge. By this point, however, his clinical condition had deteriorated. He was breathless on minimal exertion, complained of orthopnoea, and had also begun to develop significant peripheral oedema. He had a non-productive cough, but had had no chest pain. An acute hospital admission was arranged.

Examination revealed a blood pressure (BP) of 136/78 mmHg with AF on the ECG. Oxygen saturations were 93% on air with stony dullness at both bases and reduced breath sounds on auscultation. Chest X-ray (CXR) confirmed large bilateral pleural effusions (Figure 25.1). A working diagnosis of biventricular failure was postulated and as such, he was started on high-dose intravenous furosemide.

Repeat TTE demonstrated moderately impaired left ventricular function with an estimated EF of 42%. The tricuspid valve was mobile with mild TR and the mitral valve appeared to be opening well with no residual MR. There was no pericardial effusion. Routine blood tests revealed mildly raised inflammatory markers (Table 25.1). Warfarin was stopped at this stage and the patient converted to low molecular weight heparin in therapeutic doses.

Pleural fluid sampling from both sides of the chest revealed a uniformly exudative bloodstained effusion. There were no pus cells and no growth on microscopy and culture, respectively. No malignant cells were seen on cytological examination. Despite draining more than a litre from each pleural cavity through simple aspiration, the effusions quickly re-accumulated. Computed tomography pulmonary angiogram (CTPA)

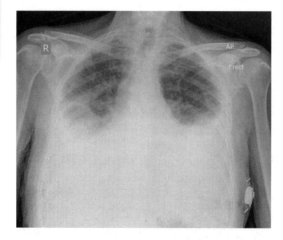

Figure 25.1 Chest radiograph on admission revealing large bilateral pleural effusions.

Table 25.1 Blood results on admission

Haematology	Biochemistry
Hb 11.7 g/dL	C reactive protein **22 mg/L**
MCV 94.3 fL	Albumin 37 g/L
White cell count 6.80×10^9/L	Bilirubin 7 micromol/L
Neutrophils 5.18×10^9/L	Alanine aminotransferase 29 IU/L
Lymphocytes **1.18×10^9/L**	
Platelets 331×10^9/L	
INR 1.2	

of the thorax was performed to rule out any other post-operative complications, but confirmed only bilateral pleural effusions with no evidence of pulmonary embolus, pulmonary or mediastinal infection, and no lung parenchymal or mesothelial masses.

A putative diagnosis of post-pericardiotomy (Dressler's) syndrome was made. Chest drains were inserted bilaterally to drain the effusions to dryness. On the right side, this resulted in subcutaneous emphysema and when removed, a small pneumothorax. This was managed conservatively and eventually settled (Figure 25.2).

Expert comment

Although the diagnosis of post-pericardiotomy syndrome is perfectly plausible here, the Dressler's syndrome may well have been caused by the initial index cardiac event which had lead to valve repair and CABG surgery.

Learning point Dressler's syndrome

Dressler first described the phenomenon of late onset pericarditis, leading to pericardial and pleural effusion in 1956 in the Journal of the American Medical Association [1]. He described ten case reports of people who had had myocardial infarctions (MIs) suffering a 'complication resembling idiopathic, recurrent, benign pericarditis'. This syndrome of late post-MI pericarditis is recognized to also affect those who are post-pericardotomy and with other forms of cardiac injury. It typically presents two to ten weeks after an MI or a pericardiotomy. It was initially estimated to have an incidence of 3–4% of MI patients, but this has vastly reduced since the onset of reperfusion therapy and, it has been postulated, because today's standard treatments like ACE inhibitors, beta-blockers, and statins have immunomodulatory effects [2,3]. Dressler's syndrome is believed to have an autoimmune aetiology caused by sensitization of myocardial cells at the time of injury. Antimyocardial antibodies have been detected [2]. Inflammation is diffuse unlike post-MI pericarditis. It is a diagnosis of exclusion and other diagnoses such as pulmonary embolism have to be considered as the population prone to Dressler's will also be at increased risk of thromboembolic disease. It is mainly self-limiting, but sometimes severe enough to warrant treatment in the form of aspirin, other non-steroidal anti-inflammatory drugs (NSAIDs) and occasionally, corticosteroids.

As the effusions, despite drainage, continued to re-accumulate, the decision was made to start a reducing course of steroids which resulted in a vast improvement in CXR appearances and clinical symptoms. Despite the resolution of his symptoms, the patient remained extremely anxious. This was exacerbated by his wife, for whom he was the main carer, being admitted to hospital.

Four days post-initiation of steroids, this anxiety appeared to take a stepwise deterioration and was now accompanied by stark paranoia. Psychiatric assessment suggested a combination of depression with some features of psychosis and the recommendation to continue on the antidepressants that had already been started earlier in the admission. A possible diagnosis of steroid psychosis was considered

Expert comment

The patient's prior carer status for his wife would have made him feel even more inadequate when his post-operative status deteriorated again secondary to Dressler's, and careful consideration would be needed to work out the best arrangements for the couple to rehabilitate together.

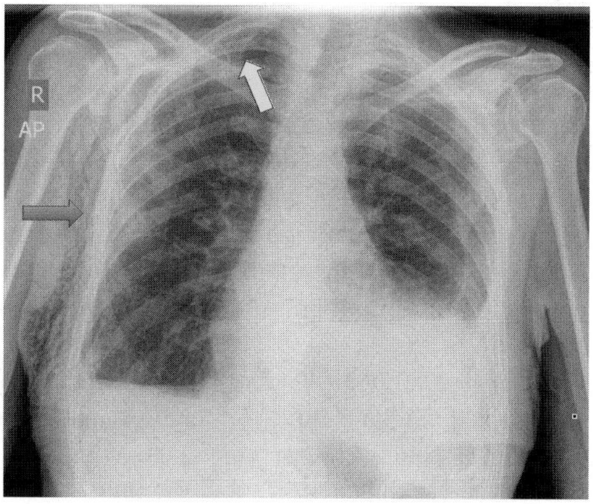

Figure 25.2 Chest radiograph post-chest drain removal demonstrating evidence of surgical emphysema (blue arrow) and a right-sided apical pneumothorax (yellow arrow).

although symptoms did not entirely correlate. The oral steroids were weaned down in any case. The patient was eventually discharged to a transitional care bed where he could be with his wife while they both continued their rehabilitation. Once home, he was again picked up by the CR service to ensure that he could continue on the programme set out for him.

Discussion

This patient was appropriately referred to the local community CR service after his surgery and completed phase one whilst still an inpatient. He then suffered setbacks both physically and mentally due to a rare complication and as such, his need for CR was even greater as it could provide the support required to overcome these barriers. However, the greatest obstacle to a full recovery could have been the question marks over his own commitment to participation; there was doubt as to whether he would actively engage in the process to allow himself to reap the full benefit.

> **Learning point** World Health Organization definition of cardiac rehabilitation
>
> 'The sum of activities required to influence favourably the underlying cause of the disease as well as to provide the best possible physical, mental, and social conditions so that they [patients] may, by their own efforts, preserve or resume when lost as normal a place as possible in the community' [4].

Patients are encouraged to be actively engaged in the CR process and become self-managers of their own illness [5]. It brings together exercise programmes, risk factor modification, psychological interventions, and patient education.

Historically, up until the 1950s, patients were prescribed extended periods of bed rest after an MI, with exercise being seen as ill-advised [6]. After this, researchers started to look at how progressive mobilization could actually be beneficial and by 1980, CR had become a standardized inpatient therapy post-infarct [6]. It has subsequently become part of ongoing outpatient treatment. The National Service Framework (NSF) for Coronary Heart Disease (CHD) has emphasized that CR, although seen as a service provided over and above those provided by primary care in the management of any chronic disease, should be seen as an integral component of both the acute stages of care and of secondary prevention [7]. It has also been expanded to include not just those who have suffered an MI, but also those who have undergone revascularization, either surgically or percutaneously.

Cardiac rehabilitation is a well established and evidence-based intervention that has led to significant reductions in both morbidity and mortality. A recent meta-analysis of 48 randomized controlled trials found that CR reduced all-cause mortality by 20% and cardiac mortality by 26% at two to five years [8]. It is cost-effective and forms part of many guidelines in the treatment of cardiovascular disease, including the NSF for CHD, Scottish Intercollegiate Guidelines Network (SIGN) guidance on cardiac rehabilitation, and NICE guidance on secondary prevention following an MI [9,10].

However, although evidence-based, the practice is constantly evolving and therefore, these guidelines have to include scope for flexibility as attitudes and knowledge changes. Recent developments have witnessed a shift towards standardization of services across the country, with the publication of the British Association for Cardiac

Expert comment

His anxiety and depression would be improved after full engagement with rehabilitation. He might, with the benefit of hindsight, have been considered for cognitive behavioural therapy in conjunction with National Institute for Health and Clinical Excellence (NICE) guidelines for the management of mild to moderate depression, but given he had an apparently severe depressive episode, psychiatric advice and medication was reasonable. An individual counselling approach should have been requested to address his pessimistic health beliefs concerning his recovery and future ability to support his wife.

Expert comment

An individually constructed rehabilitation programme should prescribe exercise within limits defined by the most limiting condition; the post-operative heart failure and Dressler's syndrome should dictate an initial lower intensity start to exercise, building the patient and his confidence up gradually to optimize benefit and compliance with the programme.

Rehabilitation (BACR) Standards and Core Components in 2007 [11]. This document sets out the six minimum standards for a CR programme to ensure that all eligible patients are offered a service that meets standards for current best practice. Despite this large weight of evidence, CR services remain patchy, often underfunded and understaffed.

> **★ Learning point** Minimum standards required for a cardiac rehabilitation programme set by the British Association for Cardiac Rehabilitation [11]
>
> 1. A coordinator who has overall responsibility for the CR service;
> 2. A CR core team of professionally qualified staff with appropriate skills and competencies to deliver the service;
> 3. A standardized assessment of individual patient needs;
> 4. Referral and access for a targeted patient population;
> 5. Registration and submission of data to the National Audit for Cardiac Rehabilitation (NACR);
> 6. A CR budget appropriate to meet the full service costs.
>
> The current best standard for CR is to provide a 'menu-driven' programme which truly allows an individualized approach to the patient's needs. This approach sets out the different services available and the patient chooses those which are relevant to them. Some of the criticism levelled at rehabilitation services in recent times has been the lack of provision for certain groups, in particular people from minority ethnic groups, women, people on low incomes, the elderly, and people with physical disabilities. The NSF for CHD also highlighted that many people who should be referred and would benefit from CR are not referred and set a target that more than 85% of people discharged from hospital with a primary diagnosis of an acute MI or after coronary revascularization are offered the service [7]. An audit in 2008 suggested this figure was closer to 47% [12].

> **★ Learning point** The four phases of cardiac rehabilitation [14]
>
> **Phase one** is delivered in hospital following an acute admission for MI or post-revascularization. An assessment is made of the patient's physical, psychological, and social needs. Advice will be given as needed on smoking cessation, physical activity (including sexual activity), diet, alcohol, return to work, return to driving, and air travel. Education about medication is also given. With shorter and shorter hospital stays, effectively delivering the first phase is challenging and also trying to rid the patient of the belief that they are 'cured'. **It is important, therefore, that a uniform message is delivered by all members of the team, including surgeons, cardiologists, nursing staff, and the CR team.**
>
> **Phase two** takes place in the community during the immediate post-discharge period. Ideally, contact is made within four working days of discharge, followed by a visit within seven working days. There is a more comprehensive assessment of the patient's needs and a review of the initial plan made in phase one. There is continuing lifestyle advice and psychological interventions. The medication is reviewed. Basic life support training is offered to all family members at this stage and planned for a time in the future.
>
> **Phase three** commences two to four weeks after the cardiac event. There are more detailed education sessions derived from the 'curriculum' set out in the BACR Standards and Core Components for Cardiac Rehabilitation 2007. A comprehensive patient profile is completed. Exercise assessment is undertaken at this point and the exercise training programme is started. Patients are encouraged to exercise at least three times a week and should have access to supervised exercise sessions for at least twelve weeks.
>
> **Phase four** concentrates on the long-term maintenance of changed behaviour. This comprises two aspects: the patient's responsibility and the continuation of healthcare provision. As indicated, referrals are made to specialist groups (if this has not already been done in an earlier phase), e.g. exercise, smoking cessation, or psychological support services. Long-term follow-up takes place in primary care with the patient's details entered onto the CHD register so that secondary prevention will be annually reviewed. Good communication between the discharging CR team and the patient's general practitioner is essential at this stage.

> **❝ Expert comment**
>
> Older patients are less likely to be referred to rehabilitation and are also less likely to take up the service than middle-aged patients; equity of access should be ensured.
>
> It is accepted that some patients will prefer a home-based rehabilitation service. Some services will be able to cater for this, but another option is to use 'The Heart Manual', a cognitive behavioural management programme produced by NHS Lothian for people with coronary heart disease [13]. It can be used as a stand-alone rehabilitation programme or can be integrated with hospital or primary care-based programmes. It is the UK's leading home-based self-management rehabilitation programme and the fourth edition is suitable for patients following an MI and revascularization, along with other cardiovascular conditions, including stable angina, heart failure, and following implantable cardioverter-defibrillator insertion.

> **❝ Expert comment**
>
> All patients should be offered a genuine choice of group or home-based programmes where at all feasible. This patient had complex needs and was best suited to a more closely supervised and encouraging programme for re-enforcement of benefit and to allow him to benefit from the company of a supportive patient and carer group. A realistic timescale for the transition to exercise from home was required in this case.

The patient in this case underwent revascularization along with valve repair. He was an anxious patient who required considerable psychological support and encouragement as he tended to be quite pessimistic about his prognosis. After initially doing well, he had effectively been rendered chair-bound due to post-operative complications. Even when this had improved, however, he became extremely reluctant to undertake any form of exercise due to lack of confidence and the belief that any form of activity would impact negatively on his physical condition. Therefore a well-constructed CR programme, with his consent, would not only focus on an exercise programme that would allow him to get back to premorbid levels of mobility, but also address his illness behaviour and beliefs and provide the psychological support to allow him to regain normal function.

> ⭐ **Learning point** DVLA guidance on driving after an acute myocardial infarction or coronary revascularization [15]
>
> Driving restrictions are set out on the DVLA website (http://www.dft.gov.uk/dvla/medical/ataglance.aspx), but in short for non-commercial drivers after percutaneous coronary intervention (PCI), patients are restricted for one week, after CABG surgery for four weeks, and after any form of ACS, inclusive of unstable angina, NSTEMI, and STEMI, depending on treatment, either one week after PCI or four weeks if no PCI was attempted or intervention was unsuccessful. Commercial drivers are restricted for at least six weeks after ACS or PCI and must meet exercise or other functional test requirements. After CABG surgery, this restriction period is extended to three months and proof of an adequate left ventricular EF is also required.

> ⭐ **Learning point** Sexual activity and the cardiovascular patient
>
> It is important to broach this subject within the CR framework. A large proportion of cardiovascular patients will experience sexual problems and problems may increase after a cardiovascular event, with concerns regarding the safety of sexual activity and other factors, including medication-induced sexual dysfunction, age-related changes in sexual response, and vascular changes associated with risk factors [16]. The patient may not want to initiate a discussion so this subject should be broached as there is an opportunity for general well-being and quality of life to be improved. NICE guidelines suggest that patients should be reassured that after recovery, sexual activity presents no greater risk than if they had never had an MI. Sexual activity can resume when they feel comfortable, usually after about four weeks [10]. A phosphodiesterase inhibitor can be used in those patients with erectile dysfunction if the MI was more than six months ago and they have been stable [10]. It should not be prescribed in those patients on long-acting nitrates and/or nicorandil as this can lead to dangerous hypotension.

> 💬 **A final word from the expert**
>
> This case represented a complex older patient, and carer, requiring combined valve and coronary surgery, whose post-operative course was complicated by heart failure and Dressler's syndrome. His CR needed particular individualization of assessment and care plan:
>
> - To ensure an understanding of his dual aetiology of heart disease and arrhythmia;
> - An appreciation of his debilitation after a prolonged post-operative course, requiring a lower intensity start to exercise ideally after a prescription-guiding exercise test;
> - A careful assessment of exercise heart rate range for prescription in AF, if persistent;
> - Hospital Anxiety and Depression (HAD) scale assessment for monitoring of his psychological issues, defining the need for particular counselling/cognitive behavioural therapy;
> - Individual goal-setting to define required but realistic functionality.
>
> *continued*

To improve compliance with rehabilitation, a genuine choice of home or group-based programmes should be offered, particularly for longer-term maintenance of active lifestyle. His experience as a carer in addition both may endanger the time he may wish give to his own rehabilitation, but can also motivate him to develop his caring skills and even take up expert patient training. The NACR finds 72% of CABG patients being referred for CR [12]. Those older than 75 years at the time of surgery have often enjoyed good health previously and may do very well, providing they learn to accept their condition, take on board the preventive measures required, including medication, and keep positive about the opportunity they have been given to make the most of their physical and mental faculties for as long as possible.

I would also suggest referral to the following publications, which serve to highlight the increasing importance of CR in the management of several facets of cardiovascular disease:

1. The latest NACR Report 2010 (reflecting 2008/2009 patient data);
2. Home-based vs centre-based CR (Cochrane systematic review and meta-analysis published in the BMJ) [17];
3. Cochrane review of exercise rehabilitation for heart failure (April 2010), encouraging the current priority of increasing referral of these patients for individualized programmes [18];
4. The first Department of Health Commissioning Guide released in October 2010, dedicated to CR.

References

1 Dressler W. A post-myocardial infarction syndrome. *JAMA* 1956; 160: 1379–1383.
2 LeWinter MM. Pericardial Disease. In: Braunwald's Heart Disease: a textbook of cardiovascular medicine. 8th ed. Philadelphia: Saunders Elsevier; 2008. p. 1849.
3 Bendjelid K, Pugin J. Is Dressler syndrome dead? *Chest* 2004; 126: 1680–1682.
4 Cardiac Rehabilitation and Secondary Prevention: Long Term Care for Patients with Ischaemic Heart Disease. WHO Regional Office for Europe: WHO Regional Office for Europe, 1993.
5 British Heart Foundation. Cardiac Rehabilitation Factfile [issued May 2005]. Available from: http://www.bhf.org.uk/healthcare-professionals/resources/factfiles.aspx#PreviousIssues.
6 Pashkow FJ. Rehabilitation after acute MI. In: Rosendorff C, editor. Essential Cardiology Principles and Practice. 2nd edition. Totowa NJ: Humana Press; 2005. p. 531–534.
7 National Service Frameworks: Coronary Heart Disease. Standard Twelve: Cardiac Rehabilitation. Available from: http://www.gmccardiacnetwork.nhs.uk/cmsupload/Coronary_Heart_Disease_NSF_2000.pdf.
8 Taylor R, Brown A, Ebrahim S, et al. Exercise-based rehabilitation for patients with coronary heart disease: systematic review and meta-analysis of randomized controlled trials. *Am J Med* 2004; 116: 682–692.
9 Scottish Intercollegiate Guidelines Network. Cardiac Rehabilitation. SIGN publication no. 57 [issued 2002]. Available from: http://www.sign.ac.uk.
10 National Institute for Health and Clinical Excellence. MI secondary prevention in primary and secondary care for patients following a myocardial infarction. Clinical guideline 48 [issued 2007]. Available from: http://www.nice.org.uk.
11 BACR Standards and Core Components for Cardiac Rehabilitation 2007. Available from: www.bcs.com/documents/BACR_Standards.pdf.
12 National Audit for Cardiac Rehabilitation. Annual Statistical Report. British Heart Foundation 2008. Available from: http://www.cardiacrehabilitation.org.uk/dataset.htm.
13 NHS Lothian. The Heart Manual. Available from: http://www.theheartmanual.com.
14 The West Midlands Cardiac Rehabilitation Standards 2009/2010. Available from: http://www.blackcountrycardiacnetwork.nhs.uk/.../wmcrSTAND0910%20(10).pdf.
15 Driver and Vehicle Licensing Agency. At a glance guide to the current medical standards of fitness to drive. Available from: http://www.dft.gov.uk/dvla/medical/ataglance.aspx.

16 Taylor HA. Sexual activity and the cardiovascular patient: guidelines. *Am J Cardiol* 1999; 84: 6N–10N.

17 Dalal HM, Zawada A, Jolly K, et al. Home-based versus centre-based cardiac rehabilitation: Cochrane systematic review and meta-analysis. *BMJ* 2010; 340: b5631.

18 Davies EJ, Moxham T, Rees K, et al. Exercise-based rehabilitation for heart failure. *Cochrane Database Syst Rev 2010*; CD003331.

INDEX

Locators in *italic* refer to expert comments.